Reduce the Fat in Your Diet
and Gain a Lean, Fit, Healthy New You!

It's easier than you think to adopt a lower-fat diet without sacrificing the foods you love. Discover the fat counts of all your favorite foods in the essential reference book for low-fat living: *The Corinne T. Netzer Fat Counter,* chock-full of the most up-to-date information available. Let Corinne T. Netzer, America's bestselling expert on the nutritional content of food, be your guide as you design a delectable, nutritious diet that's just right for you!

Books by Corinne T. Netzer

THE BRAND-NAME CALORIE COUNTER
THE BRAND-NAME CARBOHYDRATE GRAM COUNTER
THE CHOLESTEROL CONTENT OF FOOD
THE COMPLETE BOOK OF FOOD COUNTS
THE COMPLETE BOOK OF VITAMIN AND MINERALS COUNTS
THE CORINNE T. NETZER 1997 CALORIE COUNTER
THE CORINNE T. NETZER CARBOHYDRATE GRAM COUNTER
THE CORINNE T. NETZER DIETER'S DIARY
THE CORINNE T. NETZER ENCYCLOPEDIA OF FOOD VALUES
THE CORINNE T. NETZER FAT GRAM COUNTER
THE CORINNE T. NETZER FIBER COUNTER
THE CORINNE T. NETZER LOW-FAT DIARY
THE DIETER'S CALORIE COUNTER
100 LOW-FAT CHICKEN AND TURKEY RECIPES
100 LOW-FAT PASTA AND GRAIN RECIPES
100 LOW-FAT SMALL MEAL AND SALAD RECIPES
100 LOW-FAT VEGETABLE AND LEGUME RECIPES
101 LOW CHOLESTEROL RECIPES
101 LOW FAT RECIPES
101 VEGETARIAN RECIPES

THE
CORINNE T. NETZER
FAT COUNTER

Revised Edition

A Dell Book

Published by
Dell Publishing
a division of
Bantam Doubleday Dell Publishing Group, Inc.
1540 Broadway
New York, New York 10036

The trademark Dell® is registered in the U.S. Patent and Trademark
Office.

ISBN: 0-440-22055-6

Printed in the United States of America

Published simultaneously in Canada

February 1996

10 9 8 7 6 5 4

RAD

The Fat Content of Food

Fat is not funny—not eating it and not being it. The "jolly" fat man is one big lie: he's laughing in order to keep from crying.

I am not a scientist but a concerned dieter. In this book I'm going to tell you, in the simplest and most direct way I know, why you should cut down on your fat intake and how you can lose weight by doing it.

U.S. Government Recommendations

In the most far-reaching report on nutrition and health ever prepared by the United States government, the reduction of fat intake was identified as the number-one dietary priority in the country.

The report said, "If you are among the two out of three Americans who do not smoke or drink excessively, your choice of diet can influence your long-term health prospects more than any other action you might take." And it specifically points out, "Of greatest concern is our excessive intake of dietary fat and its relationship to risk for chronic diseases."

Government experts strongly recommend that the consumption of both saturated and unsaturated fats be reduced in the average American's diet.

How do these fats differ? There is a chemical distinction in the structure of each fat molecule; specifically, in the number of hydrogen atoms. When the fat is carrying as many hydrogen atoms as it can hold, it is considered *saturated* with hydrogen. When the fat contains room for more hydrogen, it is called *unsaturated*. Unsaturated fats are further divided into *mono*unsaturated and *poly*unsaturated.

Although there are exceptions, animal fats are generally more saturated than vegetable fats. Another general rule is that saturated fats are usually solid at room temperature, while unsaturated fats are usually liquid at room temperature. Fats can be made more solid by adding hydrogen. That's the difference between soft and stick margarine. The hard stick has had hydrogen added in a process called *hydrogenation*. Although there are exceptions, the more hydrogen added to a fat or oil, the more saturated and firm it becomes.

The Trouble with Fat

I doubt if there is a dieter in the United States who isn't aware of the fact that studies indicate saturated fats contribute to cardiovascular disease, particularly heart attacks and stroke. We have been bombarded with the idea that polyunsaturates are "heart-healthful" and saturates (especially animal fats, which contain cholesterol) are unhealthful. Consequently there has been a distinct decline in our consumption of red meats and eggs and an increase in the use of polyunsaturated oils. This is fine as far at it goes—but it doesn't go far enough.

Heart disease is not the only problem to be concerned about when you're eating fat. High-fat diets of *both* saturated and unsaturated fats have been tied to cancer. Studies have linked "fatty" eating to colon/rectal cancers. Former President Reagan's doctors advised him to change his diet to one lower in fat and higher in fiber to reduce his risk of developing a second colon cancer. And there is mounting evidence from international studies that too much fat in the diet leads to increased risk of breast and prostate cancers.

No one knows for certain if fat starts cancer or if it accelerates already existing cancer, but there is a definite link.

Contrary to the studies on heart disease, which point a finger at saturated fats, research indicates that unsaturated fats seem to increase cancer risk even more than saturated fats. (Fish oils may be the rare exception to the rule. Preliminary work indicates a possibility that fish oil may be helpful in lowering the risk of cardiovascular disease and cancer. But these studies are in an early stage and are by no means conclusive.)

Since high-fat diets of both kinds of fat have been linked to disease, the Surgeon General suggests—and most heart and cancer experts agree—that it's best to reduce the amount of *all* fat in the diet.

Fat and Dieting

Ounce for ounce, spoon for spoon, fat contains more calories than carbohydrates or protein. A gram of fat contains nine calories, while a gram of protein or carbohydrate has only four. Do you think a tablespoon of sugar is fattening? Just compare it to a tablespoon of butter or margarine. The sugar has about 40 calories, the fat a whopping 100! Consider this: An ounce of *any* fat is more fattening than an ounce of pasta or potato—or anything!

So, not only is fat unhealthful, fat is fattening!

The government suggests that since we now eat too much fat, we should reduce our fat to 30 percent of our caloric intake. This means that no more than 30 percent of our calories should come from fat, with no more than 10 percent from saturated fat. Indeed, such diet gurus as the late Nathan Pritikin suggest a 5 to 10 percent total intake. I have found that you can lose weight, feel good, and still not feel denied with an intake of 20 percent fat in relation to total calories.

How do you know how much fat you are having? Simple. This book is a fat-gram counter, and everything you eat is listed with its gram count. Add up the grams of fat that you consume each day and multiply by nine (the number of calories in a fat gram) and you know how many calories of fat you've had.

The 22-Gram Solution
(CTN's Low-Fat Weight-Loss Diet)

This diet is designed for you to lose weight while lowering your fat intake. The 22-Gram Solution works for me, it works for all of my friends who have tried it—and it should work for you. The principles are easy to remember and, with a little willpower, very easy to follow. Remember, not only will you be thinner—you'll be eating more healthfully.

This plan is based on a daily intake of 1000 calories, which, for most people, allows maximum weight loss without sacrificing nutrition.

You may have 1000 calories per day. If you don't already own a calorie counter, I suggest you buy one so that you can plan your meals in advance and know, without question, how many calories you're consuming.

Limit yourself to no more than 22.2 total fat grams per day. Use this book to look up each and every thing you eat and drink. You may be below 22.2 grams—in fact, that is to be encouraged—but *never* more than that amount. You may choose your own foods as long as you stay within the limit.

Have at least 1 serving of fruit and 1 serving of vegetables every day. One of the main points of low-fat dieting is to encourage intake of food with complex carbohydrates and fiber. Actually, you'll find yourself willingly adding more fruit and vegetables to your diet because they're low in fat and will help you stay within your gram goal. You'll find you're *automatically* eating more nutritiously as well as losing those pounds because you'll be limiting fatty foods.

One of the reasons this diet works so well is the hunger factor. Remember, fat has nine calories a gram while carbohydrates and protein have only four, so when you cut down on fats, you can actually eat more food, be more "filled," and not have that hungry feeling.

Vary the kinds of food you eat. It is not healthful to eat the same exact thing every day. The body needs different kinds of nutrients that can come only from different kinds of food.

If you don't vary your diet, you won't stay on it, because it will become tiresome. My friend Joy, who had never, *ever* been able to stick to a diet regimen, was successful with the 22-Gram

Solution. She was able to choose from a multitude of foods, and she didn't get bored eating the same cottage cheese and carrot sticks every day. She made a game out of making up her menus—and it worked!

I have found that if you don't vary your choices, the body eventually becomes accustomed to a sameness of input, and after a while, no matter how strict you are, the body "plateaus" (it's happened to all of us on diets) and adjusts to the input, and you stop losing weight.

The beauty of this diet is that the options are yours as long as you stick to the 1000 calories, 22.2 fat grams per day.

Walk half an hour every day (unless you're on a doctor-regulated exercise program). If you already walk, good. If you don't, start. A half hour a day is not a lot to devote to fitness, and walking is not so strenuous that you can find an excuse not to do it. Walk briskly and continuously. Walk to work, walk around the block, walk to lunch, walk around the house if it's raining—but walk. It's good for your diet and it's "heart healthy." And if you're so busy a person that you can't find half an hour in the day, then take two brisk fifteen-minute tours. Try it; you'll feel better.

The 22-Gram solution Diet Tips
- Cut *all* visible fat off meat and poultry.
- Fry nothing (it uses too much oil or fat). Bake, broil, or boil foods, or use nonstick pans.
- Poach fish. Fish has fewer calories and contains those oils that may be good for you.
- On salads, use lemon with herbs and spices added—it may not taste as good as oil but you will get used to it and it's good for you.
- Steam vegetables and use herbs and spices instead of butter or margarine to "spike" them. Experiment—go to the store and buy some spices you've never tried before and use them to top your veggies.

• When eating in a restaurant, inquire how things are prepared before you order. If a sauce is included, tell the waiter to leave it off or put it on the side. Restaurants are accustomed to dieters and no longer get upset at such requests.

• Limit your alcoholic intake. No, there's no fat there, but it's highly caloric without being nutritious. The same is true of most sweets.

• Finally, consult your doctor before going on this or any other diet.

How to Use This Book

This book is alphabetized, so there's no index. Simply look up the food you are interested in and you will find its fat-gram content.

Look up everything you eat in a day, add up the fat grams and you will get your total. Again, plan your menus in advance so that the total won't come as an awful surprise after the fact.

If you are following the 22-Gram Solution, you will not go over 22.2 total fat grams per day. However, if losing weight is not your goal, or if you do not want to go below the government-recommended 30 percent of fat in your diet, there is a simple formula for figuring out how many fat grams you should have. Take 30 percent of the calories you consume per day and divide by nine (the number of calories in a fat gram). For instance, if you have 1500 calories per day, 30 percent of 1500 is 450, and 450 divided by nine is 50—and that should be your maximum daily fat-gram intake.

If your goal is 20 percent fat in your diet, take 20 percent of your total caloric intake and divide by nine. If your calorie intake is 1500, 20 percent is 300, which divided by nine is 33.3.

No matter what your desired fat percentage is, the equation remains the same—percentage of calories divided by nine. That is how you find your maximum intake permitted, and that is the number you should not go over. And when you use this counter you won't.

Maximum Daily Grams

The following chart, based on a fat intake of 10, 20, and 30 percent, has been compiled so that you may quickly see your maximum daily allowable fat. Find the figure closest to your daily caloric intake, and do not go over the corresponding fat grams indicated—and remember, saturated fat intake should be no more than 10 percent of the total fat grams.

Maximum Daily Fat Intake

Average calories	Maximum fat grams		
	10%	20%	30%
1000	11.1	22.2	33.3
1100	12.2	24.4	36.6
1200	13.3	26.6	40.0
1300	14.4	28.8	43.3
1400	15.5	31.1	46.6
1500	16.6	33.3	50.0
1600	17.7	35.5	53.3
1700	18.8	37.7	56.6
1800	20.0	40.0	60.0
1900	21.1	42.2	63.3
2000	22.2	44.4	66.6
2100	23.3	46.6	70.0
2200	24.4	48.8	73.3
2300	25.5	51.1	76.6
2400	26.6	53.3	80.0
2500	27.7	55.5	83.3
2600	28.8	57.7	86.6
2700	30.0	60.0	90.0
2800	31.1	62.2	93.3
2900	32.2	64.4	96.6
3000	33.3	66.6	100.0

Sources of Data

The information contained in this book is based on data obtained from the United States Department of Agriculture and the various producers and processors of brand-name foods.

As we go to press, this book has the most accurate and up-to-date data available. However, food companies do sometimes change their recipes and packaging. If need be, these changes will be dealt with in future editions.

Good luck and good dieting!

C.T.N.

Abbreviations and Symbols

fl. .... fluid
gms. .... grams
lb. .... pound(s)
n.a. .... not available
oz. .... ounce(s)
pkg. .... package
pkt. .... packet
tbsp. .... tablespoon(s)
tsp. .... teaspoon(s)
tr. .... trace
w/ .... with
" .... inch(es)
* .... prepared according to basic
package directions

A

	total fat (grams)		saturated fat (grams)
Abalone, meat only:			
raw, 4 oz.	.9	....	.2
dipped in flour, fried, 4 oz.	7.7	....	1.9
Abruzzese sausage, sweet (*Cinghiale*), 1 oz.	8.0	....	3.0
Acerola, fresh:			
untrimmed, 1 lb.	1.1	....	0
trimmed, ½ cup	.1	....	0
Acerola juice, fresh, 6 fl. oz.	.5	....	0
Acorn, shelled:			
raw, 1 oz.	6.8	....	.9
dried, 1 oz.	8.9	....	1.2
Acorn flour, full-fat, 1 oz.	8.6	....	1.1
Acorn squash:			
raw, untrimmed, 1 medium, 1.3 lbs.	.4	....	.1
baked, 4 oz.	.2	....	<.1
baked, cubed, ½ cup	.1	....	tr.
boiled, mashed, ½ cup	.1	....	tr.
Adobo (*Durkee*), ¼ tsp.	0	....	0
Adzuki beans, dried:			
raw, ½ cup	.5	....	tr.
raw (*Arrowhead Mills*), ¼ cup	.5	....	0

	total fat (grams)	saturated fat (grams)
Adzuki beans, dried *(cont.)*		
boiled, ½ cup	.1	tr.
canned *(Eden)*, ½ cup	0	0
Agar, see "Seaweed"		
A la king sauce mix *(Durkee* Pouches), ½ pkg.	4.0	1.0
Ale, all brands, 12 fl. oz.	0	0
Alfalfa sprouts, raw:		
4 oz.	.8	<.1
(Arrowhead Mills), 1 cup	0	0
(Jonathan's Sprouts), 3 oz., 1 cup	.5	0
w/dill sprouts *(Jonathan's Sprouts)*, 3 oz., 1 cup	.5	0
w/radish sprouts *(Jonathan's Sprouts)*, 3 oz., 1 cup	1.5	0
Alfredo sauce, ½ cup, except as noted:		
(Five Brothers), ¼ cup	11.0	7.0
(Progresso Authentic)	27.0	15.0
refrigerated *(Contadina)*	38.0	21.0
refrigerated *(Contadina* Light)	13.0	7.0
w/mushrooms *(Five Brothers)*, ¼ cup	7.0	4.0
Alfredo sauce mix:		
(Knorr Pasta Sauce), ⅙ pkg.	1.5	0
(Lawry's Spices & Seasonings), 1½ tbsp.	1.5	1.0
(McCormick Pasta Sauce Blend), ¼ pkg.	2.5	1.5
(Spice Islands), ½ pkg.	2.5	1.5
Algae, See "Seaweed"		
Allspice, ground:		
1 tbsp.	.5	.2
1 tsp.	.2	.1
Almond, shelled, except as noted:		
dried, in shell, 4 oz.	23.7	2.3
(Dole), 1 oz.	14.0	n.a.
(Planters), 1 oz.	15.0	1.0
(Sonoma), 1.1 oz., ¼ cup	15.0	0
chopped, ¼ cup	17.0	1.6
dry-roasted, 1 oz.	14.7	1.4

	total fat (grams)	saturated fat (grams)
honey roasted (*Planters*), 1 oz.	14.0	1.0
oil-roasted, 1 oz.	16.4	1.6
sliced (*Planters Gold Measure*), 2.25-oz. pkg.	33.5	3.5
slivered (*Planters Gold Measure*), 2-oz. pkg.	31.0	2.5
toasted, 1 oz.	14.4	1.4
whole (*Sonoma*), ¼ cup	15.0	0
tamari-roasted (*Eden*), 1 oz.	12.0	1.0
Almond butter:		
1 oz.	16.8	1.6
1 tbsp.	9.5	.9
(*Roaster Fresh*), 1 oz.	16.0	1.6
honey cinnamon, 1 tbsp.	8.4	.8
Almond meal, partially defatted, 1 oz.	5.2	.5
Almond oil, 1 tbsp.	13.6	1.1
Almond paste:		
1 oz.	7.2	.7
¼ cup packed	15.4	1.5
(*Solo*), 2 tbsp.	11.0	0
Almond pastry filling (*Solo*), 2 tbsp.	2.5	.5
Almond powder:		
full fat, 1 oz.	14.7	1.4
partially defatted, 1 oz.	4.5	.4
Alum (*Durkee*), ¼ tsp.	0	0
Amaranth:		
raw, untrimmed, ½ lb.	.7	.2
raw, trimmed, ½ cup	<.1	<.1
boiled, drained, ½ cup	.1	<.1
Amaranth, whole grain, 1 cup	12.7	3.2
Amaranth entree, canned, w/garden vegetables (*Health Valley*), 1 cup	0	0
Amaranth flour (*Arrowhead Mills*), ¼ cup	1.5	0
Amaranth seeds (*Arrowhead Mills*), ¼ cup	2.0	.5
Amberjack, meat only, raw, 4 oz.	1.0	n.a.
Ambrosia (*R.W. Knudsen* Tropical Blend), 8 fl. oz.	0	0
Anasazi beans (*Arrowhead Mills*), ¼ cup	.5	0

	total fat (grams)	saturated fat (grams)
Anchovy, European, meat only, raw, 4 oz.	5.5	1.5
Anchovy, canned, in olive oil, drained:		
1.6 oz., yield from 2-oz. can	4.4	1.0
.7 oz., 5 medium	1.9	.4
Angel hair pasta, see "Pasta"		
Angel hair pasta dishes, mix:		
(*Weight Watchers Smart Ones*), 9 oz.	2.0	.5
chicken broccoli (*Lipton Golden Saute*), ⅓ cup	1.0	0
w/herbs (*Golden Grain Noodle Roni*), 1 cup*	13.0	3.5
Parmesan (*Country Inn Recipes*), 2.5 oz.	4.5	2.5
Parmesan (*Lipton Golden Saute*), ½ cup	5.0	2.0
Parmesano (*Golden Grain Noodle Roni*), 1 cup*	15.0	4.0
Angel hair pasta entree, frozen (*Lean Cuisine* Entree), 10 oz.	4.0	1.0
Anise seeds:		
1 tbsp.	1.1	n.a.
1 tsp.	.3	n.a.
Antelope, meat only, roasted, 4 oz.	3.0	1.1
Apio root, see "Celeriac"		
Apple:		
fresh:		
untrimmed, 1 lb.	1.5	.2
w/peel, 1 medium, 2¾" diameter	.5	.1
peeled, 1 medium, 2¾" diameter	.4	.1
boiled, peeled, sliced, ½ cup	.3	.1
microwaved, peeled, sliced, ½ cup	.4	.1
canned:		
all varieties (*White House*), ½ cup	0	0
rings, in heavy syrup (*Wilderness*), 2 rings	0	0
sliced (*Comstock/Wilderness*), ⅓ cup	0	0
dehydrated, uncooked, ½ cup	.2	<.1
dried:		
uncooked, 10 rings, about 2.3 oz.	.2	<.1
(*Del Monte*), ⅓ cup	0	0
(*Sonoma*), 1.4 oz., 10–12 pieces	0	0

	total fat (grams)	saturated fat (grams)
Apple, escalloped:		
canned (*White House*), ½	0	0
frozen (*Stouffer's* Side Dish), ½ of 12-oz. pkg.	3.0	tr.
Apple butter:		
2 tbsp.	0	0
(*Eden*), 1 tbsp.	0	0
(*New Morning*), 1 tbsp.	0	0
(*Smucker's*), 1 tbsp.	0	0
Apple chips (*Weight Watchers Smart Snackers*), .75 oz.	0	0
Apple cider, all brands, 8 fl. oz.	0	0
Apple cobbler, see "Cobbler"		
Apple dumpling, frozen (*Pepperidge Farm*), 3 oz.	11.0	2.5
Apple flauta, frozen (*Schwan's*), 2-oz. piece	7.0	1.0
Apple fruit square, frozen (*Pepperidge Farm*), 2.5-oz. piece	12.0	4.5
Apple juice, all brands, 8 fl. oz.	0	0
Apple pastry filling, Dutch (*Solo*), 2 tbsp.	0	0
Apple pie, see "Pie"		
Apple pie spice (*Durkee*), ¼ tsp.	0	0
Apple-almond crisp, freeze-dried* (*AlpineAire*), 1½ cups	10.0	n.a.
Apple-apricot juice (*R.W. Knudsen*), 8 fl. oz.	0	0
Apple-banana juice (*R.W. Knudsen*), 8 fl. oz.	0	0
Apple-boysenberry juice (*R.W. Knudsen*), 8 fl. oz.	0	0
Apple-cherry cider (*R.W. Knudsen*), 8 fl. oz.	0	0
Apple-cranberry juice (*R.W. Knudsen*), 8 fl. oz.	0	0
Apple-peach juice (*R.W. Knudsen*), 8 fl. oz.	0	0
Apple-raspberry juice (*R.W. Knudsen*), 8 fl. oz.	0	0
Apple-strawberry juice (*R. W. Knudsen*), 8 fl. oz.	0	0
Applesauce:		
canned or in jars:		
all varieties (*Seneca*), ½ cup	0	0

	total fat (grams)	saturated fat (grams)

Applesauce *(cont.)*

    sweetened, ½ cup or 4 oz. .... .2 .... tr.

    unsweetened, ½ cup or 4 oz. .... .1 .... tr.

    unsweetened (*Eden*), ½ cup 0 0

    freeze-dried, w/cinnamon (*AlpineAire*), 1½ cups* 8 0

Apricot:

    fresh:

        untrimmed, 1 lb. 1.7 1

        3 medium, 12 per lb. .... .4 .... tr.

        pitted, halves, ½ cup .... .3 .... tr.

    canned, ½ cup 0 0

    canned, all varieties (*Del Monte*), ½ cup 0 0

    dehydrated, uncooked, ½ cup .... .4 .... tr.

    dried:

        (*Del Monte* Sun Dried), ⅓ cup 0 0

        (*Sonoma*), 1.4 oz., 10–12 pieces 0 0

        sulfured, uncooked, halves, ½ cup .... .3 .... tr.

        sulfured, 10 halves, 1.2 oz. .... .2 .... tr.

    frozen, sweetened, ½ cup .... .1 .... tr.

Apricot kernel oil, 1 tbsp. 13.6 9

Apricot nectar, canned or bottled:

    6 fl. oz. .... .2 .... tr.

    (*Kern's*), 11.5 oz. can 0 0

    (*R.W. Knudsen*), 8 fl. oz. 0 0

Apricot pastry filling (*Solo*), 2 tbsp. 0 0

Arame, see "Seaweed"

Arby's, 1 serving:

    breakfast dishes:

        biscuit:

            plain ... . 14.9 ... 3.3

            w/bacon ... . 17.9 .... 4.3

            w/ham . ... 16.6 ... 3.9

            w/sausage ... . 31.9 .. 9.4

        croissant:

            plain .... 15.6 .... 10.4

	total fat (grams)	saturated fat (grams)
bacon and egg	30.0	15.4
ham and cheese	20.7	12.1
mushroom and cheese	37.7	15.2
sausage and egg	39.2	18.6
danish, cinnamon nut	11.0	1.0
muffin, blueberry	7.0	1.0
platter:		
scrambled egg	24.0	7.2
scrambled egg w/bacon	33.0	9.2
scrambled egg w/ham	26.2	7.9
scrambled egg w/sausage	41.0	13.3
Toastix	25.0	4.6
sandwiches:		
Arby Q	15.2	5.5
Bac'N Cheddar Deluxe	31.5	8.7
Beef'N Cheddar	26.5	7.7
chicken barbeque, grilled	13.1	3.6
chicken breast fillet	22.5	3.0
chicken Cordon Bleu	27.1	5.3
chicken deluxe, grilled	19.9	3.5
fish fillet	27.0	7.0
French dip	15.4	5.6
French Dip'N Swiss	19.0	8.8
Ham'N Cheese	14.2	5.1
Italian sub	38.8	12.8
Philly Beef'N Swiss	25.3	9.7
roast beef, giant	26.3	10.9
roast beef, junior	10.8	4.1
roast beef, regular	18.2	7.0
roast beef, super	28.3	7.6
roast beef deluxe, light	10.0	3.5
roast beef sub	32.0	11.5
roast chicken club	27.0	6.9
roast chicken deluxe, light	7.0	1.7
roast turkey deluxe, light	6.0	1.6

	total fat (grams)	saturated fat (grams)
Arby's, sandwiches *(cont.)*		
tuna sub	37.0	8.2
turkey sub	19.0	5.3
potatoes:		
baked, plain	1.9	0
baked, w/butter and sour cream	25.2	12.1
baked, Broccoli'N Cheddar	17.9	6.9
baked, deluxe	36.4	18.1
baked, Mushroom'N Cheese	26.7	5.8
cakes	12.0	2.2
fries, cheddar	21.9	9.0
fries, curly	17.7	7.4
fries, french	13.2	3.0
soups, 8 oz.:		
Boston clam chowder	10.0	4.5
cream of broccoli	7.2	3.8
lumberjack mixed vegetable	3.6	1.7
old fashioned chicken noodle	1.8	.5
potato w/bacon	8.8	4.3
Wisconsin cheese	18.0	9.0
salads:		
chef	9.5	3.9
garden	5.2	2.7
roast chicken	7.2	3.3
side	.3	<.1
sauces and dressings:		
au jus, 4 oz.	0	0
Arby's Sauce, .5 oz.	.2	0
blue cheese dressing, 2 oz.	31.2	5.8
buttermilk ranch dressing, 2 oz.	38.5	5.6
honey French dressing, 2 oz.	26.9	3.9
Horsey Sauce, .5 oz.	5.0	2.0
light Italian dressing, 2 oz.	1.1	.1
Thousand Island dressing, 2 oz.	29.2	4.3

	total fat (grams)	saturated fat (grams)
desserts:		
cheesecake	22.8	7.4
chocolate chip cookie	4.0	2.0
Polar Swirl:		
Butterfinger	18.1	8.4
Heath	21.8	5.2
Oreo	19.7	10.4
peanut butter cup	24.0	8.1
Snickers	18.8	6.7
turnover, apple	18.3	6.9
turnover, blueberry	19.0	6.3
turnover, cherry	17.8	5.3
shakes:		
chocolate	11.6	2.8
jamocha	10.5	2.5
vanilla	11.5	3.9
Arrowhead:		
raw, untrimmed, 1 lb.	1.0	n.a.
raw, 3½" diameter corm, 1.2 oz.	.1	0
boiled, drained, 1 medium corm	<.1	0
Arrowroot, powder, 1 tsp.	0	0
Arrowroot flour, 1 cup	.1	<.1
Artichoke, globe:		
fresh:		
raw, 1 medium, 11.3 oz.	.2	<.1
boiled, drained, 1 medium, 10.6 oz.	.2	<.1
boiled, trimmed, 4 oz.	.2	<.1
boiled, hearts, 3 oz., ½ cup	.1	<.1
canned or in jars:		
hearts (*Progresso*), 2 pieces	0	0
hearts (*Reese*), 2 pieces	0	0
frozen, 9-oz. pkg.	1.1	.3
frozen, hearts, boiled, drained, 4 oz.	.6	.1
Artichoke, marinated, hearts (*Progresso*), ⅓ cup	14.0	2.0
Artichoke, Jerusalem, see "Jerusalem artichoke"		

	total fat (grams)	saturated fat (grams)

Arugula, fresh:

trimmed, ½ cup 1 0

(*Frieda's*), ½ lb. 7 0

Asparagus:

fresh:

raw, untrimmed, 1 lb. 5 1

raw, 4 spears, 3.8 oz. .... .1 .... <.1

boiled, drained, 4 spears, ½" diameter base ... .2 .... <.1

boiled, drained, cuts and spears, ½ cup 3 1

canned:

(*Del Monte*), ½ cup 0 0

(*Green Giant*), ½ cup 0 0

(*Seneca*), ½ cup 0 0

(*Stokely*), ½ cup 0 0

w/liquid, 4 oz. .... .2 .... <.1

drained, 4 oz. 7 2

frozen:

cuts and spears, 10-oz. pkg. 7 1

cuts and spears, boiled, drained, 2.1 oz.,
4 spears 3 1

cuts (*Green Giant*), ½ cup 0 0

spears (*Schwan's*), 7 spears, 2.9 oz. 0 0

Asparagus bean, see "Yardlong bean"

Au jus gravy, canned, ¼ cup 1 1

Au jus gravy mix:

(*Durkee/Durkee* Roasting Bags), ⅛ pkg. 0 0

(*French's*), ⅛ pkg. 0 0

(*Knorr Gravy Classics*), ⅕ pkg. 0 0

Aubergine, see "Eggplant"

Avocado, fresh:

all varieties:

untrimmed, 1 lb. .... 51.4 .... 8.2

pulp, 1 oz. 4.3 7

pureed, ½ cup .... 17.6 .... 2.8

	total fat (grams)	saturated fat (grams)
California:		
1 medium, 8 oz.	30.0	4.5
pulp, 1 oz.	4.9	.7
pureed, ½ cup	19.9	3.0
cocktail (*Frieda's*), 1 oz.	4.6	n.a.
Avocado oil, 1 tbsp.	14.0	1.6
Avocado dip (see also "Guacamole dip"):		
(*Kraft*), 2 tbsp	4.0	3.0
(*Nalley*), 2 tbsp.	12.0	1.5

B

	total fat (grams)	saturated fat (grams)
Babassu oil, 1 tbsp.	13.6	11.0
Backfat, see "Pork backfat"		
Bacon:		
raw, 1 oz.	16.3	6.0
cooked, 4.5 oz. (1 lb. raw)	62.5	22.1
cooked, 3 slices (20 per lb.)	9.4	3.3
(*Black Label*), 2 slices, .5 oz.	7.0	2.5
(*Black Label* Center Cut), .5 oz., 3 slices	6.0	2.5
(*Black Label* Low Salt), .5 oz., 2 slices	7.0	2.5
(*Hillshire Farm* Country Smoked), 1 slice	12.0	n.a.
(*Hormel* Microwave), 1 oz.	14.0	6.0
(*Jones Dairy Farm* Slab), 2 oz.	31.0	9.0
(*Jones Dairy Farm* Sliced), .6 oz., 2 slices	8.0	3.0
(*Jones Dairy Farm* ⅛" Thick Sliced), .4-oz. slice	6.0	2.5
(*Old Smokehouse*), .5 oz., 2 slices	7.0	2.5
(*Oscar Mayer*), .4 oz., 2 cooked slices	5.0	2.0
(*Oscar Mayer* Center Cut), .5 oz., 3 cooked slices	6.0	2.0
(*Oscar Mayer* Lower Sodium), .5 oz., 2 cooked slices	5.0	2.0
(*Oscar Mayer* Thick Cut, ⅛"), 1 cooked slice	4.5	2.0

	total fat (grams)	saturated fat (grams)
(*Patrick Cudahy*), .5 oz., 2 slices	7.0	2.5
(*Patrick Cudahy* Thick Sliced), .4-oz. slice	5.0	2.0
(*Range Brand*), 2 slices, .8 oz.	9.0	3.5
(*Red Label*), .5 oz., 2 slices	7.0	2.5
(*River Rock/Sinnissippi*), .6 oz., 2 slices	8.0	3.0
(*Schwan's* Thick Sliced), 1 cooked slice	6.0	2.0
microwave (*Hormel*), .4 oz., 2 slices	5.0	2.0
turkey, see "Turkey bacon"		
Bacon, Canadian style:		
unheated, 1-oz. slice	2.0	.6
grilled, 4.9 oz. (6 oz. unheated)	11.7	4.0
(*Boar's Head*), 2 oz.	2.5	1.0
(*Hormel*), 2 oz.	3.0	1.5
(*Jones Dairy Farm* Lean Choice), 1.8 oz., 3 slices	3.0	1.0
(*Oscar Mayer*), 1.6 oz., 2 slices	2.0	1.0
(*Usinger's*), 1.9 oz.	3.9	1.3
Bacon, Irish (*Limerick*), 1-oz. piece	9.0	2.0
"Bacon," vegetarian, frozen, .6 oz., 2 strips:		
(*Morningstar Farm* Breakfast Strips)	4.5	.5
(*Worthington Stripples*)	5.0	.5
Bacon bits:		
(*Hormel*), 1 tsp.	1.5	1.0
(*Hormel* Pieces), 1 tsp.	1.5	.5
(*Oscar Mayer*), 1 tbsp.	1.5	.5
"Bacon" bits, imitation, 1 tbsp.:		
(*Concord Foods*)	1.5	0
(*Bac'n Pieces*)	1.5	0
bits or chips (*Bac★O's*)	1.0	0
bits or chips (*Durkee*)	0	0
Bacon dip, see "Bacon horseradish dip" and "Bacon onion dip"		
Bacon flavor snack:		
(*Baken-ets*), .5 oz., 9 pieces	5.0	2.0
(*Baken-ets* Cracklin'), .5 oz., 8 pieces	6.0	2.0

	total fat (grams)	saturated fat (grams)
Bacon flavor snack *(cont.)*		
hot and spicy (*Baken-ets*), .5 oz., 7 pieces	5.0	1.5
Bacon horseradish dip, 2 tbsp.:		
(*Heluva* Good)	5.0	3.0
(*Kraft/Kraft* Premium)	5.0	3.0
yogurt (*Crowley's*)	2.0	1.5
Bacon onion dip, 2 tbsp.:		
(*Knudsen's* Premium)	5.0	3.0
(*Kraft* Premium)	5.0	3.0
(*Nalley*)	11.0	2.0
sour cream (*Breakstone's*)	5.0	3.0
Bagel, 1 piece:		
(*Garden of Eatin' Bible Bagels* Original)	2.0	n.a.
(*Roman Meal* Original)	1.6	.4
all varieties, except sesame (*Pepperidge Farm* Bountiful)	1.5	0
cinnamon raisin (*Thomas'*)	1.5	0
multigrain (*Thomas'*)	1.5	0
onion or sesame (*Garden of Eatin' Bible Bagels*)	2.0	n.a.
plain, egg, or onion (*Thomas'*)	2.0	0
raisin (*Garden of Eatin' Bible Bagels*)	1.0	n.a.
sesame (*Pepperidge Farm*)	1.0	0
Bagel, frozen:		
plain (*Lender's*), 2-oz. piece	1.0	0
plain (*Lender's Big'N Crusty*), 3-oz. piece	2.0	0
blueberry (*Lender's*), 2.5 oz. piece	2.0	0
cinnamon raisin (*Lender's*), 2.5-oz. piece	1.5	0
cinnamon raisin (*Lender's Big'N Crusty*), 3-oz. piece	2.5	0
egg (*Lender's*), 2-oz. piece	1.5	0
egg (*Lender's Big'N Crusty*), 3-oz. piece	2.0	.5
garlic (*Lender's*), 2-oz. piece	1.0	0
oat bran (*Lender's*), 2.5-oz. piece	1.5	0
onion (*Lender's*), 2-oz. piece	1.5	0

	total fat (grams)	saturated fat (grams)
onion (*Lender's Big'N Crusty*), 3-oz. piece	1.5	0
poppy (*Lender's*), 2-oz. piece	1.0	0
pumpernickel (*Lender's*), 2-oz. piece	1.0	0
rye (*Lender's*), 2-oz. piece	1.0	0
sesame (*Lender's*), 2-oz. piece	1.5	0
soft (*Lender's* Original), 2.5-oz. piece	3.5	.5
Bagel chips, 1 oz.:		
cheese, three (*Pepperidge Farm*)	7.0	1.0
onion, multigrain (*Pepperidge Farm*)	3.5	0
onion, toasted, and garlic (*Pepperidge Farm*)	4.5	1.0
Bagel dog, see "Frankfurter, coated"		
Bagel pizza, see "Pizza, bagel"		
Bagel sandwich, see "Ham sandwich," "Frankfurter, coated," and "Pepperoni sandwich"		
Baked beans, canned, ½ cup, except as noted:		
(*Allens*)	1.0	.5
(*B&M* Brick Oven/Extra Hearty)	2.0	.5
(*B&M* 99% Fat Free)	1.0	0
(*Bush's Best*), 4 oz.	1.0	.5
(*Bush's Best* Homestyle), 4 oz.	1.5	.5
(*Campbell's* Lowfat)	2.0	.5
(*Campbell's* New England Style)	3.0	1.0
(*Friend's* Original/Red Kidney)	1.0	0
(*Green Giant/Joan of Arc*)	1.5	1.0
(*Heartland* Iron Kettle)	1.0	0
(*Van Camp's*)	1.5	.5
(*Van Camp's* Fat Free)	0	0
(*Van Camp's* Premium)	1.0	0
w/bacon and brown sugar (*Bush's Best*)	1.0	0
barbecue (*B&M*)	2.0	.5
barbecue (*Green Giant/Joan of Arc*)	.5	0
w/beef	4.6	2.3
brown sugar (*Van Camp's*)	3.0	1.0
w/frankfurters:		
½ cup	8.4	3.0

	total fat (grams)	saturated fat (grams)

Baked beans, w/frankfurters *(cont.)*

(*Hormel* Beans & Wieners), 7.5-oz. can	13.0	4.0
(*Hormel Kid's Kitchen* Beans & Wieners)	13.0	5.0
(*Libby's Diner*), 7.75 oz.	16.0	5.0
all varieties (*Van Camp's Beanee Weenee*), 1 cup	14.0	4.0
chili (*Van Camp's Beanee Weenee*), 7.8-oz. can	12.0	3.0
honey (*B&M*)	1.5	0
honey (*Health Valley* Fat Free), 1 cup	0	0
honey bacon flavored (*Green Giant/Joan of Arc*)	.5	0
w/onions (*Bush's Best*), 4 oz.	1.5	.5
w/onions (*Green Giant/Joan of Arc*)	1.5	.5
w/pork:		
½ cup	2.0	.8
(*Crest Top*)	1.0	.5
(*Stokely*)	1.0	n.a.
(*Wagon Master*)	1.0	.5
and jalapeños (*Trappey's*)	2.0	.5
in sweet sauce	1.8	.7
in tomato sauce	1.3	.5
in tomato sauce (*Campbell's*)	2.0	.5
in tomato sauce (*Green Giant/Joan of Arc*)	1.0	0
vegetarian:		
½ cup	.6	.1
(*Bush's Best*), 4 oz.	1.0	0
(*Stokely*)	.5	n.a.
(*Van Camp's*)	.5	0
tofu (*Health Valley* Vegetarian Cuisine), 1 cup	1.0	0
yellow eye or red kidney (*B&M*)	2.0	.5
Baking mix, whole wheat (*Hain*), ⅓ cup	1.0	0
Baking powder, 1 tsp.	0	0
Baking soda, 1 tsp.	0	0

	total fat (grams)	saturated fat (grams)
Baklava, frozen (*Apollo*), 4.4 oz., 4½ pieces	31.0	.... 5.0
Balsam pear:		
leafy tips:		
raw, untrimmed, 1 lb.	1.2	.... tr.
raw, trimmed, ½ cup	.2	 0
boiled, drained, ½ cup	.1	 0
pods:		
raw, untrimmed, 1 lb.	.6	.... tr.
raw, 5.3-oz. pod	.2	 0
boiled, drained, ½" pieces, ½ cup	.1	 0
Bamboo shoots:		
fresh:		
raw, ½" slices, ½ cup	.1	.... <.1
boiled, drained, 5-oz. shoot	.3	1
boiled, drained, ½" slices, ½ cup	.1	.... <.1
canned, drained, ⅛" slices, ½ cup	.3	1
Banana (see also "Banana, red"):		
fresh:		
untrimmed, 1 lb.	1.4	5
1 medium, 8¾" long, 6.2 oz.	.6	.... <.1
mashed, ½ cup	.5	.... <.1
dried (*Sonoma*), 2 pieces, 1.5 oz.	0	 0
Banana, baking, see "Plantain"		
Banana, red, fresh:		
1 medium, 7¼" long	.3	.... <.1
sliced, ½ cup	.2	.... <.1
Banana chips, 1 oz.	9.5	.... 8.2
Banana flavor drink mix (*Nestlé Quik*), 2 tbsp.	0	 0
Banana flavor milk drink, lowfat (*Nestlé Quik*),		
8 fl. oz.	5.0	.... 3.0
Banana nectar (*Kern's*), 11.5-oz. can	0	 0
Banana squash, baked (*Frieda's*), 1 oz.	.1	 0
Bananaberry shake (*Nestlé Killer Shakes*), 1 carton ..	15.0	.... 9.0
Barbecue sauce, 2 tbsp., except as noted:		
(*Heinz* Thick & Rich)	0	 0

	total fat (grams)	saturated fat (grams)
Barbecue sauce *(cont.)*		
(*House of Tsang Hong Kong*), 1 tsp.	0	0
all varieties:		
(*Healthy Choice*)	0	0
(*Maull's*), 2 tbsp.	0	0
except char-grill, Italian seasonings, and teriyaki (*Kraft/Kraft Thick 'N Spicy*)	0	0
char-grill or teriyaki (*Kraft*)	1.0	0
Dijon and honey(*Lawry's*)	1.0	0
honey (*Hain* Bar-B-Que), 1 tbsp.	1.0	0
honey Dijon (*KC Masterpiece*)	1.0	0
honey teriyaki (*KC Masterpiece*)	1.0	0
Italian seasonings (*Kraft*)	.5	0
(*KC Masterpiece* Original or Bold)	0	0
(*Lea & Perrins* Bold 'N Spicy)	0	0
and marinade (*Porino's*)	1.5	0
and marinade (*World Harbors Maui Mountain*), 1 tbsp.	1.0	0
original or honey mustard (*Bulls' Eye*)	0	0
Barbecue seasoning, dry:		
(*Durkee*), ¼ tsp.	0	0
(*Perc*), ¼ tsp.	<.1	0
chicken, mix (*Durkee* Pouch), ⅙ pkg.	0	0
spice, 1 tsp.	.4	<.1
Barley:		
dry, ¼ cup	1.1	.2
dry, hulless (*Arrowhead Mills*), ¼ cup	1.0	0
pearled, dry:		
¼ cup	.6	.2
(*Arrowhead Mills*), ¼ cup	.5	0
all varieties (*Quaker* Scotch), ⅓ cup	1.0	0
pearled, cooked, ½ cup	.4	<.1
Barley flour (*Arrowhead Mills*), ¼ cup	.5	0
Barley malt (*Eden*), 1 tbsp.	0	0
Barley pilaf mix (*Near East*), 1 cup*	4.0	1.0

	total fat (grams)	saturated fat (grams)
Barracuda, meat only, raw, 4 oz.	1.3	n.a.
Basil:		
fresh, 1 oz.	.2	<.1
fresh, 5 leaves or 2 tbsp. chopped	<.1	tr.
dried, crumbled, 1 tbsp.	.2	tr.
dried, crumbled, 1 tsp.	<.1	0
***Baskin-Robbins*:**		
ice cream, regular deluxe:		
Baby Ruth, chewy, ½ cup	9.0	5.0
banana nut, ½ cup	9.0	4.0
banana strawberry, ½ cup	6.0	4.0
Baseball Nut, ½ cup	8.0	4.0
black walnut, ½ cup	10.0	5.0
blackberry, Oregon, ½ cup	6.9	4.6
blackberry, Oregon, regular scoop	12.0	6.0
blueberry cheesecake, ½ cup	7.0	4.0
bubble gum, pink ½ cup	7.0	4.0
butter pecan, old fashioned, ½ cup	10.0	5.0
butter pecan, old fashioned, regular scoop	18.0	n.a.
Butterfinger, ½ cup	8.0	4.0
Butterfinger, regular scoop	15.0	n.a.
caramel chocolate crunch, ½ cup	9.0	5.0
cheesecake, cherry, ½	7.0	4.0
cheesecake, New York, ½ cup	9.0	6.0
cherries jubilee, ½ cup	6.0	4.0
cherries jubilee, regular scoop	11.0	n.a.
chunks 'n chips, ½ cup	9.0	6.0
chocolate, ½ cup	8.0	5.0
chocolate, regular scoop	14.0	n.a.
chocolate, winter white, ½ cup	8.0	5.0
chocolate, world class, ½ cup	8.0	4.0
chocolate, world class, regular scoop	14.0	n.a.
chocolate almond, ½ cup	10.0	5.0
chocolate almond, regular scoop	18.0	8.0
chocolate cake, German, ½ cup	11.0	5.0

	total fat (grams)	saturated fat (grams)

Baskin-Robbins, ice cream, regular deluxe *(cont.)*

chocolate cake, German, regular scoop	15.0	.... n.a.
chocolate chip, ½ cup	9.0	.... 5.0
chocolate chip, regular scoop	15.0	.... 10.0
chocolate chip cookie dough, ½ cup	10.0	.... 5.0
chocolate fudge, ½ cup	9.0	.... 5.0
chocolate fudge, regular scoop	15.0	.... n.a.
chocolate mousse royale, ½ cup	9.0	.... 6.0
chocolate mousse royale, regular scoop	16.0	.... n.a.
chocolate passion, triple, ½ cup	10.0	.... 6.0
chocolate ribbon, ½ cup	7.0	.... 4.0
cinnamon tax crunch, ½ cup	8.0	.... 4.0
cookies 'n cream, ½ cup	9.0	.... 6.0
cookies 'n cream regular scoop	17.0	.... n.a.
Fudge, Here Comes the, ½ cup	7.0	.... 5.0
fudge brownie, ½ cup	10.0	.... 6.0
fudge brownie, regular scoop	18.0	.... n.a.
gold medal ribbon, ½ cup	7.0	.... 4.0
Heath Bar, chunky, ½ cup	9.0	.... 6.0
Jamoca, ½ cup	7.0	.... 5.0
Jamoca, regular scoop	13.0	.... n.a.
Jamoca almond fudge, ½ cup	8.0	.... 4.0
Jamoca almond fudge, regular scoop	14.0	.... n.a.
lemon custard, ½ cup	7.0	.... 4.0
mint chocolate chip, ½ cup	9.0	.... 5.0
mint chocolate chip, regular scoop	15.0	.... n.a.
Naughty New Year's Resolution, ½ cup	11.0	.... 5.0
nutty coconut, ½ cup	11.0	.... 5.0
peach, ½ cup	6.0	.... 4.0
peach, regular scoop	11.0	.... 7.0
peanut butter, *Reese's,* ½ cup	10.0	.... 5.0
peanut butter, *Reese's,* regular scoop	18.0	.... 12.0
peanut butter 'n chocolate, ½ cup	11.0	.... 5.0
peanut butter 'n chocolate, regular scoop	20.0	.... n.a.
Peter, Peter, Pumpkin Cheezer, ½ cup	8.0	.... 5.0

	total fat (grams)	saturated fat (grams)
pistachio-almond, ½ cup	11.0	5.0
pistachio-almond, regular scoop	18.0	n.a.
pralines 'n cream, ½ cup	8.0	4.0
pralines 'n cream, regular scoop	14.0	7.0
pumpkin pie, ½ cup	6.0	4.0
Quarterback Crunch, ½ cup	9.0	6.0
rocky road, ½ cup	8.0	4.0
rocky road, regular scoop	14.0	n.a.
rum raisin, ½ cup	6.0	4.0
S'crunchous Crunch, ½ cup	8.0	5.0
S'mores, ½ cup	7.5	4.0
S'mores, regular scoop	13.0	8.0
Snickidy Doo Dah, ½ cup	8.0	5.0
strawberry, very berry, ½ cup	6.0	4.0
strawberry, very berry, regular scoop	10.0	n.a.
strawberry cheesecake, ½ cup	7.0	4.0
strawberry cheesecake, regular scoop	13.0	8.0
strawberry shortcake, ½ cup	8.0	5.0
Transylvania Twist, ½ cup	8.0	4.0
vanilla, ½ cup	8.0	5.0
vanilla, regular scoop	14.0	n.a.
vanilla, French, ½ cup	11.0	6.0
vanilla, French, regular scoop	18.0	n.a.
ice cream, light, ½ cup:		
almond buttercrunch	4.0	2.0
chocolate caramel nut	4.0	1.5
espresso 'n cream	4.0	2.5
pistachio creme chip	4.0	2.5
praline dream	4.0	1.5
raspberry, double	2.0	1.0
rocky path	4.0	1.5
ice cream, fat free, all flavors, ½ cup	0	0
ice cream, no sugar added, ½ cup:		
banana, chunky	1.5	1.0
berries 'n banana	1.0	1.0

	total fat (grams)	saturated fat (grams)

Baskin-Robbins, ice cream, no sugar added *(cont.)*

Call Me Nuts	2.0	1.0
cherry cordial	2.0	1.5
chocolate chip or chocolate chocolate chip	2.5	1.5
coconut fudge	1.5	1.0
Jamoca Swiss almond	2.5	1.5
mint, thin	2.5	1.5
pineapple coconut	1.5	1.0
raspberry revelation	1.0	.5
vanilla Swiss almond	2.0	1.5
ices and sherbets:		
daiquiri, grape, or Margarita ice, ½ cup	0	0
orange or rainbow sherbet, ½ cup	1.5	1.0
orange or rainbow sherbet, regular scoop	2.0	1.5
red raspberry sorbet, ½ cup	0	0
novelties, 1 piece:		
chillyburger, chocolate chip or mint chocolate chip	11.0	7.0
sundae bar, Jamoca almond fudge	17.0	9.0
sundae bar, peanut butter chocolate	27.0	11.0
sundae bar, pralines 'n cream	17.0	10.0
tiny toon bar, chocolate chip or mint chocolate chip	17.0	11.0
tiny toon bar, vanilla	16.0	9.0
yogurt (hard packed), ½ cup:		
brownie madness, Maui, lowfat	3.0	1.0
Boom Choco Laka	5.0	4.0
Praline, Perils of, lowfat	3.0	1.5
raspberry cheese Louise, lowfat	3.0	2.0
yogurt, lowfat, ½ cup:		
blueberry, cheesecake, or chocolate	1.5	1.0
vanilla	2.0	1.0
yogurt, nonfat or fat free, all flavors, ½ cup	0	0
fountain drinks, 1 serving, except as noted:		
Cappy Blast, w/whipped cream	10.0	7.0

	total fat (grams)	saturated fat (grams)
Cappy Blast, mocha, w/whipped cream	11.0	7.0
malt shake, vanilla ice cream	31.0	19.0
malt powder, 1 oz.	1.5	1.0
cones, 1 piece:		
cake cone	0	0
sugar cone	9.0	0
waffle cone, large	1.5	0
waffle cone, fresh baked	2.0	.5
toppings:		
butterscotch, 2 oz.	2.0	n.a.
hot fudge, 1 oz.	3.0	n.a.
hot fudge, no sugar added, 1 oz.	0	0
praline caramel or strawberry, 1 oz.	0	0
gummy bears, baby, 75 pieces	0	0
whipped cream, Rod's, 2 tsp.	2.5	1.5
Bass, meat only, 4 oz.:		
freshwater, raw	4.2	.9
freshwater, baked, broiled, or microwaved	5.4	1.1
sea, see "Sea bass"		
striped, raw	2.7	.6
striped, baked, broiled, or microwaved	6.2	1.3
Bay leaf, dried, crumbled, 1 tbsp.	.2	<.1
Bean, see specific bean listings		
Bean curd, see "Tofu"		
Bean dip, 2 tbsp.:		
(*Chi-Chi's* Fiesta)	1.5	.5
black bean:		
(*Eagle*)	1.0	0
(*Garden of Eatin' Baja*)	0	0
(*Old El Paso*)	0	0
hot:		
(*Doritos*)	1.0	0
(*Tom's*), 1.1 oz.	0	0
Mexican or onion (*Hain*)	1.0	n.a.

	total fat (grams)	saturated fat (grams)
jalapeño bean, see "Jalapeño dip"		
mild (*Eagle*)	1.5	0
red bean (*Garden of Eatin' Smoky Chipotle*)	0	0
Bean dip mix:		
black bean or Mexican (*Knorr*), ⅟₁₆ pkg.	0	0
black or pinto bean (*McCormick Collection*),		
⅛ pkg.	0	0
Bean entree, (see also "Chili" and specific listings), dry:		
country, and beef casserole, freeze-dried		
(*AlpineAire*), 1½ cups*	4.0	n.a.
Italian (*Knorr*), 1 pkg.	2.0	0
Bean salad, canned (*Green Giant*), ½ cup	0	0
Bean sauce, spicy (*House of Tsang*), 1 tsp.	0	0
Bean sprouts:		
fresh, see specific bean listings canned, 2 oz.	0	0
Beans, baked, see "Baked beans"		
Beans, refried, see "Refried beans"		
Beans and franks/weiners, see "Baked beans, w/franks"		
Béarnaise sauce mix:		
(*Knorr* Classic Sauces), ⅕ pkg.	.5	0
(*McCormick Collection*), ⅟₁₀ pkg.	0	0
Beau monde seasoning (*Spice Islands*), ¼ tsp.	0	0
Beechnuts, dried, shelled, 1 oz.	14.2	1.6
Beef, choice grade, retail trim[1], 4 oz., except as noted:		
brisket, braised:		
whole, lean and fat, 11.6 oz. (1 lb. raw)	104.1	40.8
whole, lean and fat	35.8	14.0
whole, lean only	14.5	5.2
flat half, lean and fat, 11.5 oz. (1 lb. raw)	93.1	36.0
flat half, lean and fat	32.3	12.5
flat half, lean only	11.0	3.6

---

[1]All cuts trimmed to ¼" fat, except flank steak, which is trimmed to 0" fat. For "lean only" listings, all visible fat is trimmed after cooking. (Bear in mind that a small amount of fat is always present, even in meat trimmed to 0" fat before cooking.)

	total fat (grams)	saturated fat (grams)
point half, lean and fat, 11.6 oz. (1 lb. raw) ...	112.4	44.5
point half, lean and fat	38.9	15.4
point half, lean only	17.8	6.7
brisket, corned or cured, see "Beef, corned"		
chuck, braised:		
arm, lean and fat, 9.1 oz. (1 lb. raw w/bone) ..	66.3	26.1
arm, lean and fat	29.2	11.5
arm, lean only	10.5	3.8
blade roast, lean and fat, 8.7 oz. (1 lb. raw		
w/bone)	69.0	27.5
blade roast, lean and fat	31.5	12.6
blade roast, lean only	16.3	6.3
flank steak:		
braised, lean and fat	18.6	7.8
braised, lean only	14.7	6.3
broiled, lean and fat	14.2	6.0
broiled, lean only	11.5	4.9
ground (see also "Beef patties"), 1 oz.:		
raw, extra lean	4.8	1.9
raw, lean	5.9	2.4
raw, regular	7.5	3.1
baked, extra lean, medium	18.3	7.2
baked, extra lean, well-done	18.1	7.1
baked, lean, medium or well-done	20.8	8.2
baked, regular, medium	23.7	9.3
baked, regular, well-done	24.3	9.6
broiled, extra lean, medium	18.5	7.3
broiled, extra lean, well-done	17.9	7.0
broiled, lean, medium	20.9	8.2
broiled, lean, well-done	20.0	7.9
broiled, regular, medium	23.5	9.2
broiled, regular, well-done	22.1	8.7
pan-fried, extra lean, medium	18.6	7.3
pan-fried, extra lean, well-done	18.1	7.1
pan-fried, lean, medium	21.6	8.5
pan-fried, lean, well-done	20.0	7.9

	total fat (grams)	saturated fat (grams)

Beef, ground *(cont.)*

pan-fried, regular, medium	25.6	.... 10.0
pan-fried, regular, well-done	21.5	.... 8.4

rib, whole (ribs 6–12):

broiled, lean and fat, 9.5 oz. (1 lb. raw w/bone)	79.4	.... 32.2
broiled, lean and fat	33.5	.... 13.6
broiled, lean only	15.7	.... 6.4
roasted, lean and fat, 10.2 oz. (1 lb. raw w/bone)	90.5	.... 36.5
roasted, lean and fat	35.4	.... 14.3
roasted, lean only	15.9	.... 6.4

rib, large end (ribs 6–9):

broiled, lean and fat, 9.5 oz. (1 lb. raw w/bone)	82.8	.... 33.7
broiled, lean and fat	34.9	.... 14.2
broiled, lean only	16.6	.... 6.8
roasted, lean and fat, 10.5 oz. (1 lb. raw w/bone)	94.9	.... 38.3
roasted, lean and fat	36.2	.... 14.6
roasted, lean only	16.7	.... 6.7

rib, shortrib, braised, 4 oz.:

lean and fat, 8 oz. (1 lb. raw w/bone)	94.9	.... 40.2
lean and fat	47.6	.... 20.2
lean only	20.6	.... 8.7

rib, small end (ribs 10–12):

broiled, lean and fat, 9.6 oz. (1 lb. raw w/bone)	75.1	.... 30.4
broiled, lean and fat	31.3	.... 12.7
broiled, lean only	14.3	.... 5.8
roasted, lean and fat, 9.8 oz. (1 lb. raw w/bone)	84.4	.... 34.0
roasted, lean and fat	34.3	.... 13.8
roasted, lean only	14.8	.... 5.9
rib eye, koshered (*Hebrew National*), 4 oz.	37.0	.... 17.0

	total fat (grams)	saturated fat (grams)
round, full cut:		
broiled, lean and fat, 11 oz. (1 lb. raw)	42.6	16.1
broiled, lean and fat	15.4	5.9
broiled, lean only	8.3	2.9
round, bottom:		
braised, lean and fat, 8.9 oz. (1 lb. raw)	50.6	19.0
braised, lean and fat	20.3	7.6
braised, lean only	10.7	3.6
roasted, lean and fat, 11.9 oz. (1 lb. raw)	55.3	20.8
roasted, lean and fat	18.5	7.0
roasted, lean only	9.4	3.2
round, eye of, 4 oz.:		
roasted, lean and fat, 11.7 oz. (1 lb. raw)	47.0	18.3
roasted, lean and fat	16.0	6.2
roasted, lean only	6.5	2.3
round, tip:		
roasted, lean and fat, 11.3 oz. (1 lb. raw)	47.6	18.1
roasted, lean and fat	16.9	6.4
roasted, lean only	8.3	2.9
round, top:		
braised, lean and fat, 10.2 oz. (1 lb. raw)	37.2	14.1
braised, lean and fat	14.6	5.5
braised, lean only	7.4	2.5
broiled, lean and fat, 11.5 oz. (1 lb. raw)	34.4	12.8
broiled, lean and fat	12.0	4.5
broiled, lean only	6.7	2.3
shank, crosscuts:		
simmered, lean and fat, 6.8 oz. (1 lb. raw w/bone)	28.5	11.1
simmered, lean and fat	16.6	6.5
simmered, lean only	7.2	2.6
sirloin, top:		
broiled, lean and fat, 10.8 oz. (1 lb. raw)	51.2	20.4
broiled, lean and fat	19.0	7.6
broiled, lean only	9.1	3.5
steak, see "Beef steak" and specific "Beef" listings		

	total fat (grams)	saturated fat (grams)
Beef *(cont.)*		
T-bone steak, broiled:		
lean and fat, 9 oz. (1 lb. raw w/bone)	51.9	20.9
lean and fat	24.0	9.7
lean only	11.8	4.7
tenderloin		
broiled, lean and fat, 4.1 oz. (6.1 oz. raw steak)	25.6	10.0
broiled, lean and fat	24.8	9.7
broiled, lean only	12.7	4.8
roasted, lean and fat, 11.6 oz. (1 lb. raw)	86.0	34.3
roasted, lean and fat	29.9	11.8
roasted, lean only	14.2	5.4
top loin, broiled:		
lean and fat, 6.3 oz. (9.2 oz. raw steak)	37.8	15.0
lean and fat	23.8	9.4
lean only	11.5	4.4
Beef, canned (see also specific listings), 1 oz.	4.2	1.8
Beef, corned (see also "Beef luncheon meat"):		
(*Thorn Apple Valley*), 3 oz.	14.0	n.a.
brisket, lean and fat, 11.3 oz. (1 lb. raw)	60.7	20.3
brisket, lean and fat, 4 oz.	21.5	7.2
canned (*Hormel*), 2 oz.	7.0	3.0
canned (*Libby's*), 2 oz.	7.0	3.0
Beef, corned, hash, see "Beef hash"		
Beef, dried:		
cured, 1 oz.	1.1	.5
sliced (*Hormel*), 10 slices, 1 oz.	1.5	.5
Beef, freeze-dried, diced (*AlpineAire*), ⅓ cup*	5.0	n.a.
Beef, ground, see "Beef"		
Beef, ground, seasoning (*Durkee*), ¼ pkg.	0	0
Beef, roast, see "Beef," "Beef entree," "Beef luncheon meat," and "Beef spread"		
Beef, roast, hash, see "Beef hash"		

	total fat (grams)	saturated fat (grams)
"Beef," vegetarian, canned (see also "Burger, vegetarian, canned" and "Vegetarian dishes, canned"		
(*Worthington* Savory Slices), 3 oz., 3 slices	9.0	3.5
steak (*Worthington Prime Stakes*), 3.25-oz. piece	9.0	1.5
steak (*Worthington* Vegetable Steaks), 2.5 oz., 2 pieces	1.5	.5
Swiss steak (*Loma Linda*), 3.2 oz., 1 piece	6.0	1.0
"Beef," vegetarian, frozen (see also "Burger, vegetarian, frozen" and "Vegetarian dishes, frozen"):		
(*Worthington* Beef Style Meatless), 1.9 oz., ⅜" slice	7.0	1.0
(*Worthington Stakelets*), 2.5-oz. piece	8.0	1.5
corned (*Worthington*), 2 oz., 4 slices	9.0	2.0
ground (*Worthington*), 1.9 oz., ½ cup	2.5	.5
patties (*Ken & Robert's* Veggie Burger), 2.5-oz. patty	2.0	0
pie (*Worthington*), 8-oz. pie	24.0	4.0
smoked (*Worthington*), 2 oz., 6 slices	6.0	1.0
steak (*Loma Linda* Griddle Steaks), 1.9-oz. piece	7.0	1.0
Beef dinner, frozen:		
(*Banquet*), 9.5 oz.	7.0	3.0
(*Swanson*), 11 oz.	9.0	5.0
and broccoli (*Swanson*), 10 oz.	10.0	4.0
enchilada, see "Enchilada dinner"		
meatballs, sirloin, and gravy (*The Budget Gourmet* Light & Healthy), 11 oz.	8.0	3.0
patty, w/gravy (*Banquet*), 9 oz.	20.0	8.0
patty (*Swanson Fun Feast*), 8 oz.	19.0	7.0
pepper steak (*Armour Classics*), 11 oz.	4.0	1.5
pepper steak (*Healthy Choice*), 11 oz.	5.0	2.0
pot roast, Yankee:		
(*The Budget Gourmet* Light & Healthy), 10.5 oz.	7.0	2.5
(*Healthy Choice*), 11 oz.	4.0	2.0

	total fat (grams)	saturated fat (grams)
Beef dinner, frozen, pot roast, Yankee *(cont.)*		
(*Swanson*), 11.5 oz.	7.0	4.0
(*Swanson Hungry-Man*), 16 oz.	11.0	3.0
ribs, boneless, w/barbecue sauce (*Healthy Choice*		
Generous Serving), 11 oz.	6.0	2.0
Salisbury steak:		
(*Armour Classics*), 11.25 oz.	18.0	8.0
(*Armour Classics* Lite), 11.5 oz.	7.0	4.0
(*Banquet*), 9.5 oz.	20.0	8.0
(*Banquet Extra Helping*), 19 oz.	46.0	19.0
(*Healthy Choice*), 11.5 oz.	7.0	3.0
(*Morton*), 9 oz.	9.0	4.0
(*Swanson*), 10.5 oz.	18.0	7.0
(*Swanson Hungry-Man*), 16.3 oz.	34.0	17.0
con queso (*Patio*), 11 oz.	20.0	11.0
w/mushroom gravy (*Healthy Choice Generous*		
Serving), 11 oz.	6.0	3.0
sirloin, w/red skin potato (*The Budget Gourmet*		
Light & Healthy), 11 oz.	8.0	3.0
sirloin:		
(*The Budget Gourmet* Light & Healthy Special		
Recipe), 11 oz.	7.0	3.0
w/barbecue sauce (*Healthy Choice*), 11 oz.	4.0	2.0
chopped (*Swanson*), 10.5 oz.	17.0	11.0
in wine sauce (*The Budget Gourmet* Light &		
Healthy), 11 oz.	6.0	2.0
tips (*Swanson Hungry-Man*), 15.75 oz.	16.0	6.0
teriyaki (*The Budget Gourmet* Light & Healthy),		
10.75 oz.	6.0	2.0
Beef entree, canned or packaged:		
corned or roast beef hash, see "Beef hash"		
goulash (*Hormel*), 7.5-oz. can	11.0	5.0
meatloaf, see "Meatloaf entree"		
roast:		
w/gravy (*Hormel*), 2 oz.	2.0	1.0

	total fat (grams)	saturated fat (grams)
w/gravy (*Libby's*), ⅔ cup	3.0	1.5
w/mashed potato (*Dinty Moore American Classics*), 1 bowl	5.0	2.0
tender (*Hormel Top Shelf*), 10 oz.	6.0	2.0
Salisbury steak (*Dinty Moore American Classics*), 1 cup	14.0	6.0
stew:		
(*Dinty Moore*), 1 cup	14.0	7.0
(*Dinty Moore*), 7.5-oz. can	10.0	4.0
(*Dinty Moore* Microwave Cup), 1 cup	10.0	4.0
(*Dinty Moore American Classics*), 1 bowl	13.0	6.0
(*Hormel* Micro Cup), 1 cup	9.0	4.0
(*Libby's Diner*), 7.75 oz.	20.0	5.0
(*Nalley*), 7.5 oz.	8.0	4.0
(*Nalley Big Chunk*), 7.5 oz.	12.0	6.0
(*Nalley Homestyle*), 7.5 oz.	8.0	4.0
stew, burger, hearty (*Dinty Moore* Microwave Cup), 1 cup	13.0	5.0
stew, meatball, see "Meatball entree"		
tamales, see "Tamales"		
Beef entree, freeze-dried*:		
and green peppers, onions, in sauce, w/rice (*Mountain House*), 1 cup	5.0	1.0
rotini (*AlpineAire*), 1⅓ cups	5.0	n.a.
stew with, hearty (*Mountain House*), 1 cup	2.0	1.0
Stroganoff, w/noodles (*AlpineAire*), 1½ cups	6.0	n.a.
Stroganoff sauce and, w/noodles (*Mountain House*), 1 cup	10.0	4.0
teriyaki, w/rice (*Mountain House*), 1 cup	4.0	1.0
Beef entree, frozen:		
barbecue, chopped (*Schwan's*), ½ cup	8.0	3.0
Cantonese (*The Budget Gourmet*), 9.1 oz.	8.0	3.0
casserole (*Schwan's*), 1 cup	17.0	7.0
cheeseburger, see "Beef sandwich"		

	total fat (grams)	saturated fat (grams)

Beef entree, frozen *(cont.)*
  creamed, chipped:
    (*Banquet Hot Sandwich Toppers*), 4 oz. ...... 3.0 .... 1.5
    (*Schwan's*), 1 cup ...... 17.0 .... 5.0
    (*Stouffer's*), 3.6 oz. ...... 11.0 .... 3.0
    over country biscuit (*Stouffer's*), 9 oz. ...... 29.0 .... 8.0
  enchilada, see "Enchilada"
  fingers, breaded (*Schwan's*), 5 pieces ...... 5.0 .... 2.0
  goulash (*Schwan's*), 1 cup ...... 13.0 .... 5.0
  hamburger, see "Beef sandwich"
  meatballs, see "Meatball entree"
  meatloaf, see "Meatloaf entree"
  and noodles (*Banquet* Family), 1 cup ...... 4.0 .... 2.0
  pasta, see specific pasta listings
  patty, 1 piece:
    charbroiled, w/gravy (*Banquet* Family) ...... 13.0 .... 6.0
    w/onion gravy (*Banquet* Family) ...... 14.0 .... 6.0
  pepper:
    green, steak (*Stouffer's*), 10.5 oz. ...... 9.0 .... 3.0
    Oriental (*Chun King*), 13 oz. ...... 4.0 .... 1.0
    steak (*Healthy Choice*), 9.5 oz. ...... 4.0 .... 2.0
    steak, w/rice (*The Budget Gourmet*), 10 oz. .. 8.0 .... 3.0
  pie:
    (*Banquet*), 7 oz. ...... 15.0 .... 7.0
    (*Banquet* Supreme), 7 oz. ...... 12.0 .... 5.0
    (*Morton*), 7 oz. ...... 17.0 .... 8.0
    (*Stouffer's*), 10 oz. ...... 26.0 .... 9.0
    (*Swanson*), 7 oz. ...... 19.0 .... 8.0
    (*Swanson Hungry-Man*), 14 oz. ...... 29.0 .... 14.0
  pie, hand-held, see "Steak sandwich"
  pie, shepherd's (*Schwan's*), 1 cup ...... 12.0 .... 4.0
  pot roast (*Lean Cuisine*), 9 oz. ...... 7.0 .... 1.5
  pot roast (*Stouffer's* Homestyle), 8⅞ oz. ...... 10.0 .... 3.0
  Oriental:
    (*The Budget Gourmet* Light & Healthy),
      10 oz. ...... 8.0 .... 4.0

	total fat (grams)	saturated fat (grams)
(*Lean Cuisine*), 9 oz.	8.0	3.0
(*Stouffer's Lunch Express*), 9⅝ oz.	8.0	1.5
roast, open face, w/mashed potatoes		
(*The Budget Gourmet*), 9 oz.	17.0	6.0
Salisbury steak:		
(*Banquet Hot Sandwich Toppers*), 5 oz.	16.0	7.0
(*Stouffer's* Homestyle), 9⅝ oz.	19.0	6.0
(*Weight Watchers Smart Ones*), 8.5 oz.	9.0	3.0
w/macaroni and cheese (*Lean Cuisine*), 9.5 oz.	9.0	3.5
w/whipped potatoes (*Swanson*), 9 oz.	20.0	11.0
patty (*Banquet Family*), 1 patty	14.0	6.0
sirloin (*The Budget Gourmet* Light & Healthy), 9 oz.	5.0	2.0
sandwich, see "Beef sandwich" and "Steak sandwich"		
sliced, gravy and (*Banquet Hot Sandwich Toppers*), 4 oz.	2.0	1.0
sliced, gravy and (*Banquet Family*), 2 slices	3.0	1.5
sirloin:		
in herb sauce (*The Budget Gourmet* Light & Healthy), 9.5 oz.	7.0	4.0
peppercorn (*Lean Cuisine* Cafe Classics), 8¾ oz.	7.0	1.5
roast, supreme (*The Budget Gourmet*), 9 oz.	13.0	6.0
sirloin cheddar melt (*The Budget Gourmet*), 9.4 oz.	21.0	10.0
sirloin tips, w/vegetables (*The Budget Gourmet*), 10 oz.	14.0	6.0
stew (*Banquet Family*), 1 cup	4.0	2.0
Stroganoff (*The Budget Gourmet* Light & Healthy), 8.75 oz.	7.0	4.0
Stroganoff (*Stouffer's*), 9¾ oz.	20.0	7.0
tips, w/gravy (*Schwan's*), 1 cup	6.0	2.5

	total fat (grams)	saturated fat (grams)
Beef entree, frozen *(cont.)*		
tips, w/mushroom gravy (*Healthy Choice*), 9.5 oz. ..	6.0	.... 2.0
Beef gravy, canned:		
¼ cup	1.4	7
(*Franco-American*), 2 oz., ¼ cup	2.0	.... 1.0
(*Swanson*), ¼ cup	2.0	.... 1.0
Beef hash, canned:		
corned beef:		
(*Dinty Moore* Microwave Cup), 1 cup	22.0	.... 9.0
(*Libby's*), 1 cup	36.0	.... 17.0
(*Mary Kitchen*), 1 cup	24.0	.... 10.0
(*Mary Kitchen*), 7.5-oz. can	22.0	.... 9.0
(*Nalley*), 7.5 oz.	34.0	.... 16.0
roast beef:		
(*Libby's*), 1 cup	33.0	.... 13.0
(*Mary Kitchen*), 1 cup	24.0	.... 10.0
(*Mary Kitchen*), 7.5-oz. can	21.0	.... 9.0
Beef jerky, see "Beef stick"		
Beef liver, see "Liver"		
Beef luncheon meat, 2 oz., except as noted:		
corned (see also "Beef, corned"):		
(*Hansel 'n Gretel Healthy Deli*)	3.0	.... 1.0
(*Healthy Choice*), 1 oz.	1.0	.... <1.0
(*Hebrew National* Deli Express)	3.0	.... 1.0
(*Hebrew National* Rounds)	2.0	.... 1.0
(*Hillshire Farm* Deli Select), 1 slice	<1.0	.... n.a.
(*Hormel*), 1 oz.	3.0	.... 1.0
(*Hormel Light & Lean* Deli)	2.0	.... 1.0
brisket (*Boar's Head* 1st Cut)	3.0	.... 1.5
dried, see "Beef, dried"		
pastrami, see "Pastrami"		
roast:		
(*Boar's Head* Deluxe Custom Cut)	4.0	.... 1.5
(*Healthy Choice*)	2.0	.... 1.0
(*Healthy Choice* Deli Meats), 1 oz.	1.0	.... <1.0

	total fat (grams)	saturated fat (grams)
(*Hillshire Farm* Deli Select), 1 slice	<1.0	.... n.a.
(*Hormel Light & Lean* Deli), 3 oz.	2.5	.... 1.0
(*Oscar Mayer Deli-Thin*), 1.8 oz., 4 slices	1.5	5
(*Thumann's*), 1 oz.	1.5	.... n.a.
round (*Boar's Head* Custom Cut No Salt)	4.0	.... 1.5
round, eye, Cajun seasoned (*Boar's Head*) ...	2.5	.... 1.5
round, eye, pepper seasoned (*Boar's Head*) ..	3.0	.... 1.5
round, top, choice (*Boar's Head* No Salt/Deluxe Low Sodium)	3.0	.... 1.5
seasoned (*Hansel 'n Gretel Healthy Deli*)	2.0	5
seasoned, Italian (*Hansel 'n Gretel Healthy Deli*)	1.5	5
sliced, 1 oz.	.9	4
smoked (*Hillshire Farm* Deli Select), 1 slice	<1.0	.... n.a.
Beef marinade, see "Beef seasoning"		
Beef patties, frozen:		
(*Schwan's*), 4-oz. patty	23.0	.... 9.0
pizza (*Schwan's*), 3.5-oz. patty	26.0	.... 11.0
stuffed, w/cheddar (*Schwan's* Beef Pattie Melt), 4-oz. patty	27.0	.... 15.0
Beef pie, see "Beef entree, frozen"		
Beef sandwich, frozen, 1 piece:		
barbecue (*Hormel Quick Meal* BBQ)	16.0	.... 6.0
w/cheese (*Kid Cuisine*)	7.0	.... 4.0
cheeseburger:		
(*Hormel Quick Meal*)	20.0	.... 9.0
bacon (*Hormel Quick Meal*)	23.0	.... 10.0
chili (*Hormel Quick Meal*)	23.0	.... 10.0
mini (*Jimmy Dean*)	5.0	.... n.a.
hamburger (*Hormel Quick Meal*)	15.0	.... 6.0
hamburger, mini (*Jimmy Dean*)	4.0	.... n.a.
Reuben, pocket (*Weight Watchers*)	6.0	.... 2.0
steak, see "Beef steak"		
Beef sausage, see "Sausage" and "Summer sausage"		

	total fat (grams)	saturated fat (grams)
Beef seasoning (see also specific listings):		
(*Perc*), ¼ tsp.	<.1	0
marinade (*Durkee*), ⅒ pkg.	0	0
marinade (*Lawry's* Spices & Seasonings), ¾ tsp.	0	0
Beef spread, canned, roast		
(*Underwood*), 2 oz., ¼ cup	11.0	4.5
Beef steak (see also "Beef"), frozen:		
(*Schwan's Big Sam*), 6-oz. steak	7.0	3.0
breaded, cubed (*Schwan's*), 4-oz. steak	20.0	9.0
chopped (*Schwan's*), 5.3-oz. steak	31.0	13.0
dinner (*Schwan's*), 7-oz. steak	32.0	13.0
sandwich, Phili style (*Schwan's*), 3 slices	5.0	2.5
sirloin (*Schwan's* Ball Tip), 6-oz. steak	12.0	5.0
sirloin (*Schwan's* Filet), 4-oz. steak	6.0	3.0
Beef stew, see "Beef entree"		
Beef stew seasoning:		
(*French's*), ⅑ pkg.	0	0
(*Lawry's* Spices & Seasonings), 2 tsp.	0	0
mix (*Durkee* Pouch), ⅒ pkg.	0	0
Beef stick, 1 piece:		
(*Boar's Head*)	9.0	3.5
(*Rustlers Roundup*)	6.0	2.5
(*Tombstone/Tombstone/Snappy Sticks*)	10.0	4.5
jerky, 1-oz. piece	3.7	1.7
jerky (*Rustlers Roundup*)	2.0	1.0
Beef stock base (*Spice Islands*), 2 tsp.	0	0
Beef Stroganoff entree, see "Beef entree"		
Beef Stroganoff hors d'oeuvre, frozen		
(*Pepperidge Farm* Kit), 1 filled shell	29.0	12.0
Beef tallow, 1 tbsp.	12.8	6.4
Beefalo, meat only:		
roasted, 12 oz. (1 lb. raw)	21.5	9.1
roasted, 4 oz.	7.2	3.0
Beer, regular or light, all brands, 12 fl. oz.	0	0

	total fat (grams)	saturated fat (grams)
Beerwurst (see also "Salami, beer"):		
beef, 1 oz.	8.3	3.4
pork, 1 oz.	5.3	1.8
Beet:		
fresh:		
raw, untrimmed, 1 lb.	.4	.1
raw, 2 medium, 2" diameter, 8.6 oz.	.2	<.1
boiled, drained, 2 medium, 2" diameter	.1	tr.
boiled, drained, sliced, ½ cup	<.1	0
canned, ½ cup:		
regular, Harvard or pickled	.1	tr.
all varieties (*Del Monte*)	0	0
all varieties (*Green Giant*)	0	0
all varieties (*Greenwood*)	0	0
all varieties (*Seneca*)	0	0
all varieties (*Stokely*)	0	0
Beet greens, fresh:		
raw, untrimmed, 1 lb.	.2	<.1
raw, 1" pieces, ½ cup	<.1	0
boiled, drained, 1" pieces, ½ cup	.1	<.1
Berries, see specific listings		
Berries, mixed, frozen (*Stilwell* Festival of Berries),		
1¼ cups	0	0
Berry drink or juice, all varieties and brands, 8 fl. oz.	0	0
Biscotti, see "Cookie"		
Biscuit (see also "Cracker" and "Roll"):		
(*Arnold* Old Fashioned), 2 pieces	5.0	1.0
(*Awrey's* Round or Square), 2"-piece, 1 oz.	3.0	1.0
(*Awrey's* Square/Country), 3"-piece, 2 oz.	5.0	1.0
Biscuit, refrigerated or frozen:		
(*Ballard Extra Lights Oven Ready*), 3 pieces	2.0	0
(*Big Country Butter Tastin'*), 1 piece	4.0	1.0
(*Grands!* HomeStyle), 1 piece	9.0	2.5
(*Pillsbury* Country), 3 pieces	4.0	0
baking powder (*1869* Brand), 1 piece	5.0	1.5

	total fat (grams)	saturated fat (grams)

Biscuit, refrigerated or frozen *(cont.)*

butter (*Grands!*), 1 piece	10.0	2.5
butter (*Pillsbury*), 3 pieces	2.5	0
buttermilk:		
(*Ballard Extra Lights Oven Ready*), 3 pieces	2.0	0
(*Big Country*), 1 piece	4.0	1.0
(*1869* Brand), 1 piece	5.0	1.5
(*Grands!*), 1 piece	10.0	3.0
(*Hungry Jack* Flaky), 2 pieces	7.0	1.5
(*Pillsbury*), 3 pieces	4.0	0
(*Pillsbury* Tender Layer), 3 pieces	7.0	5.0
cinnamon raisin:		
(*Grands!*), 1 piece	8.0	2.0
w/icing (*Schwan's*), 1 piece	15.0	9.0
flaky:		
(*Grands!*), 1 piece	9.0	2.0
(*Hungry Jack*), 2 pieces	7.0	1.5
(*Hungry Jack Butter/Honey Tastin'*),		
2 pieces	7.0	1.5
fluffy (*Hungry Jack*), 2 pieces	8.0	2.0
fluffy (*Pillsbury Good 'N Buttery*), 1 piece	5.0	1.0
garlic and cheese (*Pepperidge Farm*), 1 piece	6.0	2.5
Southern style:		
(*Big Country*), 1 piece	4.0	1.0
(*Grands!*), 1 piece	10.0	2.5
(*Hungry Jack* Flaky), 2 pieces	7.0	1.5
Biscuit mix (*Arrowhead Mills*), ¼ cup	1.0	0
Biscuit sandwich, see specific sandwich listings		
Black bean dip, see "Bean dip"		
Black beans:		
dry, ¼ cup	.7	.2
dry, boiled, ½ cup	.5	.1
canned, ½ cup:		
(*Eden* Organic)	0	0
(*Green Giant/Joan of Arc*)	0	0

	total fat (grams)	saturated fat (grams)
(*Old El Paso*)	1.0	0
(*Progresso*)	1.0	0
(*Stokely*)	.5	0
Western (*Health Valley* Vegetarian Cuisine), 1 cup	1.0	0
turtle, dry (*Arrowhead Mills*), ¼ cup	.5	0
turtle, canned (*Hain*), 4 oz.	1.0	0
Black beans, mix, instant (*Fantastic Foods International*), ⅓ cup	.5	0
Black beans, refried, see "Refried beans"		
Black beans, tofu (*Health Valley* Vegetarian Cuisine), 1 cup	1.0	0
Black beans and rice, see "Rice dishes, mix"		
Blackberry:		
fresh, 1 pint	1.5	tr.
fresh, trimmed, ½ cup	.3	0
canned (*Allens*), ⅔ cup	.5	0
canned, in syrup (*Wilderness*), ½ cup	0	0
frozen (*Stilwell*), 1 cup	0	0
Blackeye peas:		
fresh, dry, or canned, see "Cowpeas"		
frozen (*Stilwell*), ½ cup	1.0	0
Blintzes, frozen, 4.4 oz., 2 pieces:		
apple (*Empire* Kosher)	5.5	1.5
blueberry or cherry (*Empire* Kosher)	4.0	1.0
cheese (*Empire* Kosher)	6.0	2.0
potato (*Empire* Kosher)	6.0	1.5
Bloody Mary mixer, 8 fl. oz.:		
regular/rich and spicy (*Mr. & Mrs. "T"*)	0	0
regular (*Tabasco*)	.3	.1
spicy (*Tabasco*)	.4	.1
Blueberry:		
fresh, 1 pint	1.5	tr.
fresh, ½ cup	.3	0
canned, in syrup (*Wilderness*), ½ cup	0	0

	total fat (grams)	saturated fat (grams)

Blueberry *(cont.)*

frozen (*Stilwell*), 1 cup	0	....	0
dried (*Sonoma*), 1 cup	0	....	0
freeze-dried (*AlpineAire*), 1 oz.	.5	....	0

Blueberry nectar (*R. W. Knudsen*), 8 fl. oz. 0 0

Blueberry pastry filling (*Solo*), 2 tbsp. 0 0

Blueberry-cranberry drink (*Cran•Blueberry*),

8 fl. oz.	0	....	0

Bluefish, meat only:

raw, 4 oz.	4.8	....	1.1
baked, broiled, or microwaved, 4 oz.	6.2	....	1.3

Boar, wild, meat only:

roasted, 12 oz. (1 lb. raw)	14.9	....	4.4
roasted, 4 oz.	5.0	....	1.5

Bockwurst, 1 link, 7 links per lb. .... 8.6 .... 3.3

Bok choy, see "Cabbage, Chinese"

Bologna, 2 oz., except as noted:

(*Boar's Head*)	13.0	....	4.5
(*Boar's Head* Lower Sodium)	13.0	....	5.0
(*Healthy Choice*)	2.0	....	1.0
(*Hansel 'n Gretel Healthy Deli*)	2.5	..	1.0
(*Hillshire Farm* Deli Select Light), 1 slice	1.0	....	n.a
(*Hillshire Farm* Flavor Pack Light), .7-oz. slice	2.0	....	n.a.
(*Hillshire Farm* Large or Ring), 1 oz.	8.0	....	n.a.
(*Oscar Mayer*), 1-oz. slice	8.0	....	3.0
(*Oscar Mayer Healthy Favorites*), 1.6 oz.,			
2 slices	1.0	....	0
(*Oscar Mayer* Light), 1-oz. slice	4.0	....	1.5
(*Oscar Mayer* Wisconsin Made Ring)	16.0	....	6.0
(*Patrick Cudahy*)	15.0	....	6.0
(*Thorn Apple Valley*), 1-oz. slice	8.9	....	n.a.
(*Thumann's*), 1 oz.	7.5	..	n.a.

beef:

1-oz. slice	8.1	....	3.4
(*Boar's Head*)	13.0	...	4.0

	total fat (grams)	saturated fat (grams)
(*Healthy Choice*)	2.0	1.0
(*Hebrew National*)	16.0	6.0
(*Hebrew National* Lean)	6.0	2.0
(*Hebrew National* Reduced Fat)	12.0	5.0
(*Hebrew National* Wide Bulk Deli)	15.0	6.0
(*Hormel Light & Lean* Deli)	1.5	.5
(*Oscar Mayer*), 1-oz. slice	8.0	4.0
(*Oscar Mayer* Light), 1-oz. slice	4.0	1.5
(*Thorn Apple Valley*), 1-oz. slice	9.0	n.a.
w/turkey and pork (*Healthy Choice* Deli), 1 oz.	1.0	<1.0
beef, Lebanon, 1 oz.	3.7	1.7
beef and pork, 1-oz. slice	8.0	3.0
chicken, see "Chicken bologna"		
garlic (*Boar's Head*)	13.0	4.5
(*Oscar Mayer*), 1.4-oz. slice	12.0	4.0
ham, see "Ham bologna"		
pork, 1-oz. slice	5.6	2.0
turkey, see "Turkey bologna"		
"Bologna," vegetarian, frozen (*Worthington Bolono*), 2 oz., 3 slices	3.5	1.0
Bonito, meat only:		
Caribbean, raw, 4 oz.	4.8	n.a.
Japanese, raw, 4 oz.	2.3	n.a.
Borage:		
raw, 1" pieces, ½ cup	.3	0
boiled, drained, 4 oz.	.9	0
Bouillon, see "Soup"		
Bouillon cube:		
all varieties (*Herb-Ox*), 1 cube or pkt.	0	0
beef or chicken (*Knorr*), ½ cube	1.5	.5
fish flavor (*Knorr*), ½ cube	1.0	0
vegetarian vegetable (*Knorr*), ½ cube	1.0	0
Bourguignon recipe mix (*Knorr*), ⅙ pkg.	1.0	.5
Bow tie pasta entree, frozen, and chicken (*Lean Cuisine* Cafe Classics), 9.5 oz.	6.0	1.5

	total fat (grams)	saturated fat (grams)
Boysenberry:		
fresh, see "Blackberry"		
canned, in syrup (*Wilderness*), ½ cup	0	0
frozen, unsweetened, ½ cup	.2	0
Boysenberry juice, 6 fl. oz.	0	0
Boysenberry nectar (*R. W. Knudsen*), 8 fl. oz.	0	0
Brains, braised or simmered:		
beef, 13.8 oz. (1 lb. raw)	49.0	11.4
beef, 4 oz.	14.2	3.3
lamb, 12.25 oz. (1 lb. raw)	35.3	9.0
lamb, 4 oz.	11.5	2.9
pork, 13.5 oz. (1 lb. raw)	36.3	8.2
pork, 4 oz.	10.8	2.4
veal, 12 oz. (1 lb. raw)	32.6	n.a.
veal, 4 oz.	10.9	n.a.
Bran, see "Cereal" and specific grain listings		
Bratwurst:		
(*Boar's Head*), 4 oz.	25.0	11.0
(*Hillshire Farm* Fully Cooked), 2 oz.	16.0	n.a.
(*Schwan's*), 3.3-oz. link	23.0	11.0
fresh, smoked, or spicy (*Hillshire Farm*), 2 oz.	17.0	n.a.
light (*Hillshire Farm*), 2 oz.	11.0	n.a.
pork, cooked, 3-oz. link	22.0	7.0
pork and beef, cooked, 2.5-oz. link	19.5	7.0
Braunschweiger, 2 oz., except as noted:		
(*Boar's Head* Lite Liverwurst)	8.0	5.0
(*Hillshire Farm*), 1 oz.	8.0	n.a.
(*Jones Dairy Farm* Chub)	12.0	4.0
(*Jones Dairy Farm* Chub Light)	6.0	2.0
(*Jones Dairy Farm* Chunk)	16.0	5.0
(*Jones Dairy Farm* Chunk Light)	6.0	2.0
(*Oscar Mayer* Sliced), 1-oz. slice	9.0	3.0
(*Thorn Apple Valley*), 1 oz.	7.0	n.a.
(*Thumann's* Liverwurst), 1 oz.	7.0	n.a.
(*Usinger's* Low Fat)	5.0	2.0

	total fat (grams)	saturated fat (grams)
pork, 1 oz.	9.1	3.1
sliced (*Jones Dairy Farm*), 1.2-oz. slice	10.0	3.0
sliced, 1.6 oz., 2 slices	13.0	4.0
spread:		
(*Oscar Mayer* Liver Sausage)	17.0	6.0
(*Oscar Mayer* German Brand)	18.0	6.0
(*Oscar Mayer* Sandwich Spread)	10.0	3.5
w/bacon or onion (*Jones Dairy Farm* Club)	12.0	4.0
Brazil nut:		
in shell, 4 oz.	36.1	8.8
shelled, 1 oz., 6 large or 8 medium kernels	18.8	4.6
Bread, 1 slice, except as noted:		
apple walnut or apple walnut swirl (*Pepperidge Farm*)	2.0	.5
(*Arnold/Brownberry Bran'nola* Original)	2.0	0
bran (see also specific grains and listings):		
(*Arnold/Brownberry* Light Country), 2 slices	1.5	0
honey (*Pepperidge Farm*)	1.0	0
whole (*Brownberry* Natural)	1.0	0
buttermilk (*Arnold*)	1.5	0
chapati (*Garden of Eatin' Chapati*)	.5	0
cinnamon or cinnamon swirl (*Pepperidge Farm*)	2.5	.5
cranberry (*Arnold*)	1.0	0
date nut (*Thomas'*), 1 oz.	2.0	0
flatbread, see "Crackers"		
French (see also "Rolls"):		
stick (*Arnold/Francisco*), 1 oz.	1.0	0
twin (*Brownberry/Francisco* International), 1-oz. slice	1.0	0
golden swirl (*Pepperidge Farm* Vermont)	2.5	1.0
grain (see also specific listings):		
(*Brownberry* Hearth)	1.5	0
(*Roman Meal* Original Round Top)	1.0	0
(*Roman Meal* Sun Grain Premium)	1.5	0
7 (*Pepperidge Farm* Hearty)	1.5	0

	total fat (grams)	saturated fat (grams)

Bread, grain *(cont.)*

7 (*Pepperidge Farm* Light), 3 slices	1.0	0
7 (*Roman Meal* Light), 2 slices	1.1	0
7 (*Roman Meal* Premium)	1.0	0
7, white (*Arnold Bran'nola*)	2.0	0
9 (*Pepperidge Farm* Whole Grain)	1.0	0
12 (*Brownberry* Natural), 2 slices	2.5	0
12 (*Roman Meal*)	1.5	0
crunchy (*Pepperidge Farm* Whole Grain)	1.5	0
nutty (*Brownberry Bran'nola*)	2.5	0
w/oat bran (*Roman Meal* Original)	1.0	0
hazelnut poppyseed (*Roman Meal*)	4.0	.5
honey oat bran (*Roman Meal* Premium)	1.0	0
honey nut and oat bran (*Roman Meal* Premium)	1.5	0
honey wheatberry:		
(*Arnold*)	1.0	0
(*Pepperidge Farm* Hearty)	1.5	0
(*Roman Meal* Premium)	1.0	0
Italian (see also "Rolls"):		
(*Arnold/Brownberry Bakery* Light)	1.0	0
(*Arnold/Francisco* Sliced, 1 lb.), 2 slices	1.0	0
(*Brownberry/Francisco* International Thick Sliced), 2 slices	1.0	0
(*Savoni's*)	.5	0
stick (*Arnold/Francisco*), 1 oz.	1.0	0
stick, sliced (*Francisco*), 2 slices	1.0	0
nan, garlic or whole wheat (*Garden of Eatin'* Naan), 2.5-oz. piece	4.0	1.0
nut, health (*Brownberry* Natural)	1.5	0
oat:		
(*Arnold Bran'nola* Country)	2.5	.5
(*Roman Meal* Premium)	1.0	0
crunchy (*Pepperidge Farm* Hearty)	2.0	0
oat bran (*Roman Meal* Light), 2 slices	1.0	0

	total fat (grams)	saturated fat (grams)
oatmeal:		
(*Brownberry* Natural)	1.0	0
(*Arnold/Brownberry Bakery* Light), 2 slices	1.0	0
(*Pepperidge Farm*)	1.0	0
(*Pepperidge Farm* Light Style), 3 slices	1.0	0
soft (*Brownberry*)	1.5	0
soft (*Pepperidge Farm*)	.5	0
thin sliced (*Pepperidge Farm*)	1.0	0
orange raisin (*Brownberry*)	1.0	0
pita (sandwich pocket):		
(*Sahara* Original), 2-oz. pita	1.0	0
(*Sahara* Original), 1-oz. pita	0	0
(*Sahara* Original Large), 3-oz. pita	1.0	0
oat bran (*Sahara*), 2-oz. pita	1.0	0
onion (*Sahara*), 2-oz. pita	.5	0
sourdough (*Sahara*), 2-oz. pita	.5	0
white (*Pepperidge Farm* Wholesome Choice), 1 pita	1.0	0
white, mini (*Pepperidge Farm* Wholesome Choice), 1 pita	0	0
whole wheat (*Sahara*), 2-oz. pita	1.0	0
whole wheat (*Sahara*), 1-oz. pita	.5	0
whole wheat and rye (*Garden of Eatin' Pita Pockets*), 1 pita	2.0	.5
potato (*Arnold* Country)	2.0	0
potato, russet (*Pepperidge Farm* Hearty)	1.5	.5
pumpernickel:		
(*Arnold/August Bros.*)	1.0	0
(*Arnold/Levy's*)	.5	0
(*Pepperidge Farm* Classic Dark)	1.0	.5
(*Pepperidge Farm* Party), 8 slices	1.5	0
rye (*Brownberry* Natural)	.5	0
raisin (*Arnold Sunmaid*)	1.0	0
raisin cinnamon:		
(*Arnold/Brownberry*)	1.0	0
(*Monk's*)	1.0	0

	total fat (grams)	saturated fat (grams)
Bread, raisin cinnamon *(cont.)*		
(*Pepperidge Farm*)	1.5	0
raisin walnut (*Brownberry*)	2.5	0
rye:		
(*Arnold* Deli)	.5	0
(*August Bros.* 1 lb.)	1.0	0
(*Brownberry* Hearth)	1.5	0
dill (*Arnold*), 2 slices	1.0	0
dill (*Brownberry* Natural)	1.0	0
Dijon (*Arnold* Real Jewish)	1.0	0
Dijon (*Pepperidge Farm* Thin), 2 slices	1.5	.5
onion (*Pepperidge Farm*)	1.0	.5
party (*Pepperidge Farm* Party), 8 slices	1.5	0
pumpernickel (*Arnold/August Bros.* Rye N'Pump)	1.0	0
seeded (*Arnold/Levy's* Real Jewish)	1.0	0
seeded (*Brownberry* Natural Caraway)	1.0	0
seeded or seedless (*August Bros.*)	1.0	0
seeded or seedless (*Arnold* Real Jewish Melba Thin), 2 slices	1.0	0
seeded or seedless (*Pepperidge Farm* Jewish)	1.0	.5
seedless (*Arnold* Real Jewish)	1.0	0
seedless (*Levy's* Real Jewish, 1 lb.)	.5	0
seedless (*August Bros.* Thin), 2 slices	1.0	0
seedless (*Brownberry* Natural)	1.0	0
seedless (*Brownberry* Natural Thin), 2 slices	1.0	0
soft (*Arnold* Country)	1.0	0
soft (*Arnold Bakery* Light), 2 slices	1.0	0
soft (*Brownberry Bakery* Light)	0	0
soft, seeded or unseeded (*Arnold Bakery*)	1.0	0
sandwich (*Roman Meal* Original), 2 slices	1.5	.2
sourdough:		
(*Arnold/August Bros.*)	1.0	0
(*Arnold Bakery* Light), 2 slices	1.0	0

	total fat (grams)	saturated fat (grams)
(*Arnold/Brownberry/Francisco*)	1.0	0
(*Parisian*)	0	0
(*Pepperidge Farm* Light), 3 slices	1.0	0
(*Roman Meal* Whole Grain Premium)	1.0	0
baguette or loaf (*Boudin Sourdough*), 2 oz.	1.0	0
brown and serve (*Francisco*), 1 oz.	.5	0
stick, sliced (*August Bros.*), 2 slices	1.0	0
stick, sliced (*Brownberry/Francisco* International)	0	0
sub loaf (*Arnold Francisco*), 1 oz.	.5	0
sunflower and bran (*Monk's*)	2.0	0
toast, Texas (*August Bros.*)	3.0	.5
Vienna:		
(*Pepperidge Farm* Thick Slice)	1.0	0
(*Pepperidge Farm* Light), 3 slices	1.0	.5
sliced (*Arnold/Francisco*)	1.0	0
wheat (see also "wheat, whole" below):		
(*Arnold Brick Oven* 8 oz.), 2 slices	2.5	.5
(*Arnold Brick Oven* 1 lb.), 2 slices	3.0	.5
(*Arnold Brick Oven* 2 lb.)	2.0	0
(*Arnold Sunny Valley*), 2 slices	1.5	0
(*Arnold/Brownberry* Country)	1.5	0
(*Brownberry* Natural)	1.0	0
(Arnold/Brownberry Premium Light), 2 slices	1.0	0
(*Brownberry* Hearth)	1.0	0
(*Pepperidge Farm/Pepperidge Farm* Natural)	1.5	0
(*Pepperidge Farm* Family)	1.0	0
(*Pepperidge Farm* Light), 3 slices	1.0	0
(*Pepperidge Farm* Very Thin), 3 slices	2.0	.5
(*Roman Meal* Light /Light Hearty), 2 slices	1.0	0
(*Roman Meal* Premium Natural)	1.0	.2
(*Thomas'* Lite)	1.0	<1.0
apple honey (*Brownberry*)	1.0	0
cracked (*Pepperidge Farm* Thin)	1.0	0
dark (*Arnold/Brownberry Bran'nola*)	2.0	0
golden (*Arnold/Brownberry Bakery* Light)	0	0

	total fat (grams)	saturated fat (grams)

Bread, wheat *(cont.)*

hearty (*Arnold/Brownberry/Bran'nola*)	3.0	.5
sesame (*Pepperidge Farm* Hearty Slices)	1.5	0
soft (*Arnold Brick Oven/Brownberry*)	2.0	0
(*wheatberry (Roman Meal* Light), 2 slices	.9	.1

wheat, whole:

(*Arnold* Stone Ground 100% 2 lb.), 2 slices	1.5	0
(*Arnold* Stone Ground 100% 1 lb. 4 oz.)	1.0	0
(*Pepperidge Farm* 100% Whole Grain)	1.0	0
(*Pepperidge Farm* Thin)	1.0	0
(*Roman Meal* 100%)	1.0	0
(*Roman Meal* Light), 2 slices	.8	.1
soft (*Pepperidge Farm*)	.5	0
stoneground (*Monk's*)	1.0	0

white:

(*Arnold Brick Oven* 8 oz./1 lb.), 2 slices	2.5	0
(*Arnold Brick Oven* 2 lb.)	1.5	0
(*Arnold Sunny Valley*), 2 slices	1.5	0
(*Arnold/Brownberry* Country)	1.5	0
(*Brownberry* Natural), 2 slices	1.5	0
(*Monk's* Enriched)	1.0	0
(*Pepperidge Farm* Hearty Country)	1.0	0
(*Pepperidge Farm* Thin Enriched/Large Family)	1.5	0
(*Pepperidge Farm* Very Thin), 3 slices	1.5	0
(*Roman Meal* Light), 2 slices	1.0	0
sandwich (*Pepperidge Farm*), 2 slices	2.0	.5
soft (*Arnold* Country)	1.5	0
soft (*Brownberry*)	1.5	0
toasting (*Pepperidge Farm*)	3.0	1.0

Bread, canned, brown, plain or raisin

(*B&M/Friends*), 2 oz., ½" slice	.5	0

Bread, frozen or refrigerated:

(*Pillsbury Pipin' Hot*), ⅙ loaf	.5	0
cheese, cheddar, two (*Pepperidge Farm*), ⅙ loaf	11.0	5.0

	total fat (grams)	saturated fat (grams)
cheese, Monterey jack w/jalapeño (*Pepperidge Farm*), 1/6 loaf	10.0	4.0
cornbread twists (*Pillsbury*), 1 piece	6.0	1.5
French loaf (*Pillsbury*), 1/5 loaf	1.0	0
garlic:		
(*Pepperidge Farm*), 1/6 loaf	10.0	3.0
five cheese (*Schwan's*), 1 piece, 3.4 oz.	20.0	6.0
mozzarella (*Pepperidge Farm*), 1/6 loaf	10.0	5.0
parmesan (*Pepperidge Farm*), 1/6 loaf	7.0	2.0
sourdough (*Pepperidge Farm*), 1/6 loaf	9.0	2.5
wheat, honey (*Schwan's*), 2 oz., 1/8 loaf	1.5	0
wheat, stone-ground (*Schwan's*), 2 oz., 1/8 loaf	1.5	0
white (*Rich's*), 2.2 oz., about 1" slice	2.0	0
white (*Schwan's*), 2 oz., 1/8 loaf	1.5	0
Bread, mix (see also "Bread, sweet, mix"):		
beer (*Aunt Patsy's Pantry/Buckeye*), 1/14 pkg.	1.0	0
bran, multi (*Buckeye*), 1/12 pkg.	1.0	0
cheddar cheese (*Dromedary*), 1/9 pkg.	2.5	1.5
cornbread, see "Bread, sweet, mix"		
herb, Italian (*Dromedary*), 1/9 pkg.	2.5	1.5
kamut (*Arrowhead Mills*), 1/3 cup	1.0	0
mixed grain:		
(*Arrowhead Mills LifeBread*), 1/4 cup	.5	0
(*Arrowhead Mills* Multi Grain), 1/3 cup	1.0	0
rye (*Arrowhead Mills*), 1/3 cup	.5	0
sourdough (*Aunt Patsy's Pantry/Buckeye*), 1/14 pkg.	0	0
sourdough (*Dromedary*), 1/9 pkg.	2.0	1.0
spelt (*Arrowhead Mills*), 1/3 cup	1.0	0
white:		
(*Arrowhead Mills*), 1/3 cup	.5	0
(*Dromedary* Country), 1/9 pkg.	1.0	.5
crusty (*Pillsbury*), 1/12 pkg.	2.0	0
wheat (*Dromedary* Stoneground), 1/9 pkg.	2.0	1.0
wheat, cracked (*Pillsbury*), 1/12 pkg.	2.0	0

	total fat (grams)	saturated fat (grams)

Bread mix *(cont.)*

whole wheat (*Arrowhead Mills*), ⅓ cup 1.0 0

whole wheat (*Aunt Patsy's Pantry/Buckeye*),
 ¹⁄₁₄ pkg. 0 0

Bread, sweet, mix, ¹⁄₁₂ pkg., except as noted:

(*Buckeye*), ¹⁄₁₆ pkg. 0 0

apple cinnamon (*Pillsbury*) .... 6.0 .... 1.0

banana (*Pillsbury*) .... 6.0 .... 1.0

blueberry (*Pillsbury*) .... 6.0 .... 1.0

carrot (*Pillsbury*) .... 5.0 .... 1.0

cinnamon raisin (*Backstreet Breads*), 3 tbsp. 0 0

cornbread:

 (*Arrowhead Mills*), ¼ cup 1.0 0

 (*Aunt Jemima's Easy*), ⅓ cup .... 4.0 .... 1.0

 (*Aunt Patsy's Pantry/Buckeye*) 0 0

 (*Ballard*), ¹⁄₁₈ pkg. .... 2.5 .... 1.0

 (*Dromedary*), ¹⁄₁₀ pkg. .... 2.5 .... 1.0

cranberry (*Pillsbury*) .... 4.0 .... 1.0

date (*Pillsbury*) .... 4.0 .... 1.0

date nut (*Dromedary*) .... 7.0 .... 2.0

gingerbread (*Betty Crocker*), ⅛ pkg. .... 7.0 .... 2.0

 (*Dromedary*), ⅙ pkg. .... 4.0 .... 1.0

gingerbread (*Pillsbury*), ⅛ pkg. .... 5.0 .... 1.5

lemon poppy seed (*Backstreet Breads*), 3 tbsp. 5 0

mandarin orange poppy seed (*Backstreet Breads*),
 3 tbsp. 5 0

nut (*Pillsbury*) .... 6.0 .... 1.0

oatmeal raisin (*Pillsbury*) .... 7.0 .... 1.0

pumpkin (*Pillsbury*) .... 6.0 .... 1.0

Bread crisps snack, 1 oz.:

cinnamon-raisin swirled (*Pepperidge Farm*) 5.0 5

garlic-butter swirled (*Pepperidge Farm*) .... 8.0 .... 1.5

Bread crumbs:

lemon herb (*Progresso*), ¼ cup 1.0 0

plain or Italian (*Arnold*), ½ oz. .... <1.0 0

	total fat (grams)	saturated fat (grams)
plain, Italian, or tomato basil (*Progresso*), ¼ cup	1.5	0
seasoned, (*Contadina*), ⅓ cup	1.5	0
Bread cubes (see also "Croutons" and "Stuffing"):		
unseasoned (*Arnold*), 2 cups	3.0	.5
Bread shell, Italian:		
(*Boboli*), ½ of 6" shell	3.0	1.0
(*Boboli*), ⅛ of 12" single shell	3.0	1.0
(*Boboli* Thin Crust), ⅕ shell	3.5	1.0
Bread sticks:		
plain:		
(*Barbara's*), 8 sticks	3.0	n.a.
(*Stella D'Oro*), 1 piece	1.0	n.a.
(*Stella D'Oro* Fat Free Deli/Grissini/Traditional), 2 pieces	0	0
(*Stella D'Oro* Fat Free Grissini), 1 piece	0	0
(*Stella D'Oro* Fat Free Traditional), 1 piece	0	0
(*Stella D'Oro* Sodium Free), 2 pieces	2.0	n.a.
brown and serve (*Pepperidge Farm,* 1 piece	1.5	.5
cheddar (*Pepperidge Farm* Thin), 6 oz., 7 pieces	2.5	1.0
garlic (*Stella D'Oro*), 1 piece	.8	n.a.
garlic (*Stella D'Oro* Fat Free Deli/Grissini/Traditional), 1 piece	0	0
Italian (*Barbara's*), 1 oz.	3.0	n.a.
onion (*Pepperidge Farm* Thin), 6 oz., 7 pieces	2.0	0
onion (*Stella D'Oro*), 1 piece	1.0	n.a.
sesame:		
(*Barbara's*), 1 oz.	4.0	n.a.
(*Pepperidge Farm* Thin), 6 oz., 7 pieces	1.5	0
(*Stella D'Oro*), 1 piece	2.0	n.a.
(*Stella D'Oro* Sodium Free), 1 piece	2.5	n.a.
wheat (*Stella D'Oro*), 1 piece	1.0	n.a.
Bread sticks, refrigerated (*Pillsbury*), 1 piece	2.5	.5

	total fat (grams)	saturated fat (grams)

Bread stuffing, see "Stuffing"

Breadfruit:

| ¼ small, approximately 3.4 oz. | .2 | 0 |
| trimmed, ½ cup | .3 | 0 |

Breadfruit seeds:

raw, South American cultivar, in shell, 4 oz.	4.3	1.2
raw, South American cultivar, shelled, 1 oz.	1.6	.4
boiled, Pacific area cultivar, shelled, 1 oz.	.7	.2
roasted, South American cultivar, shelled, 1 oz.	.8	.2

Breakfast dishes, see specific listings

Breakfast bar, see "Granola and cereal bars"

Broad beans:

fresh:

raw, untrimmed, 1 lb.	2.6	.6
raw, trimmed, ½ cup	.4	.1
boiled, drained, 4 oz.	.6	.2
dry, ¼ cup	.6	.1
dry, boiled, ½ cup	.3	.1
canned, (*Progresso* Fava), ½ cup	.5	0

Broccoli:

fresh:

raw, untrimmed, 1 lb.	1.0	.2
raw, 1 spear, 8.7 oz.	.5	.1
boiled, drained, chopped, ½ cup	.2	<.1
freeze-dried, chopped (*AlpineAire*), ½ cup*	.2	0

frozen:

spears, 10-oz. pkg.	1.0	.2
(*Schwan's*), 2.2-oz. spear	0	0
(*Stilwell*), 4 florets	0	0
cut (*Stilwell*), ½ cup	0	0
cuts or spears (*Green Giant/Green Giant Harvest Fresh*), ½ cup	0	0
in butter sauce (*Green Giant*), ½ cup	1.5	0
in cheese sauce (*Green Giant*), ⅔ cup	2.5	1.0

	total fat (grams)	saturated fat (grams)
Broccoli, combinations, frozen:		
in butter sauce, ¾ cup:		
cauliflower, carrots, corn and peas (*Green Giant*)	2.0	1.5
pasta, peas, corn & peppers (*Green Giant*)	2.5	1.0
in cheese sauce, ⅔ cup:		
(*Green Giant*)	2.5	1.0
w/cauliflower and carrots (*Green Giant*)	2.5	1.5
stir-fry (*Green Giant Create-A-Meal*), 2⅓ cup	3.5	.5
Broccoli pastry, frozen, w/cheese (*Pepperidge Farm*), 3.7-oz. piece	14.0	4.5
Broiling spice (*Durkee* Broil 'n Grill), ¼ tsp.	0	0
Brown gravy mix:		
(*Durkee*), ¼ pkg.	.5	0
(*French's*), ¼ pkg.	.5	0
(*Hain*), ¼ pkg.	0	0
(*Knorr Gravy Classics*), ⅙ pkg.	.5	0
(*McCormick*), ¼ pkg.	.5	0
(*Pillsbury*), 2 tsp.	0	0
(*Weight Watchers*), ¼ pkg.	0	0
herb (*Durkee/French's*), ¼ pkg.	0	0
mushroom or onion (*Durkee*), ¼ pkg.	0	0
and onion (*Knorr Gravy Classics* Lyonnaise), ⅕ pkg.	.5	0
vegetarian (*Loma Linda Gravy Quik*), 1 tbsp.	.2	0
Brown sauce, spicy (*House of Tsang*), 1 tsp.	0	0
Brownie:		
(*Drake's* Old Fashioned), 1.25-oz. piece	5.0	2.0
(*Health Valley* Fat Free), 1 piece	0	0
(*Hostess Brownie Bites*), 5 pieces	14.0	4.0
(*Hostess* Light), 2 pieces	5.0	2.0
fudge nut (*Awrey's* Sheet), 2" × 2" piece	16.0	1.0
fudge nut, iced (*Awrey's* Sheet), 2" × 2" piece	17.0	3.0
fudge walnut (*Tastykake*), 1 piece	17.0	4.0
w/walnuts (*Hostess Brownie Bites*), 5 pieces	15.0	4.0

	total fat (grams)	saturated fat (grams)

Brownie, refrigerated, fudge (*Pillsbury*), 1.4 oz.,

| ⅟₂₀ pkg. | 6.0 | 1.5 |

Brownie dessert, frozen:

a la mode (*Sweet Celebrations*), 6.4 oz. piece	4.0	1.0
w/chocolate frosting (*Sweet Celebrations*),		
1.25-oz. piece	2.5	1.0
peanut butter fudge (Sweet Celebrations), 1.2 oz.	2.5	.5

Brownie mix, 1 piece*:

chocolate, deluxe (*Pillsbury*)	7.0	1.5
cream cheese swirl (*Pillsbury*)	9.0	2.5
fudge:		
(*Betty Crocker*)	9.0	2.0
(*Betty Crocker* Lowfat)	2.5	.5
(*Betty Crocker* Supreme)	9.0	2.0
(*Pillsbury*, 15 oz.)	6.0	1.0
(*Pillsbury*, 21.5 oz.)	8.0	1.5
(*Pillsbury Lovin' Lites*)	3.5	1.0
cookies n' cream (*Betty Crocker*)	10.0	2.0
hot (*Pillsbury*)	7.0	2.0
peanut butter w/*Reese's Pieces* (*Betty Crocker*)	10.0	3.0
walnut (*Pillsbury*)	9.0	1.5
white chocolate swirl (*Betty Crocker*)	8.0	2.5

Browning sauce:

| (*Gravymaster*), ¼ tsp. | 0 | 0 |
| and flavoring (*Brown Kwik*), ¼ tsp. | 0 | 0 |

Brussels sprouts:

fresh:		
raw, untrimmed, 1 lb.	1.2	.3
raw or boiled, 1 sprout, .7 oz.	.1	<.1
boiled, drained, ½ cup	.4	.1
frozen:		
10-oz. pkg.	1.2	.2
boiled, drained, ½ cup	.3	.1

	total fat (grams)	saturated fat (grams)
(*Stilwell*), 3 oz., 6 medium	0	0
in butter sauce (*Green Giant*), ⅔ cup	1.5	1.5
Buckwheat, whole grain, ¼ cup	1.5	.3
Buckwheat flour:		
¼ cup	.9	.2
(*Arrowhead Mills*), ¼ cup	1.0	0
Buckwheat groats:		
roasted, dry, ¼ cup	1.1	.2
roasted, cooked, ½ cup	.6	.2
toasted, dry (*Arrowhead Mills*), ¼ cup	1.0	0
Bulgur:		
dry, ¼ cup	1.0	.1
dry (*Arrowhead Mills*), ¼ cup	.5	0
cooked, ½ cup	.2	<.1
Bulgur pilaf mix (*Casbah*), 1 oz. dry or ½ cup*	0	0
Bun, see "Roll"		
Bun, sweet (see also "Roll, sweet"):		
apple or pineapple cheese (*Entenmann's* Fat Free), 1 piece	0	0
cinnamon (*Entenmann's*), 2.2-oz. piece	10.0	6.0
honey:		
(*Aunt Fanny's*), 3-oz. piece	20.0	5.0
(*Aunt Fanny's* Large), 4-oz. piece	29.0	7.0
(*Morton*), 2.3-oz. piece	10.0	2.5
applesauce filled (*Aunt Fanny's*), 3.2-oz. piece	17.0	4.0
banana or chocolate creme (*Aunt Fanny's*), 3.2-oz. piece	18.0	4.0
glazed (*Hostess*), 2.7-oz. piece	19.0	9.0
glazed or iced (*Tastykake*), 3.3-oz. piece	17.0	4.0
iced (*Aunt Fanny's*), 3-oz. piece	18.0	4.0
iced (*Hostess*), 3.4-oz. piece	20.0	9.0
mini (*Hostess*), 1.33-oz. piece	8.0	2.0
raspberry filled (*Aunt Fanny's*), 3.2-oz. piece	17.0	5.0

	total fat (grams)		saturated fat (grams)

Bun, sweet, honey *(cont.)*
    vanilla creme filled (*Aunt Fanny's*),
        3.2-oz. piece .... 18.0 .... 4.0

Burbot, meat only, 4 oz.:
    raw 9 2
    baked, broiled, or microwaved 1.2 2

Burdock root:
    raw, 1 medium, 7.3 oz. 1 0
    boiled, drained, 1" pieces, ½ cup 1 0

Burger, vegetarian, canned (see also "Vegetable dishes"):
    (*Loma Linda Redi-Burger*), 3 oz., ⅝" slice .... 10.0 .... 1.5
    (*Loma Linda Vege-Burger*), ¼ cup 1.5 5
    (*Worthington*), ¼ cup 2.0 0

Burger, vegetarian, frozen (see also "Vegetable burger"
    and "Vegetarian dishes, frozen"), 2.3-oz. patty,
    except as noted:
    (*Loma Linda Redi-Burger*), 3 oz., ⅝" slice .... 10.0 .... 1.5
    (*Loma Linda Sizzle Burger*), 2.5-oz. patty .... 12.0 .... 1.5
    (*Morningstar Farms Better'n Burgers*),
        2.8-oz. patty 0 0
    (*Morningstar Farm Garden Vege Patties*),
        2.4-oz. patty 4.0 5
    (*Morningstar Farms Grillers*) .... 7.0 .... 1.0
    (*Morningstar Farms Prime*) .... 5.0 .... 1.5
    (*Natural Touch Okra Patty*) .... 12.0 .... 2.0
    (*Natural Touch Vegan Burger*) 0 0
    (*Natural Touch Vege Burger*) .... 6.0 .... 1.0
    (*Worthington Fri-Pats*) .... 6.0 .... 1.0
    (*Worthington Prosage Patties*), 1.4-oz. patty ..... 7.0 .... 2.0

Burger, vegetarian, mix:
    (*Fantastic Foods Nature's Burger Original*),
        ¼ cup 3.0 0
    (*Loma Linda Patty Mix*), ⅓ cup 1.0 0
    (*Worthington Granburger*), 3 tbsp. 5 0

	total fat (grams)	saturated fat (grams)
barbecue (*Fantastic Foods* Nature's Burger), ⅓ cup	1.5	0
chunk (*Loma Linda Vita-Burger*), ¼ cup	1.5	.5
granules (*Loma Linda Vita-Burger*), 3 tbsp.	1.0	0
Burger King, 1 serving:		
breakfast:		
Croissan'wich, w/bacon, egg, and cheese	24.0	8.0
Croissan'wich, w/ham, egg, and cheese	22.0	7.0
Croissan'wich, w/sausage, egg, and cheese	41.0	14.0
French toast sticks	27.0	7.0
hash browns	12.0	3.0
jam, grape, or strawberry *A.M. Express*	0	0
burgers, chicken, and sandwiches:		
cheeseburger	19.0	9.0
cheeseburger, double	36.0	17.0
cheeseburger, double, w/bacon	39.0	18.0
chicken sandwich	43.0	9.0
chicken sandwich, *BK Broiler*	29.0	6.0
Chicken Tenders, 6 pieces	12.0	3.0
fish sandwich, *BK Big Fish*	43.0	8.0
hamburger	15.0	6.0
Whopper	39.0	11.0
Whopper, w/cheese	46.0	16.0
Whopper, double	56.0	19.0
Whopper, double, w/cheese	63.0	24.0
Whopper Jr.	24.0	8.0
Whopper Jr., w/cheese	28.0	10.0
salads and side dishes:		
chicken salad, broiled, w/out dressing	10.0	5.0
garden salad, w/out dressing	5.0	3.0
french fries, medium	20.0	5.0
onion rings	14.0	2.0
side salad, w/out dressing	3.0	2.0
Burger King dressings, 2 tbsp., 1.1 oz.:		
bleu cheese	16.0	4.0

	total fat (grams)	saturated fat (grams)
Burger King dressings *(cont.)*		
French	10.0	2.0
Italian, reduced calorie light	.5	0
ranch	19.0	4.0
Thousand Island	12.0	3.0
condiments and sauces:		
A.M. Express dip, 1 oz.	0	0
barbecue, honey, or sweet and sour dipping		
sauce, 1 oz.	0	0
Bull's Eye barbecue sauce, ½ oz.	0	0
mayonnaise, 1 oz.	23.0	3.0
ranch dipping sauce, 1 oz.	17.0	3.0
tartar sauce, 1 oz.	19.0	3.0
desserts and shakes:		
apple pie, Dutch	15.0	3.0
chocolate, strawberry, or vanilla shake,		
medium	7.0	4.0
Burrito (see also "Burrito, breakfast"), frozen:		
(*Schwan's*), 4.3-oz. piece	13.0	3.0
bean and cheese (*Old El Paso*), 5-oz. piece	9.0	4.5
bean and cheese (*Patio*), 5-oz. piece	5.0	2.0
beef (*Hormel Quick Meal*), 4-oz. piece	13.0	6.0
beef, nacho, mini (*Patio Britos*), 6 oz.,		
10 pieces	18.0	n.a.
beef and bean:		
(*Patio*), 5-oz. piece	7.0	3.0
chili, green (*Patio*), 5-oz. piece	5.0	1.5
chili, red (*Patio*), 5-oz. piece	5.0	2.0
hot or medium (*Old El Paso*), 5-oz. piece	10.0	4.0
medium or mild (*Healthy Choice Quick Meal*),		
5.4 oz.	7.0	3.0
mild (*Old El Paso*), 5-oz. piece	9.0	3.0
mini (*Patio Britos*), 6 oz., 10 pieces	19.0	7.0
cheese (*Hormel Quick Meal*), 4-oz. piece	6.0	2.0

	total fat (grams)	saturated fat (grams)
cheese, nacho, mini (*Patio Britos*), 6 oz., 10 pieces	13.0	4.0
chicken:		
(*Patio*), 5-oz. piece	4.0	1.5
con queso (*Healthy Choice Quick Meal*), 5.4 oz.	8.0	2.0
spicy, mini (*Patio Britos*), 6 oz., 10 pieces	16.0	4.0
chili, red (*Hormel Quick Meal*), 4-oz. piece	11.0	4.5
chili, red (*Patio*), 5-oz. piece	6.0	2.0
pizza, cheese or sausage (*Old El Paso*), 3.5-oz. piece	9.0	4.0
pizza, pepperoni (*Old El Paso*), 3.5-oz. piece	10.0	5.0
Burrito, breakfast, frozen:		
(*Schwan's Bright Starts*), 4-oz. piece	17.0	4.5
(*Swanson*), 3.5-oz. piece	12.0	4.0
Burrito mix:		
(*Old El Paso*), 1 tortilla and seasoning	3.5	.5
filled (*Old El Paso*), 1 piece*	7.0	3.0
Burrito seasoning mix:		
(*Durkee* Pouches), 1/10 pkg.	1.0	0
(*Lawry's* Spices & Seasonings), 1 tbsp.	.5	0
(*Old El Paso*), 1/8 pkg.	0	0
Butter (see also "Butter, light"):		
regular, salted or unsalted:		
1 stick or 4 oz.	92.0	57.2
1 tbsp.	11.4	7.1
1 tsp.	3.8	2.4
(*Land O'Lakes*), 1 tbsp.	11.0	7.0
whipped, salted or unsalted:		
½ cup or 1 stick	61.3	38.2
1 tbsp.	7.6	4.7
1 tsp.	3.8	2.4
whipped, salted (*Land O'Lakes*), 1 tbsp.	7.0	4.5
whipped, unsalted (*Land O'Lakes*), 1 tbsp.	7.0	5.0

	total fat (grams)	saturated fat (grams)

Butter, light (see also "Margarine"), 1 tbsp.:

    stick, salted or unsalted (*Land O'Lakes*) .... 6.0 .... 4.0

    whipped, salted (*Land O'Lakes*) .... 3.5 .... 2.5

Butter oil, 1 tbsp. .... 12.7 .... 7.9

Butter salt (*Durkee*), ½ tsp. 0 0

Butter sprinkles (*Smart Seas*), ¾ tsp. 0 0

Butterbeans, see "Lima bean"

Butterbeans, speckled, frozen (*Stilwell*), ½ cup 0 0

Butterbur:

    raw, untrimmed, 1 lb. 2 0

    boiled, drained, 4 oz. .... <.1 0

    canned, chopped, ½ cup 1 0

***Butterfinger* flavor milk drink, lowfat** (*Nestlé Quik*)

    8 fl. oz. .... 5.0 .... 3.0

Butterfish, meat only, 4 oz.:

    raw .... 9.1 .... n.a.

    baked, broiled, or microwaved .... 11.7 .... n.a.

Buttermilk, see "Milk"

Butternut, dried:

    in shell, 4 oz. 17.5 4

    shelled, 1 oz. 16.2 4

Butternut squash:

    fresh:

        raw, untrimmed, 1 lb. 4 1

        raw, cubed, ½ cup .... .1 .... <.1

        baked, 4 oz. or ½ cup cubes .... .1 .... <.1

    frozen, 12-oz. pkg. 3 1

    frozen, boiled, drained, mashed, ½ cup .... .1 .... <.1

Butterscotch, see "Candy"

Butterscotch chips, baking:

    (*Guittard*), 33 pieces, about .5 oz. .... 4.5 .... 4.0

    (*Nestlé Toll House Morsels*), 1 tbsp. .... 4.0 .... 4.0

	total fat (grams)	saturated fat (grams)

Butterscotch topping, 2 tbsp.:

	total fat (grams)	saturated fat (grams)
(*Kraft*)	1.5	1.0
(*Mrs. Richardson's*)	1.0	.5
caramel (*Smucker's*)	1.0	.5
and caramel (*Smucker's* Fat Free)	0	0
caramel fudge (*Mrs. Richardson's*)	1.5	1.5

C

	total fat (grams)		saturated fat (grams)
Cabbage, fresh:			
raw, 5¾"-diameter head, 2.5 lbs.	1.6	....	.2
raw, shredded, ½ cup	.1	....	tr.
boiled, drained, 4 oz.	.3	....	<.1
boiled, drained, shredded, ½ cup	.2	....	<.1
Cabbage, Chinese, fresh:			
bok-choy:			
raw, untrimmed, 1 lb.	.8	....	.1
raw, shredded, ½ cup	.1	....	tr.
boiled, drained, shredded, ½ cup	.1	....	<.1
napa, raw (*Frieda's*), 1 oz.	<.1	....	0
pe-tsai:			
raw, untrimmed, 1 lb.	.8	....	.2
raw, shredded, ½ cup	.1	....	<.1
boiled, drained, shredded, ½ cup	.1	....	<.1
Cabbage, red:			
fresh:			
raw, untrimmed, 1 lb.	.9	....	.1
raw, shredded, ½ cup	.1	....	<.1
boiled, drained, shredded, ½ cup	.2	....	<.1
canned, sweet and sour (*Greenwood*), ½ cup	0	....	0

	total fat (grams)	saturated fat (grams)

Cabbage, savoy, fresh:

raw, untrimmed, 1 lb.	.4	<.1
raw, shredded, ½ cup	<.1	tr.
boiled, drained, shredded, ½ cup	.1	tr.

Cabbage, stuffed, entree, frozen (*Lean Cuisine*),

| 9.5 oz. | 7.0 | 1.5 |

Cabbage, swamp, see "Swamp cabbage"

Cacciatore sauce, see "Cooking sauce" and "Chicken seasoning/sauce mix"

| **Caesar salad,** fresh (*Dole* Complete), 3.5 oz. | 14.0 | 1.5 |

Cajun seasoning, meat, poultry, or fish (*Durkee* Spices), ¼ tsp.

| | 0 | 0 |

Cake:

all varieties (*Entenmann's* Fat Free), 1 serving	0	0
angel food (*Hostess*), ⅙ cake	3.0	1.5
apple streusel (*Awrey's*), 2" x 2" piece	9.0	1.0
banana, iced (*Awrey's* Sheet), 2" x 2" piece	8.0	2.0
banana crunch (*Entenmann's*), ⅛ cake	9.0	2.0
Black Forest (*Awrey's* 4-Layer Torte), 1/14 cake	21.0	7.0

carrot:

(*Entenmann's*), ⅛ cake	16.0	3.5
cream cheese iced (*Awrey's* 3-Layer), 1/12 cake	23.0	5.0
supreme, iced (*Awrey's* Sheet), 2" x 2" piece	12.0	3.0

chocolate:

w/out icing (*Awrey's* Sheet), 2" x 2" piece	3.0	1.0
double (*Awrey's* 4-Layer Torte), 1/14 cake	15.0	4.0
double (*Awrey's* 3-Layer), 1/12 cake	14.0	4.0
double (*Awrey's* 2-Layer), 1/12 cake	11.0	3.0
double, iced (*Awrey's* Sheet), 2" x 2" piece	6.0	2.0
fudge (*Entenmann's*), ⅙ cake	14.0	5.0
German (*Awrey's* 3-Layer), 1/12 cake	18.0	6.0
German, iced (*Awrey's* Sheet), 2" x 2" piece	9.0	3.0
white iced (*Awrey's* 2-Layer), 1/12 cake	15.0	5.0

	total fat (grams)	saturated fat (grams)

Cake *(cont.)*

coconut butter cream (*Awrey's* Sheet), 2" x 2" .... 9.0 .... 3.0

coffee cake:

    (*Awrey's* Long John), 1/12 cake .... 8.0 .... 2.0

    caramel nut (*Awrey's*), 1/12 cake .... 8.0 .... 2.0

    cheese (*Entenmann's*), 1/9 cake .... 8.0 .... 3.5

    cheese filled crumb (*Entenmann's*), 1/8 cake ... 10.0 .... 4.0

    crumb (*Entenmann's*), 1/10 cake .... 12.0 .... 3.0

crumb, all butter French (*Entenmann's*), 1/8 cake .. 10.0 .... 6.0

crunch, Louisiana (*Entenmann's*), 1/9 cake .... 13.0 .... 3.5

danish pastry cake (see also "Danish pastry"):

    cinnamon fibert ring (*Entenmann's*), 1/6 ring .. 17.0 .... 3.0

    pecan ring (*Entenmann's*), 1/8 ring .... 15.0 .... 3.0

    raspberry twist (*Entenmann's*), 1/8 twist ...... 11.0 .... 3.0

    walnut ring (*Entenmann's*), 1/8 ring .... 14.0 .... 3.0

devil's food, marshmallow iced (*Entenmann's*),

    1/6 cake .... 18.0 .... 5.0

devil's food, white iced (*Awrey's* Sheet),

    2" x 2" piece .... 8.0 .... 3.0

golden, thick fudge (*Entenmann's*), 1/6 cake ...... 16.0 .... 4.0

lemon (*Awrey's* 3-Layer), 1/12 cake .... 19.0 .... 5.0

loaf, all butter (*Entenmann's*), 1/6 loaf .... 10.0 .... 6.0

marble loaf (*Entenmann's*), 1/8 loaf .... 10.0 .... 6.0

Neapolitan (*Awrey's* 4-Layer Torte), 1/14 cake ..... 22.0 .... 7.0

orange (*Awrey's* 3-Layer), 1/12 cake .... 17.0 .... 4.0

orange, frosty, iced (*Awrey's* Sheet), 2" x 2" piece ... 8.0 .... 2.0

panettone (*Dal Forno*), 2 oz., 1/9 cake .... 8.0 .... 3.8

peanut butter (*Awrey's* 4-Layer Torte), 1/14 cake ... 22.0 .... 5.0

pistachio (*Awrey's* 4-Layer Torte), 1/14 cake ...... 22.0 .... 7.0

pound (*Hostess*), 1/5 cake .... 16.0 .... 4.0

pound, golden (*Awrey's*), 1/12 cake .... 5.0 .... 1.0

raisin loaf (*Entenmann's*), 1/8 loaf .... 9.0 .... 2.0

raisin spice, iced (*Awrey's* Sheet), 2" x 2" piece ... 8.0 .... 2.0

raspberry nut (*Awrey's*), 1/16 cake .... 16.0 .... 3.0

	total fat (grams)	saturated fat (grams)
sour cream chip and nut loaf (*Entenmann's*), ⅛ loaf	14.0	4.0
sponge, w/out icing (*Awrey's* Sheet), 2" x 2" piece	3.0	1.0
strawberry supreme (*Awrey's* 4-Layer Torte), 1/14 cake	12.0	3.0
strudel, apple (*Entenmann's*), ¼ strudel	14.0	3.5
walnut (*Awrey's* 4-Layer Torte), 1/14 cake	19.0	4.0
yellow:		
w/out icing (*Awrey's* Sheet), 2" x 2" piece	3.0	1.0
coconut iced (*Awrey's* 3-Layer), 1/12 cake	21.0	7.0
lemon iced (*Awrey's* 2-Layer), 1/12 cake	17.0	5.0
milk chocolate iced (*Awrey's* 2-Layer), 1/12 cake	17.0	5.0
white iced (*Awrey's* Sheet), 2" x 2" piece	9.0	3.0
Cake, frozen:		
Boston cream (*Pepperidge Farm*), ⅛ cake	9.0	2.5
Boston cream (*Mrs. Smith's*), ⅛ cake	5.0	1.5
brownie cheesecake (*Weight Watchers*), 3.5 oz.	6.0	2.0
carrot (*Oregon Farms*), ⅙ cake	15.0	2.5
carrot, deluxe (*Pepperidge Farm*), ⅛ cake	16.0	4.0
cheesecake:		
(*Baby Watson*), 3 oz.	20.0	14.0
almond amaretto (*Sweet Celebrations*), 3 oz.	5.0	2.5
chocolate chip (*Sara Lee* Original), ¼ cake	21.0	14.0
strawberry (*Sweet Celebrations*), 3.9 oz.	5.0	2.0
triple chocolate (*Sweet Celebrations*), 3.15 oz.	5.0	2.5
chocolate fudge:		
double (*Sweet Celebrations*), 2.75 oz.	4.5	1.0
layer (*Pepperidge Farm*), ⅙ cake	16.0	5.0
stripe (*Pepperidge Farm*), ⅙ cake	14.0	3.0
chocolate, German, layer (*Pepperidge Farm*), ⅙ cake	16.0	4.0
chocolate mousse (*Pepperidge Farm*), ⅛ cake	10.0	3.0
coconut (*Sara Lee*), ⅛ cake	14.0	12.0

	total fat (grams)	saturated fat (grams)

Cake, frozen *(cont.)*

coconut, layer (*Pepperidge Farm*), ⅙ cake	14.0	4.0
devil's food, layer (*Pepperidge Farm*), ⅙ cake	14.0	5.0
golden, layer (*Pepperidge Farm*), ⅙ cake	14.0	3.0
lemon mousse (*Pepperidge Farm*), ⅛ cake	12.0	4.0
pineapple cream (*Pepperidge Farm*), ⅑ cake	10.0	3.0
pound (*Sara Lee*), ¼ cake	16.0	9.0
pound, all butter (*Pepperidge Farm*), ⅕ cake	13.0	7.0
strawberry cream (*Pepperidge Farm*), ⅑ cake	9.0	3.0
strawberry shortcake (*Sweet Celebrations*), 6.5 oz.	1.5	.5
strawberry stripe, layer (*Pepperidge Farm*), ⅙ cake	13.0	4.0
vanilla, layer (*Pepperidge Farm*), ⅙ cake	13.0	2.5

Cake mix*, 1/12 cake, except as noted:

angel food (*Pillsbury Moist Supreme*)	0	0
angel food (*Pillsbury Plus*), 1/10 cake	0	0
banana (*Pillsbury Moist Supreme*)	11.0	2.5
banana (*Pillsbury Plus*)	11.0	2.5
butter recipe (*Pillsbury Moist Supreme*)	12.0	6.0
butter recipe (*Pillsbury Plus*)	12.0	6.0
carrot:		
(*Betty Crocker SuperMoist*), 1/10 cake	13.0	3.0
(*Pillsbury Moist Supreme*)	12.0	2.5
(*Pillsbury Plus*)	12.0	3.0
cheesecake (*Jell-O* No Bake), ⅙ cake	5.0	3.0
chocolate:		
(*Pillsbury Moist Supreme*)	11.0	2.5
(*Pillsbury Plus*)	12.0	3.0
butter recipe (*Pillsbury Moist Supreme*)	13.0	7.0
butter recipe (*Pillsbury Plus*)	13.0	7.0
caramel nut (*Pillsbury Bundt*), 1/16 cake	18.0	3.5
dark (*Pillsbury Moist Supreme*)	11.0	2.5
dark (*Pillsbury Plus*)	12.0	3.0
double swirl (*Betty Crocker SuperMoist*)	12.0	3.0

	total fat (grams)	saturated fat (grams)
fudge (*Betty Crocker SuperMoist*)	11.0	3.0
German (*Pillsbury Moist Supreme*)	11.0	2.5
German (*Pillsbury Plus*)	11.0	2.5
swirl w/peanut butter (*Betty Crocker SuperMoist*), 1/12 cake	10.0	2.5
chocolate chip (*Pillsbury Moist Supreme*)	10.0	3.0
chocolate chip (*Pillsbury Plus*)	10.0	3.0
cinnamon streusel (*Pillsbury Streusel Swirl*), 1/16 cake	11.0	2.5
coffee (*Aunt Jemima's* Easy Mix), 1/3 cup dry	5.0	1.0
devil's food:		
(*Betty Crocker SuperMoist*)	12.0	3.0
(*Pillsbury Lovin' Lites*), 1/10 cake	5.0	2.0
(*Pillsbury Moist Supreme*)	14.0	3.0
(*Pillsbury Moist Supreme Lovin' Lites*), 1/10 cake	5.0	2.0
(*Pillsbury Plus*)	14.0	3.0
fudge:		
hot, double (*Pillsbury Bundt*), 1/16 cake	16.0	5.0
swirl (*Pillsbury Moist Supreme*)	10.0	2.5
swirl (*Pillsbury Plus*)	12.0	3.0
triple brownie (*Betty Crocker*), 1/9 cake	12.0	5.0
Funfetti (*Pillsbury Moist Supreme*)	9.0	2.0
Funfetti (*Pillsbury Plus*)	9.0	2.0
gingerbread (*Pillsbury*), 1/9 cake	5.0	1.0
lemon:		
(*Pillsbury Moist Supreme*)	13.0	3.0
(*Pillsbury Plus*)	13.0	3.0
pineapple upside-down (*Betty Crocker*), 1/6 cake	15.0	4.0
pound, golden (*Betty Crocker*), 1/8 cake	13.0	3.5
pound (*Dromedary*), 1/8 pkg.	10.0	3.0
strawberry:		
(*Pillsbury Moist Supreme*)	11.0	2.5
(*Pillsbury Plus*)	11.0	2.5
cream cheese (*Pillsbury Bundt*), 1/16 cake	17.0	4.5

	total fat (grams)	saturated fat (grams)
Cake mix*, strawberry *(cont.)*		
swirl (*Betty Crocker SuperMoist*), 1/10 cake	12.0	3.0
vanilla		
French (*Pillsbury Moist Supreme*), 1/10 cake	13.0	3.0
French (*Pillsbury Plus*)	15.0	3.5
sunshine (*Pillsbury Moist Supreme*)	12.0	3.0
sunshine (*Pillsbury Plus*)	12.0	3.0
white:		
(*Pillsbury Lovin' Lites*), 1/10 cake	5.0	1.5
(*Pillsbury Moist Supreme*)	11.0	2.5
(*Pillsbury Moist Supreme Lovin' Lites*),		
1/10 cake	5.0	1.5
(*Pillsbury Plus*)	11.0	2.5
and fudge swirl (*Pillsbury Moist Supreme*)	10.0	2.5
and fudge swirl (*Pillsbury Plus*)	10.0	2.5
yellow		
(*Betty Crocker SuperMoist*),	11.0	6.0
(*Pillsbury Lovin' Lites*), 1/10 cake	5.0	1.5
(*Pillsbury Moist Supreme*)	10.0	2.5
(*Pillsbury Moist Supreme Lovin' Lites*),		
1/10 cake	5.0	1.5
(*Pillsbury Plus*)	11.0	2.5
Cake, snack (see also "Pastry pocket," "Pie, snack," "Donut" and other specific listings):		
almond twirl (*Aunt Fanny's*), 1-oz. piece	4.0	.5
apple puffs (*Entenmann's*), 3-oz. piece	12.0	3.0
(*Aunt Fanny's* Dunkin' Stix), 1.4-oz. piece	11.0	4.0
(*Aunt Fanny's* Dunkin' Stix), 1.65-oz. piece	13.0	5.0
banana:		
(*Hostess Suzy Q's*), 2-oz. piece	10.0	1.0
(*Hostess Twinkies*), 2.7 oz., 2 pieces	13.0	1.5
(*Tastykake Creamies*), 1.5-oz. piece	7.0	1.5
twins (*Little Debbie*), 2.2-oz. pkg.	10.0	2.0
Boston creme (*Drake's*), 1 piece, 1.5 oz.	8.0	3.0

	total fat (grams)	saturated fat (grams)

butterscotch iced:

(Tastykake Krimpets), 3 oz., 3 pieces	8.0	2.0
(Tastykake Krimpets), 2 oz., 2 pieces	5.0	1.5
cheesecake, New York (*Boar's Head*), 4-oz. piece	30.0	18.0
cherry (*Aunt Fanny's* Dunkin' Stix), 1.4-oz. piece	11.0	3.0
cherry cordial (*Little Debbie*), 1.3-oz. pkg.	8.0	1.5

chocolate:

(Aunt Fanny's Dunkin' Stix), 1.4-oz. piece	12.0	3.0
(Drake's Devil Dogs), 1.6-oz piece	7.0	3.0
(Drake's Ring Dings) 1.5-oz. piece	10.0	4.0
(Drake's Ring Dings), 2.7 oz., 2 pieces	18.0	6.5
(Drake's Ring Dings), 2.5 oz., 2 pieces	16.0	6.0
(Drake's Ring Dings Family Pack), 2.7 oz., 2 pieces	14.0	7.0
(Hostess Choco Licious), 1.5-oz. piece	6.0	2.5
(Hostess Choco-Diles), 1.8-oz. piece	10.0	7.0
(Hostess Ding Dongs), 1.3-oz. piece	9.0	6.0
(Hostess Ho-Hos), 1-oz. piece	6.0	4.0
(Hostess Suzy Q's), 2-oz. piece	9.0	4.0
(Little Debbie), 2.1-oz. pkg.	12.0	2.5
(Little Debbie Choco-Cake), 2.2-oz. pkg.	14.0	3.0
(Little Debbie Choco-o-Jels), 1.2-oz. pkg.	7.0	1.5
(Tastykake Creamies), 1.5-oz. piece	7.0	2.0
(Tastykake Juniors), 3.3-oz. piece	13.0	2.5
(Tastykake Kandy Kakes), 2.7 oz., 4 pieces	17.0	10.0
(Tastykake Kandy Kakes), 2 oz., 3 pieces	13.0	8.0
chip (*Little Debbie*), 2.4-oz. pkg.	15.0	3.0
fingers (*Aunt Fanny's*), 3 oz., 2 pieces	10.0	4.0
roll (*Drake's Yodels*), 2.2 oz., 2 pieces	16.0	6.0
twins (*Little Debbie*), 2.4-oz. pkg.	9.0	1.5
cinnamon twirl (*Aunt Fanny's*), 1-oz. piece	4.0	.5

coconut:

(Hostess Sno Balls), 1.6-oz. piece	5.0	2.5
(Little Debbie), 2.2-oz. pkg.	13.0	3.0
(Tastykake Juniors), 3.3-oz. piece	8.0	4.0
(Tastykake Kandy Kakes), 2.7 oz., 4 pieces	17.0	13.0

	total fat (grams)	saturated fat (grams)

Cake, snack, coconut *(cont.)*

(*Tastykake Kandy Kakes*), 2 oz., 3 pieces	13.0	.... 10.0
rounds (*Little Debbie*), 1.2-oz. pkg.	7.0	.... 2.5
twirl (*Aunt Fanny's*), 1-oz. piece	4.0	.... 1.0
coffee cake:		
(*Drake's Cakes*), 1.1-oz. piece	6.0	.... 2.0
(*Drake's Cakes*), 2.3-oz. piece	11.0	.... 5.0
apple streusel (*Little Debbie*), 2-oz. pkg.	7.0	.... 1.0
cinnamon crumb (*Hostess* 97% Fat Free), 1.8 oz., 2 pieces	1.0	 0
crumb (*Hostess*), 2 pieces, 1.9 oz.	8.0	.... 3.0
creme filled (see also specific snack cake listings):		
(*Tastykake Kreme Krimpies*), 3 oz., 3 pieces ..	12.0	.... 2.5
(*Tastykake Kreme Krimpies*), 2 oz., 2 pieces ..	8.0	.... 1.5
(*Tastykake* Witchy Good Treats), 2.7 oz., 2 pieces	11.0	.... 2.0
cupcake (*Tastykake Kreme Kup*), 2 pieces	6.0	.... 1.5
cupcake, butter cream iced:		
(*Tastykake*), 2.25 oz., 2 pieces	8.0	.... 2.0
mini (*Tastykake*), 2 oz., 4 pieces	7.0	.... 2.0
mini (*Tastykake*), 1 oz., 2 pieces	4.0	.... 1.0
cupcake, chocolate:		
(*Aunt Fanny's*), 3 oz., 2 pieces	12.0	.... 5.0
(*Hostess*), 1.6-oz. piece	5.0	.... 2.5
(*Tastykake*), 2.2 oz., 2 pieces	6.0	.... 1.5
(*Tastykake*), 3.25 oz., 3 pieces	9.0	.... 2.5
(*Tastykake Tasty Too*), 2 pieces	3.0	.... 1.0
creme filled (*Hostess* Lights), 1.4-oz. piece ...	1.5	 0
creme filled (*Drake's Yankee Doodles*), 2 oz., 2 pieces	9.0	.... 4.0
creme filled (*Drake's Yankee Doodles*), 3 oz., 3 pieces	12.0	.... 5.0
creme filled (*Tastykake Koffee Kake*), 2 oz., 2 pieces	9.0	.... 2.0

	total fat (grams)	saturated fat (grams)
creme filled, mini (*Tastykake* Koffee Kake), 4 pieces	9.0	1.5
cupcake, chocolate iced, creme filled:		
(*Tastykake*), 2.25 oz., 2 pieces	8.0	2.0
mini (*Tastykake*), 2 oz., 4 pieces	7.0	2.0
mini (*Tastykake*), 1 oz., 2 pieces	4.0	1.0
vanilla, mini (*Tastykake*), 2 oz., 4 pieces	8.0	1.5
vanilla, mini (*Tastykake*), 1 oz., 2 pieces	4.0	1.0
cupcake, creme filled (*Tastykake* Koffee Kake), 1 oz., 2 pieces	4.0	1.0
cupcake, orange (*Aunt Fanny's*), 3 oz., 2 pieces	12.0	4.0
cupcake, orange (*Hostess*), 1.5-oz. piece	5.0	2.0
cupcake, vanilla:		
(*Tastykake Tasty Too*), 2 pieces	4.0	1.5
creme filled (*Drake's Sunny Doodles*), 2 oz., 2 pieces	8.0	4.0
creme filled (*Drake's Sunny Doodles*), 3 oz., 3 pieces	13.0	6.0
devil's food:		
(*Hostess Twinkies*), 2.7 oz., 2 pieces	12.0	5.0
creme-filled (*Little Debbie*), 1.6-oz. pkg.	8.0	1.5
squares (*Little Debbie*), 2.2-oz. pkg.	13.0	3.0
donuts, see "Donuts"		
(*Drake's Funny Bones*), 2.5 oz., 2 pieces	12.0	5.0
frosty (*Tastykake Kandy Kakes*), 2.7 oz., 4 pieces	15.0	11.0
frosty (*Tastykake Kandy Kakes*), 2 oz., 3 pieces	11.0	8.0
fruit (*Hostess* Fruit Loaf), 3.8-oz. piece	10.0	1.0
fudge:		
crispy bar (*Little Debbie*), 1.1-oz. pkg.	10.0	2.5
macaroon (*Little Debbie*), 1-oz. pkg.	8.0	4.0
rounds (*Little Debbie*), 1.2-oz. pkg.	6.0	1.0
glazed (*Entenmann's Popems*), 2 oz., 6 pieces	11.0	2.5
glazed, chocolate (*Entenmann's Popems*), 1.8 oz., 4 pieces	10.0	2.5

	total fat (grams)	saturated fat (grams)

Cake, snack *(cont.)*

golden, creme-filled:

(*Hostess Twinkies*), 1.4-oz. piece .... 4.0 .... 2.0

(*Hostess Twinkies* Light), 1.4-oz. piece 1.5 0

(*Little Debbie*), 1.5-oz. pkg. .... 7.0 .... 2.0

(*Hostess Baseball*), 1.7-oz. piece .... 3.0 .... 1.0

(*Hostess Dessert Cups*), 1-oz. piece 1.5 0

(*Hostess L'il Angels*), 1-oz. piece .... 2.0 .... 1.0

(*Hostess Tiger Tails*), 1.5-oz. piece .... 6.0 .... 2.5

jelly filled:

(*Tastykake*), 3 oz., 3 pieces .... 4.0 .... 1.0

(*Tastykake*), 2 oz., 2 pieces 3.0 5

(*Tastykake Tasty Too*), 2.1 oz., 2 pieces ...... 1.5 .... 1.0

lemon (*Little Debbie* Stix), 1.5-oz. pkg. .... 10.0 .... 2.5

lemon filled (*Tastykake Tasty Too*), 1.2 oz.,

2 pieces .... 2.0 .... 1.5

marshmallow supreme (*Little Debbie*),

1.1-oz. pkg. .... 5.0 .... 1.0

mint (*Little Debbie Sprints*), 1.5-oz pkg. .... 13.0 .... 3.0

peanut butter:

(*Tastykake Kandy Kakes*), 2.7-oz., 4 pieces ... 19.0 .... 9.0

(*Tastykake Kandy Kakes*), 2 oz., 3 pieces .... 14.0 .... 7.0

(*Tastykake Kandy Kakes*), 1.3 oz., 2 pieces ... 10.0 .... 4.0

bar (*Little Debbie*), 1.9-oz. pkg. .... 15.0 .... 2.5

and jelly sandwich (*Little Debbie*), 1.1-oz. pkg. .. 5.0 .... 1.0

wafer (*Little Debbie Nutty Bar*), 2-oz. pkg. .... 17.0 .... 3.0

peanut cluster (*Little Debbie*), 1.4-oz. pkg. .... 11.0 .... 2.0

pecan twirl (*Aunt Fanny's*), 1-oz. piece 4.0 5

pound cake:

(*Aunt Fanny's*), 2.5-oz. piece .... 10.0 .... 3.0

(*Drake's*), 2.5-oz. piece .... 12.0 .... 7.0

(*Tastykake* Juniors), 3-oz. piece .... 13.0 .... 5.0

pumpkin (*Little Debbie Delights*), 1.2-oz. pkg. .... 5.0 .... 1.0

raspberry fingers (*Aunt Fanny's*), 3 oz., 2 pieces .. 8.0 .... 4.0

spice (*Little Debbie*), 2.5-oz. pkg. .... 15.0 .... 3.0

	total fat (grams)	saturated fat (grams)
sprinkled (*Tastykake* Creamies), 2.7 oz., 2 pieces	11.0	1.5
sprinkled (*Tastykake* Creamies), 1.3 oz., 1 piece	6.0	.5
strawberry:		
filled (*Hostess Twinkies*), 1.6-oz. piece	3.0	1.0
iced (*Tastykake*), 3 oz., 3 pieces	8.0	1.5
iced (*Tastykake*), 2 oz., 2 pieces	5.0	1.0
Swiss roll (*Little Debbie*), 2.2-oz. pkg.	12.0	3.0
(*Tastykake* Dunkin Stix), 1.4-oz. piece	11.0	4.0
(*Tastykake Koffee Kake* Juniors), 2.5-oz. piece	9.0	1.5
vanilla:		
(*Little Debbie*), 2.6-oz. pkg.	16.0	3.0
(*Tastykake* Creamies), 1.5-oz. piece	8.0	1.5
fingers (*Aunt Fanny's*), 3 oz., 2 pieces	10.0	4.0
zebra cake (*Little Debbie*), 2.6-oz. pkg.	16.0	3.0
Cake, snack, frozen:		
Black Forest (*Pepperidge Farm*), 2.5-oz. cake	10.0	2.0
brownie, hot fudge (*Pepperidge Farm*), 3-oz. cake	18.0	9.0
cheesecake, strawberry (*Pepperidge Farm*), 4-oz. cake	8.0	4.0
chocolate, German (*Pepperidge Farm*), 2.3-oz. cake	13.0	4.0
coffee, cinnamon streusel (*Weight Watchers*), 2.25-oz. cake	3.5	1.0
Mississippi mud pie (*Pepperidge Farm*), 2.6-oz. cake	17.0	3.0
Cake, snack, mix, ⅑ cake*:		
banana, vanilla frosted (*Pillsbury Microwave*)	7.0	2.0
carrot, cream cheese frosted (*Pillsbury Microwave*)	7.0	2.0
chocolate, fudge frosted (*Pillsbury Microwave*)	7.0	2.0
cupcake, chocolate or yellow, frosted (*Pillsbury Funfetti Microwave*)	7.0	2.0
Cake frosting, see "Frosting"		

	total fat (grams)	saturated fat (grams)

Calamari, see "Squid"

Candy:

(*Aero*), 1.4-oz. bar	13.0	7.0
all flavors (*Pez* Refill Regular/Sugar Free), .3-oz. roll	0	0
almond clusters (*Ghirardelli*), 3 pieces, 1.3 oz.	16.0	4.0
(*Baby Ruth*), 2.1-oz. bar	12.0	7.0
(*Baby Ruth* Fun Size), 2 mini bars	9.0	5.0
(*Brock's* Candy Rolls/Glitters), .5 oz., 2 rolls	0	0
(*Brock's* Tootsie Midgees), 2-oz. pkg.	4.0	1.0
butter mints (*Kraft*), 7 pieces	0	0
butter rum (*Pearson Nips*), 2 pieces	1.5	1.5
(*Butterfinger*), 2.1-oz. bar	11.0	6.0
(*Butterfinger* Fun Size), 2 mini bars	8.0	4.0
(*Butterfinger BB's*), 1.7-oz. bag	10.0	7.0
butterscotch (*Brock's* Discs), 3 pieces, .6 oz.	0	0
candy corn (*Brock's*), 21 pieces, 1.4 oz.	0	0
caramel:		
(*Brocks* Dots), 3 pieces, 1.4 oz.	3.0	1.0
(*Kraft*), 5 pieces	3.0	1.0
(*Pearson Nips*), 2 pieces	1.5	1.5
(*Sugar Babies*), 1.7 oz.	2.0	2.0
(*Sugar Daddy*), 1.7 oz.	2.5	2.5
chocolate coated (*Pom Poms*), 1.58 oz.	6.0	4.5
caramel cookie bar, see "Cookie"		
cherry:		
dark chocolate coated (*Cella*), 1 oz., 2 pieces	4.0	3.0
milk chocolate coated (*Cella*), 1 oz., 2 pieces	4.0	2.5
chocolate cordial or jubilee (*Andes* Thins), 1.3 oz., 8 pieces	13.0	11.0
chocolate, assorted (*Hershey* Miniatures), 1.5 oz., 5 pieces	14.0	8.0
chocolate, dark (see also "Chocolate, semisweet," below, and "Chocolate, baking"):		
(*Dove*), ¼ of 6-oz. bar	14.0	8.0

	total fat (grams)	saturated fat (grams)
(*Dove* Miniatures), 7 pieces, 1.5 oz.	14.0	8.0
(*Dove* Singles), 1.3-oz. bar	12.0	7.0
(*Ghirardelli*), 1.25-oz. bar	11.0	6.0
(*Ghirardelli*), ½ of 3-oz. bar	14.0	8.0
(*Ghirardelli* Square), ⅜-oz. piece	3.0	2.0
(*Hershey's Special Dark*), 1.3 oz., 3 blocks	12.0	7.0
w/almonds (*Ghirardelli*), ½ of 3-oz. bar	15.0	7.0
w/raspberries (*Ghirardelli*), ½ of 3-oz. bar	13.0	8.0
chocolate, milk:		
(*Cadbury/Dairy Milk*), 1.4 oz., 9 blocks	12.0	8.0
(*Dove*), ¼ of 6-oz. bar	13.0	8.0
(*Dove* Miniatures), 7 pieces, 1.5 oz.	13.0	8.0
(*Dove* Singles), 1.3-oz. bar	12.0	7.0
(*Ghirardelli*), 1.25-oz. bar	11.0	7.0
(*Ghirardelli*), ½ of 3-oz. bar	14.0	8.0
(*Ghirardelli* Block), 1 oz.	8.0	5.0
(*Hershey's*), 1.5 oz., 3 blocks	12.0	7.0
(*Hershey's Hugs/Kisses*), 1.4 oz., 8 pieces	12.0	8.0
(*Hershey's* Nuggets), 1.4 oz., 4 pieces	12.0	8.0
(*Symphony*), 1.4 oz., 4 blocks	13.0	8.0
(*Nestlé*), 1.45-oz. bar	13.0	7.0
w/almonds (*Cadbury*), 1.4 oz., 9 blocks	13.0	7.0
w/almonds (*Ghirardelli*), 2.1-oz. bar	21.0	11.0
w/almonds (*Ghirardelli*), ½ of 3-oz. bar	15.0	7.0
w/almonds (*Hershey's*), 3 blocks, 1.3 oz.	13.0	6.0
w/almonds (*Hershey's Hugs*), 1.4 oz., 9 pieces	13.0	6.0
w/almonds (*Hershey's* Nuggets), 1.4 oz., 4 pieces	13.0	6.0
w/almonds (*Hershey's Kisses*), 1.3 oz., 8 pieces	13.0	7.0
w/almonds and toffee (*Symphony*), 1.4 oz., 4 blocks	14.0	7.0
w/caramel (*Caramello*), 1.4 oz., 5 blocks	9.0	6.0

	total fat (grams)	saturated fat (grams)

Candy, chocolate, milk *(cont.)*

w/crisp rice (*Ghirardelli*), 2.1-oz. bar	17.0	10.0
w/crisp rice (*Ghirardelli*), 2.5-oz. bar	20.0	12.0
w/crisps (*Nestlé Buncha Crunch*), 1.4-oz. bag	10.0	5.0
w/crisps (*Nestlé Crunch*), 1.4-oz. bar	12.0	7.0
w/crisps (*Nestlé Crunch* Fun Size), 4 bars	10.0	6.0
w/crisps and nuts (*100 Grand*), 1.5-oz. bar	8.0	5.0
w/fruit and nuts (*Cadbury*), 1.4 oz., 9 blocks	11.0	6.0
w/fruit and nuts (*Nestlé Chunky*), 1.4 oz. bar	11.0	6.0
w/honey and almond nougat (*Toblerone*), ⅓ of 3.5-oz. bar	10.0	6.0
w/macadamias (*Ghirardelli*), 1.25-oz. bar	13.0	6.0
w/macadamias (*Ghirardelli*), 2.5-oz. bar	26.0	13.0
mint (*Hershey's* Cookies 'n' Mint Nuggets), 1.4 oz., 4 pieces	10.0	5.0
w/pecans (*Ghirardelli*), ½ of 3-oz. bar	16.0	7.0
w/peanuts (*Mr. Goodbar*), 1.3 oz., 3 blocks	14.0	6.0
w/toffee (*Ghirardelli*), ½ of 3-oz. bar	13.0	8.0
chocolate, milk or mint (*Ghirardelli* Square), ⅜-oz. piece	3.0	2.0
chocolate, milk, candy coated:		
(*M&M's*), 1.5 oz.	9.0	5.0
(*M&M's* Fun Size), .75-oz. bag	4.0	2.5
(*M&M's* King Size), ½ of 3.2-oz. bag	9.0	6.0
(*M&M's* Singles), 1.7-oz. bag	10.0	6.0
almond (*M&M's*), 1.5 oz.	12.0	4.0
almond (*M&M's* Singles), 1.3-oz. bag	11.0	3.5
mint (*M&M's*), 1.5 oz.	9.0	5.0
mint (*M&M's* Singles), 1.7-oz. bag	10.0	6.0
peanut (*M&M's*), 1.5 oz.	11.0	4.0
peanut (*M&M's* Fun Size), .75-oz. bag	5.0	2.0
peanut (*M&M's* King Size), ½ of 3.3-oz. bag	12.0	5.0
peanut (*M&M's* Singles), 1.7-oz. bag	13.0	5.0
peanut butter (*M&M's*), 1.5 oz.	12.0	8.0

	total fat (grams)	saturated fat (grams)
peanut butter (*M&M's* Fun Size), .7-oz. bag ...	6.0	4.0
peanut butter (*M&M's* Singles), 1.6-oz. bag ...	13.0	8.0
chocolate, candy-coated, semisweet (*M&M's*), .5 oz.	3.5	2.0
chocolate, coconut (*Andes* Toasted Coconut Thins), 1.3 oz., 8 pieces	13.0	11.0
chocolate mint:		
(*Ghirardelli*), 2.1-oz. bar	19.0	11.0
(*Ghirardelli*), ½ of 3-oz. bar	14.0	8.0
(*Pearson Nips*), 2 pieces	1.5	1.5
chocolate, nut and honey (*Andes* Thins), 1.3 oz., 8 pieces	13.0	10.0
chocolate, truffle filled (*La Trufflina*), 1.3 oz., 3 pieces	15.0	10.0
chocolate, parfait (*Pearson Nips*), 2 pieces ...	2.0	2.0
chocolate wafers, milk or mint (*Ghirardelli*), 1.5 oz., 11 pieces	12.0	7.0
cinnamon (*Brock's* Discs), .6 oz., 3 pieces ...	0	0
coconut (*Brock's* Mountains), 1.4 oz., 4 pieces ...	6.0	5.0
coffee (*Pearson Nips*), 2 pieces	1.5	1.5
fruit (*Brock's* Fruit Basket/Kisses), .6 oz., 3 pieces ..	0	0
fruit chews:		
(*Starburst* Original), ⅓ of 1.2-oz. bag	3.0	.5
(*Starburst* Original Singles), 2-oz. stick	5.0	1.0
(*Starburst* Original), 8 pieces	3.0	.5
(*Starburst* California Fruits), 8 pieces	3.0	.5
(*Starburst* California Fruits Singles), 2-oz. stick	4.5	1.0
(*Starburst* Strawberry Fruits), 8 pieces	3.0	.5
(*Starburst* Strawberry Fruits), 2-oz. stick	5.0	1.0
(*Starburst* Tropical Fruits), 8 pieces	3.0	.5
(*Starburst* Tropical Fruits Singles), 2-oz. stick ...	5.0	1.0
fruit-flavored:		
(*Skittles* Original), 1.5 oz.	2.0	0
(*Skittles* Original Fun Size), 3 pieces, 1.6 oz. ..	2.0	0

	total fat (grams)	saturated fat (grams)

Candy, fruit-flavored *(cont.)*

(*Skittles* Original King Size), ½ of 1.3-oz. bag ...	1.5	0
(*Skittles* Original Singles), 2.2-oz. bag	2.5	.5
(*Skittles* Tropical), 1.5 oz.	1.5	0
(*Skittles* Tropical Fun Size), 1.4 oz., 2 pieces ..	1.5	0
(*Skittles* Tropical Singles), 2.2-oz. bag	2.5	.5
(*Skittles* Wild Berry), 1.5 oz.	1.5	0
(*Skittles* Wild Berry Fun Size), 1.4 oz., 2 pieces	1.5	0
(*Skittles* Wild Berry Singles), 2.2-oz. bag	2.5	.5
fudge (*Kraft* Fudgies), 5 pieces	5.0	2.5
gum, chewing, all varieties and brands, 1 piece ...	0	0
gum drops, all flavors, 1 oz.	0	0
gummed (*Brock's* Gummy Bears/Squirms), 15 pieces	0	0
gummed, fruit (*Jujyfruits*), 1.4 oz., 15 pieces	0	0
hard:		
all flavors (*LifeSavers/LifeSavers Holes*), 1 oz.	0	0
all flavors (*Pez*), 1 roll	0	0
butter and cream (*Brock's*), .5 oz., 2 pieces ...	1.0	.5
mixed (*Brock's*), .6 oz., 3 pieces	0	0
jelly beans, all flavors, 1 oz.	0	0
lemon drops (*Brock's*), .5 oz., 3 pieces	0	0
licorice:		
(*Pearson Nips*), 2 pieces	1.5	1.5
(*Tom's* Red Twist), 2 oz.	0	0
(*Twizzlers*), 1.5 oz., 4 pieces	.5	0
bits (*Switzer*), 1.4 oz., about 11 pieces	0	0
candy coated (*Good & Plenty*), ¼ of 7-oz. box	0	0
lollipop, all flavors (*LifeSavers*), 1 piece	0	0
lollipop (*Tootsie Roll*), .6-oz. pop	0	0
(*Mars* Almond Bar Fun Size), 1.3 oz.	10.0	3.0
(*Mars* Almond Bar), 1.76-oz. bar	13.0	4.0

	total fat (grams)	saturated fat (grams)
marshmallow (*Brock's* Circus Peanuts), 6 pieces ..	0	0
marshmallow, all varieties (*Kraft*), 1 oz.	0	0
(*Milky Way* Fun Size), 1.4 oz., 2 bars	7.0	3.5
(*Milky Way* King Size), ⅓ of 1.2-oz. bar	6.0	3.0
(*Milky Way* Miniatures), 5 pieces	7.0	4.0
(*Milky Way* Singles), 2.15-oz. bar	11.0	5.0
(*Milky Way* Dark Fun Size), .7-oz. bar	3.0	1.5
(*Milky Way* Dark Miniature), 5 pieces	7.0	4.0
(*Milky Way* Dark Singles), 1.76-oz. bar	8.0	4.5
mint:		
(*Andes* Creme de Menthe Thins), 1.3 oz.,		
8 pieces	13.0	12.0
(*Brock's* Starlight), .6 oz., 3 pieces	0	0
(*Kraft* Party Mints), 7 pieces	0	0
all varieties (*LifeSavers/LifeSavers Holes*),		
1 oz.	0	0
chocolate (*Andes* Thins), 1.3 oz., 8 pieces	13.0	11.0
chocolate coated (*Junior Mints*), 1.6 oz.	4.0	2.5
mixed (*Andes* Thins), 1.3 oz., 8 pieces	13.0	11.0
orange (*Andes* Thins), 1.3 oz., 8 pieces	13.0	12.0
parfait (*Andes* Thins), 1.3 oz., 8 pieces	13.0	11.0
party (*Brock's*), .5 oz., 9 pieces	0	0
(*Nestlé Turtles*), 2 pieces	9.0	3.0
non pareils (*Ghirardelli*), 10 pieces	9.0	5.0
non pareils (*Nestlé Sno-Caps*), 2.3-oz. box	13.0	8.0
nougat, vanilla, chocolate coated (*Charleston Chew*),		
1.9-oz. bar	7.0	6.0
(*Oh Henry!*), 1.8-oz. bar	9.0	4.0
orange (*Brock's* Slices), 1.5 oz., 4 pieces	0	0
peanut, chocolate covered (*Goobers*), 1.4-oz. bag ..	13.0	5.0
peanut brittle, 1.5 oz.	6.0	1.0
peanut brittle (*Kraft*), 5 pieces	5.0	1.0
peanut butter (*Snickers* Singles), 2-oz. bar	20.0	7.0
peanut butter crunch (*Brock's*), .6 oz., 3 pieces ...	2.0	n.a.
peanut butter parfait (*Pearson Nips*), 2 pieces	2.0	2.0

	total fat (grams)	saturated fat (grams)

Candy *(cont.)*

peanut clusters (*Ghirardelli*), 1.3 oz., 3 pieces	15.0	.... 5.0
pecan brittle (*Dewey's* Gourmet), 1.5 oz.	9.0	.... 2.0

raisins:

chocolate coated (*Raisinets*), 1⅝-oz. bag	8.0	.... 4.0
yogurt coated, vanilla (*Del Monte*), 1-oz. bag ..	3.0	.... 3.0
yogurt coated, strawberry (*Del Monte*), .9-oz. bag	3.0	.... 2.5
(*Snickers* Fun Size), 1.4 oz., 2 bars	9.0	.... 4.0
(*Snickers* King Size), ⅓ of 1.2-oz. bar	8.0	.... 3.0
(*Snickers* Miniature), 4 pieces	8.0	.... 3.0
(*Snickers* Singles), 2.1-oz. bar	14.0	.... 5.0
(*Snickers Munch* Singles), 1.4-oz. bar	15.0	.... 3.5
sour balls (*Brock's*), .6 oz., 3 pieces	0	 0
spearmint (*Brock's* Leaves), 1.4 oz., 4 pieces	0	 0
spice (*Brock's* Drops), 1.4 oz., 12 pieces	0	 0
(*3 Musketeers* Fun Size), 2 bars	4.0	.... 2.5
(*3 Musketeers* Singles), 2.1-oz. bar	8.0	.... 4.0
toffee (*Brock's*), 1.5 oz., 6 pieces	5.0	.... 1.5
toffee crunch chocolate (*Andes* Thins), 1.3 oz., 8 pieces	12.0	.... 11.0
(*Tootsie Roll*), 1 oz.	2.0	 0
(*Tootsie Roll* Midgees), 1.4 oz., 6 pieces	3.0	5

Cane syrup, 1 tbsp.	0	 0

Cannellini beans, see "Kidney beans"

Canelloni entree, frozen, cheese (*Lean Cuisine*),

9⅛ oz.	8.0	.... 3.5

Canola oil:

1 tbsp.	14.0	.... 1.0
(*Hain*), 1 tbsp.	14.0	.... 1.0
(*Smart Beat*), 1 tbsp.	14.0	.... 1.0
w/vitamin E (*Hollywood*), 1 tbsp.	14.0	.... 1.0

Cantaloupe:

untrimmed, 1 lb.	.6	 0

	total fat (grams)	saturated fat (grams)
½ of 5"-diameter melon	.7	0
pulp, cubed, ½ cup	.2	0
Capers:		
(*Krinos*), 1 tbsp.	0	0
drained (*Progresso*), 1 tbsp.	0	0
Capon, see "Chicken"		
Caponata, see "Eggplant appetizer"		
Cappuccino, iced:		
hot, see "Coffee, flavored, mix"		
coffee, mocha, or vanilla		
(*Maxwell House Cappio*), 8 fl. oz.	2.5	1.5
Carambola:		
fresh:		
untrimmed, 1 lb.	1.5	tr.
1 medium, 4.7 oz.	.4	0
pulp, cubed, ½ cup	.2	0
dried (*Sonoma*), 1.4 oz., 7–9 pieces	0	0
Caramel, see "Candy"		
Caramel topping:		
(*Kraft*), 2 tbsp.	0	0
(*Mrs. Richardson's* Fat Free), 2 tbsp.	0	0
hot (*Smucker's*)	3.0	.5
Caraway seeds:		
1 tbsp.	1.0	<.1
1 tsp.	.3	tr.
Carbonara sauce mix (*Knorr* Pasta Sauces),		
⅛ pkg.	2.0	.5
Cardamom:		
ground, 1 tbsp.	.4	<.1
ground or seeds, 1 tsp.	.1	tr.
Cardoon:		
raw, untrimmed, 1 lb.	.2	<.1
raw, shredded, ½ cup	.1	<.1
boiled, drained, 4 oz.	.1	<.1
Caribou, meat only, roasted, 12 oz. (1 lb. raw)	15.0	5.8

	total fat (grams)	saturated fat (grams)

Carissa:

untrimmed, 1 lb. .... 5.1 .... n.a.

sliced, ½ cup .... 1.0 .... tr.

Carne asada seasoning (*Lawry's* Spices & Seasoning), 1 tsp. 0 0

Carob flavor drink mix, dry, 3 tsp. .... tr. .... tr.

Carob flour, ½ cup .... .2 .... tr.

Carp, meat only:

raw, 4 oz. .... 6.4 .... 1.2

baked, broiled, or microwaved, 4 oz. .... 8.1 .... 1.6

Carrot:

fresh:

raw, trimmed, 4 oz. .... .2 .... tr.

raw, 1 medium, 7½" long, or ½ cup
shredded .... .1 .... <.1

boiled, drained, 1 medium or ½ slices .... .1 .... <.1

canned, ½ cup:

(*Allen/Crest Top*) 5 0

all cuts (*Seneca*) 0 0

all cuts (*Stokely*) 0 0

sliced (*Del Monte*) 0 0

sliced (*Green Giant*) 0 0

whole, baby (*Green Giant LeSueur*) 0 0

freeze-dried (*AlpineAire*), ½ cup∗ 3 0

frozen:

all cuts, 10-oz. pkg. 6 1

cut, baby (*Green Giant Harvest Fresh*),
⅔ cup 0 0

whole, baby (*Green Giant Select*), ¾ cup 0 0

whole, baby (*Schwan's*), 13 pieces, 2.9 oz. ... 0 0

whole, baby, or crinkle cut (*Stilwell*), ⅔ cup .. 0 0

Carrot chips:

(*Hain/Hain* No Salt Added), 1 oz. .... 9.0 .... n.a.

barbeque (*Hain*), 1 oz. .... 8.0 .... n.a.

	total fat (grams)	saturated fat (grams)
Carrot juice, canned:		
6 fl. oz.	.3	.1
(*Hain/Hollywood*), 1 can	1.0	0
Casaba:		
untrimmed, 1 lb.	.3	tr.
pulp, cubed, ½ cup	.1	0
Cashew:		
(*Eagle* Lightly Salted), 1 oz., 19 pieces	14.0	3.0
(*Frito-Lay*), 1½ oz.	22.0	4.0
dry-roasted:		
1 oz., about 18 medium kernels	13.2	2.6
whole and halves, ½ cup	31.8	6.3
(*Planters* Lightly Salted), 1 oz.	14.0	3.0
honey-roasted (*Eagle*), 1 oz., 18 pieces	14.0	3.0
honey-roasted (*Planters*), 1 oz.	12.0	2.0
oil-roasted:		
1 oz., about 18 medium kernels	13.7	2.7
(*Planters/Planters* Fancy), 1 oz.	14.0	3.0
halves (*Planters* Lightly Salted), 1 oz.	13.0	2.5
and peanuts, see "Nuts, mixed"		
Cashew butter:		
1 tbsp.	7.9	1.6
(*Roaster Fresh*), 1 oz.	14.0	2.9
Catfish, meat only, 4 oz.:		
farmed, raw	8.6	2.0
farmed, baked, broiled, or microwaved	9.1	2.0
wild, raw	3.2	.8
wild, baked, broiled, or microwaved	3.2	.8
Catfish, frozen:		
fillet:		
breaded (*Delta Pride*), 3.9 oz.	4.0	1.0
breaded (*Schwan's*), 4 oz., 1½ pieces	7.0	1.0
Cajun marinated (*Delta Pride*), 3.9 oz.	6.0	1.5
Italian (*Delta Pride*), 3.9 oz.	6.0	1.5
lemon pepper marinated (*Delta Pride*), 3.9 oz.	8.0	2.0
shank (*Delta Pride* Classics), 3.9 oz.	3.0	.5

	total fat (grams)	saturated fat (grams)
Catfish, frozen fillet *(cont.)*		
steaks (*Delta Pride*), 3.9 oz.	9.0	2.0
strips (*Delta Pride*), 3.9 oz.	4.5	1.0
fingers, breaded (*Schwan's*), 4 pieces	6.0	1.5
nuggets (*Delta Pride*), 3.9 oz.	8.0	2.0
nuggets, breaded (*Delta Pride*), 3.9 oz.	7.0	1.5
strips, breaded (*Delta Pride*), 3.9 oz.	6.0	1.5
Catsup:		
1 tbsp.	.1	<.1
(*Brooks* Rich & Tangy), 1 tbsp.	0	0
(*Del Monte*), 1 tbsp.	0	0
(*Healthy Choice*), .5 oz.	0	0
(*Heinz*), 1 tbsp.	0	0
(*Hunt's*), 1 tbsp.	0	0
(*Smucker's*), 1 tbsp.	0	0
w/horseradish (*Gold's*), 1 tbsp.	0	0
Cauliflower:		
fresh:		
raw, untrimmed, 1 lb.	.3	<.1
raw, green (*Dole*), ⅕ medium head	0	0
raw, 3 florets or ½ cup pieces	.1	<.1
boiled, drained, 3 florets or ½ cup pieces	.1	<.1
frozen:		
10-oz. pkg.	.8	.1
(*Stilwell*), 1 cup	0	0
cuts (*Green Giant*), 1 cup	0	0
in cheese sauce (*Green Giant*), ½ cup	2.5	.5
Cauliflower, pickled, in jars, 1 oz.	0	0
Cavatelli entree, frozen (*Celentano*), 3.2 oz., about ⅔ cup	1.5	.5
Caviar, granular (see also "Roe"):		
black or red, 1 oz.	5.0	n.a.
black or red, 1 tbsp.	2.9	n.a.
carp (*Krinos* Tarama), 1 tbsp.	.5	.5
Caviar spread, see "Taramosalata"		

	total fat (grams)	saturated fat (grams)

Cayenne, see "Pepper"

Celeriac:

raw, untrimmed, 1 lb.	1.2	tr.
raw, trimmed, ½ cup	.2	0
boiled, drained, 4 oz.	.2	0

Celery, fresh:

raw, untrimmed, 1 lb.	.6	.1
raw, 7½" stalk or ½ cup diced	.1	<.1
boiled, drained, 4 oz. or ½ cup diced	.1	<.1

Celery, dried:

flakes, 1 tsp.	.5	<.1
seeds, 1 tbsp.	1.6	.1
seeds, 1 tsp.	.5	<.1

Celery root or knob, see "Celeriac"

Celery salt:

| 1 tsp. | .4 | <.1 |
| (*Durkee/Spice Islands*), ¼ tsp. | 0 | 0 |

Cellophane noodles, see "Noodle, Chinese"

Celtus, 1 oz. | .1 | 0 |

Cereal, ready-to-eat, dry:

amaranth flakes (*Arrowhead Mills*), 1 cup	2.0	0
amaranth flakes (*Health Valley*), ¾ cup	0	0
(*Banana Nut Crunch*), 1 cup	6.0	1.0
(*Barbara's Frosted Funnies*), 1 cup	0	0
(*Barbara's Startoons* Cocoa), 1 cup	.5	0
(*Barbara's Startoons* Honey), 1 cup	0	0
(*Blueberry Morning*), 1¼ cups	3.5	.5

bran (see also "oat bran," below):

(*All-Bran/All-Bran* Extra Fiber), ½ cup	1.0	0
(*Bran Buds*), ⅓ cup	1.0	0
(*Bran'Nola* Original), ½ cup	3.0	.5
(*Nabisco 100% Bran*), ⅓ cup	.5	0
(*Quaker* Crunchy), ¾ cup	1.0	0
flakes (*Arrowhead Mills*), 1 cup	1.0	0
flakes (*Kellogg's Complete*), ¾ cup	.5	0

	total fat (grams)	saturated fat (grams)

Cereal, ready-to-eat, bran *(cont.)*

flakes (*Malt-O-Meal*), ¾ cup	1.0	0
flakes (*New Morning*), 1 cup	1.0	n.a.
flakes (*Post*), ⅔ cup	.5	0
flakes (*Ralston*), ¾ cup	1.0	0
frosted (*Kellogg's Frosted Bran*), ¾ cup	0	0
frosted (*Malt-O-Meal*), 1 cup	.5	0
w/fruit (*Kellogg's Fruitful Bran*), 1¼ cup	1.0	0
w/apple or raisins (*Health Valley* Organic), ¾ cup	0	0
w/raisins (*Barbara's*), 1 cup	1.0	0
w/raisins (*Bran'Nola*), ½ cup	3.0	.5
w/raisins (*Erewhon*), 1 cup	.5	0
w/raisins (*Kellogg's*), 1 cup	1.0	0
w/raisins (*Malt-O-Meal*), 1¼ cup	1.0	0
w/raisins (*New Morning*), 1 cup	.5	0
w/raisins (*Post*), 1 cup	1.0	0
w/raisins (*Ralston* Raisin Bran), ¾ cup	1.0	0
w/raisins, multi-bran (*New Morning*), 1 cup	.5	0
unprocessed (*Quaker*), ⅓ cup	0	0
corn:		
all varieties, except peanut butter (*Cap'n Crunch*), ¾ cup	1.5	0
(*Cap'n Crunch* Peanut Butter), ¾ cup	2.5	.5
(*Corn Chex*), 1¼ cups	0	0
(*Erewhon* Honey Crisp Corn), 1 cup	2.5	0
(*Honeycomb*), 1½ cups	0	0
(*Kellogg's Corn Pops*), 1 cup	0	0
(*Kellogg's Nut & Honey Crunch*), 1¼ cup	4.0	1.0
(*Post Toasties*), 1 cup	0	0
flakes (*Arrowhead Mills*), 1 cup	0	0
flakes (*Barbara's*), 1.1 oz., 1 cup	0	0
flakes (*Erewhon*), 1¼ cups	2.5	0
flakes (*Health Valley*), ¾ cup	0	0
flakes (*Kellogg's Corn Flakes*), 1 cup	0	0

	total fat (grams)	saturated fat (grams)
flakes (*New Morning*), 1 cup	1.0	0
flakes (*Ralston*), 1¼ cups	0	0
flakes, frosted (*Kellogg's Frosted Flakes*), ¾ cup	0	0
flakes, frosted (*Quaker* Kids Favorites), ¾ cup	0	0
flakes, frosted (*Ralston Frosted Flakes*), ¾ cup	0	0
flakes or sugar frosted (*Malt-O-Meal*), 1 cup	0	0
puffed (*Arrowhead Mills*), 1 cup	0	0
puffed (*Health Valley*), 1 cup	0	0
puffs (*Popeye Jeepers*), 1⅓ cup	.5	0
apple (*Arrowhead Mills* Apple Corns), 1 cup	1.5	0
cocoa (*Pebbles*), ¾ cup	1.0	1.0
cocoa (*Ralston Crunchies*), ¾ cup	1.0	0
cocoa-flavored (*Malt-O-Meal*), ¾ cup	1.0	0
maple (*Arrowhead Mills* Maple Corns), 1 cup	3.0	.5
fiber flakes (*Health Valley*), ¾ cup	0	0
(*Heartland*), ¼ cup	4.0	n.a.
(*Golden Crisp*), ¾ cup	0	0
granola, see "mixed/multigrain," below		
honey clusters and flakes, all varieties (*Health Valley*), ¾ cup	0	0
kamut:		
flakes (*Arrowhead Mills*), 1 cup	1.0	0
flakes (*Erewhon*), ⅔ cup	0	0
puffed (*Arrowhead Mills*), 1 cup	0	0
(*New Morning Kamutios*), 1 cup	1.0	0
millet, puffed (*Arrowhead Mills*), 1 cup	.5	0
mixed/multigrain:		
all varieties (*Fruit & Fibre*), 1 cup	3.0	.5
(*Apple Jacks/Apple Raisin Crisp*), 1 cup	0	0
(*Barbara's High-5*), ¾ cup	.5	0
(*Cookie Crisp*), 1 oz., 1 cup	1.5	0
(*Double Chex*), 1¼ cups	0	0

	total fat (grams)	saturated fat (grams)

Cereal, ready-to-eat, mixed/multigrain *(cont.)*

(*Erewhon Apple Stroodles*), ¾ cup	.5	0
(*Erewhon Aztec/Super O's*), 1 cup	0	0
(*Erewhon Banana O's*), ¾ cup	0	0
(*Erewhon Galaxy Grahams*), ¾ cup	.5	0
(*Graham Chex*), 1 cup	1.5	0
(*Grape-Nuts*), ½ cup	1.0	0
(*Grape-Nuts*), ¾ cup	1.0	0
(*Kellogg's Crispix*), 1 cup	0	0
(*Kellogg's Double Dip Crunch*), ¾ cup	0	0
(*Kellogg's Just Right* Crunchy Nuggets), 1 cup	1.5	0
(*Kellogg's Froot Loops*), 1 cup	1.0	.5
(*Kellogg's Mueslix*), ⅔ cup	3.0	0
(*Kellogg's Mueslix Golden Crunch*), ¾ cup ...	5.0	1.0
(*Kellogg's Product 19*), 1 cup	0	0
(*Malt-O-Meal* Fruit & Frosted O's), 1 cup	1.0	0
(*Multi-Bran Chex*), 2 oz., 1¼ cups	2.0	0
(*Quaker Life*), ¾ cup	1.5	0
(*Ralston Crisp Crunch*), ¾ cup	1.0	0
(*Ralston Nutty Nuggets*), ½ cup	1.5	0
(*Team* Flakes), 1¼ cups	0	0
(*Uncle Sam*), 1 cup	5.0	.5
almond (*Almond Delight*), 1 cup	3.0	0
almond raisin (*Kellogg's Nutri-Grain*), 1¼ cup	3.0	0
almond raisin (*New Morning Crunchy*), 1 cup	2.0	0
blueberry (*Ralston Cranberry Muesli*), 1 cup ..	2.5	1.5
cinnamon (*Kellogg's* Mini Buns), ¾ cup	.5	0
cinnamon (*Quaker Life*), 1 cup	2.0	0
cranberry (*Ralston Cranberry Muesli*), ¾ cup	3.0	0
flakes (*Arrowhead Mills* Multi Grain), 1 cup ...	1.5	0
flakes (*Kellogg's Healthy Choice*), 1 cup	0	0

	total fat (grams)	saturated fat (grams)
frosted, all varieties (*Kellogg's Pop-Tarts Crunch*), ¾ cup	1.0	0
fruit (*Ralston Fruit Rings*), ¾ cup	1.0	0
fruit and nut (*Kellogg's Just Right*), 1 cup	1.5	0
granola:		
all varieties (*Health Valley* Fat Free), ¾ cup	0	0
(*Heartland* Original), ½ cup	11.0	1.5
w/almonds (*Sun Country*), ½ cup	9.0	1.5
hearty (*C.W. Post*), ⅔	9.0	1.0
low fat (*Heartland*), ½ cup	3.0	1.0
low fat (*Kellogg's*), ½ cup	3.0	.5
raisin (*Heartland*), ½ cup	10.0	1.5
raisin and date (*Sun Country*), ½ cup	8.0	1.0
w/raisins, low fat (*Kellogg's*), ½ cup	3.0	1.0
peach (*Ralston Peach Muesli*), ¾ cup	3.0	0
peach, honey roasted (*Kellogg's Temptations*), 1 cup	2.5	0
pecan, crunchy (*Great Grains*), ⅔ cup	6.0	1.0
puffed (*Arrowhead Mills* Crispy Puffs), 1 cup	1.0	0
puffed, w/honey (*Arrowhead Mills*), 1 cup	0	0
raisin (*Erewhon Raisin Grahams*), 1 cup	1.0	0
w/raisins (*Quaker* Lowfat 100% Natural), ½ cup	3.0	1.0
raisins, dates, pecans (*Great Grains*), ⅔ cup	5.0	.5
raisins, oat, almonds (*Kellogg's Healthy Choice*), 1 cup	2.0	0
raspberry (*Ralston Raspberry*) Muesli), ¾ cup	3.0	0
strawberry (*Ralston Strawberry Muesli*), 1 cup	3.0	1.5
squares (*Kellogg's Healthy Choice*), 1¼ cup	1.0	0
vanilla almond (*Kellogg's Temptations*), ¾ cup	2.0	1.0

	total fat (grams)	saturated fat (grams)

Cereal, ready-to-eat *(cont.)*

oat bran:

(*Health Valley Oat Bran O's*), ¾ cup	0	0
(*Kellogg's Common Sense*), ¾ cup	1.0	0
(*Kellogg's Cracklin' Oat Bran*), ¾ cup	8.0	3.0
(*New Morning Ultimate*), 1 cup	2.0	n.a.
almond crunch (*Health Valley*), ½ cup	4.0	0
flakes (*Arrowhead Mills*), 1 cup	2.0	1.0
flakes or w/raisins (*Health Valley*), ¾ cup	0	0

oats:

(*Alpha-Bits*), 1 cup	1.0	0
(*Arrowhead Mills Nature O's*), 1 cup	2.0	.5
(*Barbara's Breakfast O's*), 1 cup	2.0	0
(*Kellogg's Nut & Honey Crunch O's*), ¾ cup	2.5	0
(*Malt-O-Meal*), 1 cup	2.0	0
(*New Morning Oatios*), 1 cup	1.0	0
(*Popeye Oat'mmms*), 1 cup	2.0	.5
(*Popeye Oat'mmms* Toasted), 1 cup	1.5	0
(*Quaker* Oat Squares), 1 cup	3.0	.5
(*Quaker* Toasted Oatmeal), 1 pouch	.5	0
(*Ralston Magic Stars*), ¾ cup	1.0	0
(*Ralston Tasteeos*), 1¼ cups	2.5	0
w/almonds (*Honey Bunches of Oats*), ¾ cup	3.0	.5
apple cinnamon (*Malt-O-Meal*), ¾ cup	2.0	0
apple cinnamon (*Ralston Tasteeos*), 1 cup	1.5	0
apple cinnamon (*New Morning Oatios*), 1 cup	1.5	0
cinnamon (*Quaker* Oat Squares), 1 cup	2.5	.5
honey (*Quaker* 100% Natural), ½ cup	8.0	3.5
honey, roasted (*Honey Bunches of Oats*), ¾ cup	1.5	.5
honey-almond (*New Morning Oatios*), 1 cup	1.0	0
honey-graham (*Quaker Oh!s*), ¾ cup	2.0	.5
honey and nut (*Malt-O-Meal*), ¾ cup	1.0	0

	total fat (grams)	saturated fat (grams)
honey nut (*Quaker* Toasted Oatmeal), 1 pouch	2.5	.5
honey nut (*Ralston Tasteeos*), 1 cup	1.5	0
honey and raisins (*Quaker* 100% Natural), ½ cup	8.0	3.5
w/marshmallows (*Alpha-Bits*), 1 cup	1.0	0
w/marshmallows (*Malt-O-Meal Mateys*), 1 cup	1.0	0
rice:		
(*Apple Cinnamon Rice Krispies*), ¾ cup	0	0
(*Erewhon Poppets*), 1 cup	1.0	0
(*Kellogg's Cocoa Krispies*), ¾ cup	.5	0
(*Kellogg's Frosted Krispies*), ¾ cup	0	0
(*Kellogg's Rice Krispies*), 1¼ cup	0	0
(*Kellogg's Rice Krispies Treats*), ¾ cup	1.5	0
(*New Morning* Crispy Rice), 1 cup	1.0	n.a.
(*Ralston Crisp Rice*), 1¼ cups	0	0
(*Rice Chex*), 1 cup	0	0
brown (*New Morning* Brown Rice), 1 cup	1.0	n.a.
brown, crisp (*Health Valley*), 1 cup	0	0
brown, crispy (*Erewhon/Erewhon* No Salt), 1 cup	0	0
crisps (*Barbara's*), 1 cup	1.0	0
crispy or puffed (*Malt-O-Meal*), 1 cup	0	0
cocoa (*Ralston* Crispy Rice), 1 cup	1.0	0
w/marshmallow (*Kellogg's Fruity Marshmallow Krispies*), ¾ cup	0	0
puffed (*Arrowhead Mills*), 1 cup	0	0
puffed (*Quaker* Puffed Rice), 1 box	0	0
toasted (*Kellogg's Special K*), 1 cup	0	0
spelt flakes (*Arrowhead Mills*), 1 cup	1.0	0
wheat (see also "bran," above):		
(*Kellogg's Nutri-Grain* Golden Wheat), ¾ cup	.5	0
(*Nabisco Frosted Wheat Bites*), 1 cup	1.0	0

	total fat (grams)	saturated fat (grams)

Cereal, ready-to-eat, wheat *(cont.)*

(*Wheat Chex*), ¾ cup	1.0	0
all fruit varieties (*Fruit Wheats*), ¾ cup	.5	0
biscuits, frosted (*Kellogg's Frosted Mini-Wheats*), 1 cup	1.0	0
biscuits, fruit-filled, all varieties (*Kellogg's Squares*), ¾ cup	1.0	0
flakes (*Erewhon*), 1 cup	.5	0
flakes, multivitamin (*Ralston* Whole Grain), 1 cup	1.0	0
puffed (*Arrowhead Mills*), 1 cup	.5	0
puffed (*Kellogg's Smacks*), ¾ cup	.5	0
puffed (*Quaker*), 1 box	0	0
puffed, regular or frosted (*Malt-O-Meal*), 1 cup	0	0
shredded (*Barbara's*), 2 biscuits	1.0	0
shredded (*Barbara's* Spoonfuls), ¾ cup	1.5	0
shredded (*Nabisco*), 2 biscuits	.5	0
shredded (*Nabisco Shredded Wheat 'N Bran*), 1¼ cups	1.0	0
shredded (*Quaker*), 3 biscuits	1.5	.5
w/fruit (*Erewhon Fruit'n Wheat*), ¾ cup	1.5	0
w/raisins (*Kellogg's Nutri-Grain*), ¾ cup	1.0	0

Cereal, freeze-dried*, granola:

w/blueberries, milk (*Mountain House*), ⅓ cup	4.0	2.0
blueberry or strawberry honey, milk (*AlpineAire*), 1 cup	11.0	n.a.

Cereal, hot or cooking (see also specific grains), uncooked, except as noted:

barley (*Erewhon* Barley Plus), ¼ cup	1.0	0
barley flakes, rolled (*Arrowhead Mills*), ⅓ cup	1.0	0
bulgur (*Arrowhead Mills*), ¼ cup	.5	0
corn grits, see "Corn grits"		
kamut flakes, rolled (*Arrowhead Mills*), ⅓ cup	1.0	0

	total fat (grams)	saturated fat (grams)
mixed grain:		
(*Mother's* Multigrain), ½ cup	1.5	0
(*Pritikin*), 1 pkt.	1.5	0
4 grain plus flax (*Arrowhead Mills*), ¼ cup	2.0	0
7 grain (*Arrowhead Mills*), ⅓ cup	1.5	0
7 grain, wheat free (*Arrowhead Mills*), ¼ cup	1.5	0
multi-bran, apple cinnamon (*Roman Meal*), ⅓ cup	2.2	.3
oats, wheat, rye, bran, flax (*Roman Meal*), ⅓ cup	1.5	.2
wheat, rye, bran, flax (*Roman Meal*), ⅓ cup	.5	0
oat bran:		
(*Arrowhead Mills*), ⅓ cup	2.5	0
(*Quaker*), ½ cup	3.0	1.0
w/toasted wheat germ (*Erewhon*), ⅓ cup	2.5	.5
oatmeal:		
(*Maypo*), ½ cup mix	2.0	0
(*Mother's*), ½ cup	3.0	1.0
(*Quaker* Old Fashioned), ½ cup	3.0	.5
(*Quaker* Instant Low Sodium), 1 pkt.	2.5	.5
(*Quaker* Quick), ½ cup	3.0	.5
apple cinnamon (*Erewhon* Instant), 1 pkt.	2.0	.5
apple raisin spice (*Pritikin*), 1 pkt.	2.5	.5
apple raisin walnut (*Quaker* Instant), 1 pkt.	2.5	.5
w/apples & cinnamon (*Quaker* Instant), 1 pkt.	1.5	.5
blueberry fruit & cream (*Quaker* Instant), 1 pkt.	2.5	.5
bran (*Mother's*), ½ cup	3.0	.5
w/added bran (*Erewhon* Instant), 1 pkt.	2.5	.5
cinnamon graham cookie (*Quaker* Instant), 1 pkt.	2.5	.5
cinnamon spice (*Quaker* Instant), 1 pkt.	2.0	0
cinnamon toast (*Quaker* Instant), 1 pkt.	2.0	0
honey nut (*Quaker* Instant), 1 pkt.	3.0	.5
maple/brown sugar (*Quaker* Instant), 1 pkt.	2.0	.5

	total fat (grams)	saturated fat (grams)

Cereal, hot or cooking, oatmeal *(cont.)*

maple spice (*Erewhon* Instant), 1 pkt.	2.0	.5
peaches and cream (*Quaker* Instant), 1 pkt.	2.0	.5
raspberry (*Quaker* Instant), 1 pkt.	3.0	.5
raisin, date, and walnut (*Quaker* Instant), 1 pkt.	2.5	.5
raisins, dates, and walnuts (*Erewhon* Instant), 1 pkt.	2.5	.5
raisin spice (*Quaker* Instant), 1 pkt.	2.0	.5
strawberries & cream (*Quaker* Instant), 1 pkt.	2.0	.5
strawberries 'n stuff (*Quaker* Instant), 1 pkt.	2.0	.5
oats, rolled, flakes (*Arrowhead Mills*), ⅓ cup	2.5	0
oats, steel cut (*Arrowhead Mills*), ¼ cup	3.0	.5
oats and wheat, ⅓ cup:		
w/coconut, almonds, honey (*Roman Meal*)	6.0	3.0
w/dates, raisins, almonds (*Roman Meal*)	1.7	.3
potato flakes (*Arrowhead Mills*), ⅓ cup	0	0
rice:		
(*Arrowhead Mills Rice & Shine*), ¼ cup	1.0	0
ambergrain (*Lundberg Family Farms*), ⅓ cup	1.5	0
cream (*Erewhon*), ¼ cup	1.0	.1
creamy, cinnamon raisin (*Lundberg Family Farms*), ⅓ cup	1.5	0
creamy, honey almond (*Lundberg Family Farms*), ⅓ cup	3.5	0
rye, cream of (*Roman Meal*), ⅓ cup	1.0	0
soybean grits (*Arrowhead Mills*), ¼ cup	6.0	1.0
wheat:		
(*Arrowhead Mills Bear Mush*), ¼ cup	1.0	0
(*Malt-O-Meal*), 3 tbsp.	0	0
(*Maltex*), ⅓ cup	.5	0
chocolate (*Malt-O-Meal*), ⅓ cup	.5	0
cracked (*Arrowhead Mills*), ¼ cup	.5	0
farina (*Pillsbury*), ⅔ cup cooked	0	0

	total fat (grams)	saturated fat (grams)
flakes, rolled (*Arrowhead Mills*), 1/3 cup	.5	0
maple brown sugar (*Malt-O-Meal*), 1/3 cup	0	0
toasted (*Wheatena*), 1/3 cup mix	1.0	0
whole (*Mother's* Natural), 1/2 cup	1.0	0
Cereal bars, see "Granola and cereal bars"		
Cereal crumbs (*Kellogg's* Corn Flakes), 2 tbsp.	0	0
Cervelat, see "Summer sausage" and "Thuringer cervelat"		
Charcoal seasoning (*Durkee* Spices), 1/4 tsp.	0	0
Chapati, see "Bread"		
Cheddarwurst:		
(*Hillshire Farm* Bun Size), 4 oz.	18.0	n.a.
links (*Hillshire Farm*), 4 oz.	17.0	n.a.
lite (*Hillshire Farm*), 2.7 oz. link	15.0	n.a.
Cheese (see also "Cheese, fat-free or nondairy," "Cheese food," and "Cheese product"), 1 oz., except as noted:		
American, processed:		
(*Boar's Head* Loaf)	9.0	6.0
(*Hoffman's* Colored or White)	9.0	6.0
(*Hoffman's* Colored Slices), .6-oz. slice	5.0	3.5
reduced fat (*Alpine Lace*)	6.0	4.0
reduced fat (*Alpine Lace* Slices), .7-oz. slice	3.0	2.0
w/bacon (*Hoffman's* Chees'N Bacon)	7.0	5.0
(*Bel Paese* Regular or Flavored)	10.0	4.0
(*Bel Paese* Medallions), .75 oz.	5.5	3.5
blue:		
(*Hoffman's* Danish)	8.0	6.0
(*Kraft* Cold Pack)	8.0	6.0
1 oz.	8.2	5.3
crumbled, 1/2 cup not packed	19.4	12.6
crumbled (*Kraft*)	8.0	6.0
brick:		
1 oz.	8.4	5.3
1" cube	5.1	3.2
(*Kraft*)	9.0	6.0

	total fat (grams)	saturated fat (grams)

Cheese *(cont.)*

Brie	7.9	n.a
butterkase, regular or smoked (*Boar's Head*)	9.0	6.0
Camembert	6.9	4.3
Camembert, 1" cube	4.1	2.6
caraway	8.3	n.a.

cheddar:

(*Dorman* Bar New York Colored/White)	9.0	5.0
(*Dorman* Bar Reduced Fat	5.0	3.0
(*Heluva* Good Very Low Sodium)	9.0	6.0
(*Hoffman's* New York/Vermont)	9.0	6.0
mild, sharp, or extra sharp (*Heluva* Good Sticks)	9.0	5.0
mild, medium and sharp (*Kraft*)	9.0	6.0
mild and sharp (*Kraft* ⅓ Less Fat)	5.0	3.5
mild and sharp (*Weight Watchers* Reduced Sodium), 1 oz.	5.0	3.0
nacho blend w/peppers (*Kraft*)	9.0	6.0
reduced fat (*Alpine Lace*)	4.5	3.0
reduced fat, mild (*Heluva* Good)	6.0	3.5
sharp, reduced fat (*Cracker Barrel*)	5.0	3.0
sharp, slicing (*Boar's Head*)	9.0	5.0
sharp, super (*Hoffman's*), 1.1-oz. slice	10.0	7.0
sharp, super, white (*Hoffman's*)	9.0	6.0
shredded (*Heluva* Good), 1 oz. or ¼ cup	9.0	5.0
shredded (*Kraft*), 1 oz. or ¼ cup	8.0	5.0
shredded, finely (*Kraft*), 1 oz. or ¼ cup	10.0	6.0
shredded, mild (*Kraft* ⅓ Less Fat), 1 oz. or ¼ cup	6.0	4.0
shredded w/Monterey Jack (*Kraft* Taco Cheese), 1 oz. or ¼ cup	8.0	6.0
shredded, sharp, reduced fat (*Cracker Barrel*)	5.0	3.0
smokey sharp (*Hoffman's*)	9.0	6.0

	total fat (grams)	saturated fat (grams)
cheddar, double Glouster (*Boar's Head*)	10.0	6.0
cheddar curds (*Heluva* Good)	9.0	5.0
Cheshire	8.7	n.a.
colby:		
(*Dorman* Sandwich Slice), 1.1-oz. slice	10.0	6.0
(*Heluva* Good)	9.0	6.0
(*Hoffman's* Mild/Medium)	9.0	6.0
(*Kraft*)	9.0	6.0
(*Kraft* ⅓ Less Fat)	5.0	3.5
colby and Monterey jack (*Kraft*)	9.0	6.0
colby and Monterey jack, shredded (*Kraft*),		
1 oz. or ¼ cup	10.0	6.0
reduced fat (*Alpine Lace*)	5.0	3.0
colby jack (*Heluva* Good)	9.0	6.0
colby jack (*Hoffman's*)	9.0	6.0
cottage, creamed, ½ cup:		
4% large or small curd (*Breakstone's*)	5.0	3.5
4% large or small curd (*Crowley/Axelrod*)	6.0	3.5
4% (*Friendship* California Style)	5.0	3.0
4% large or small curd (*Knudsen*)	5.0	3.5
4% large or small curd (*Sealtest*)	5.0	3.5
2% (*Friendship* Pot Style)	2.5	1.5
2% (*Weight Watchers*)	2.0	1.5
2% large or small curd (*Breakstone's*)	2.5	1.5
2% small curd (*Knudsen*)	2.5	1.5
2% small curd (*Sealtest*)	2.5	1.5
1% (*Friendship* Lowfat)	1.0	.5
1% (*Light n' Lively*)	1.5	1.0
1% (*Weight Watchers*)	1.0	.5
1% small curd (*Crowley/Axelrod*)	1.5	1.0
w/garden salad, 1% (*Light n' Lively*)	1.5	1.0
w/peach, 1.5% (*Knudsen*)	1.5	1.0
w/peach and pineapple, 1% (*Light 'n Lively*)	1.0	1.0
w/pineapple, 1% (*Crowley/Axelrod* Lowfat)	1.5	1.0
w/pineapple, 1% (*Friendship* Lowfat)	1.0	.5

	total fat (grams)	saturated fat (grams)
Cheese, cottage, creamed *(cont.)*		
w/pineapple, 4% *(Crowley/Axelrod)*	4.5	2.5
w/pineapple, 4% *(Friendship)*	4.0	2.5
w/pineapple, 1.5% *(Knudsen)*	1.5	1.0
w/strawberry, 1.5% *(Knudsen)*	1.5	1.0
w/tropical fruit, 1.5% *(Knudsen)*	2.0	1.5
cottage, dry curd, 4 oz.	.5	.3
cottage, dry curd *(Breakstone's)*, ¼ cup	0	0
cottage, dry curd *(Crowley/Axelrod)*, ½ cup	.5	0
cottage or cream, nonfat or nondairy, see "Cheese, fat free or nondairy"		
cream:		
3-oz. pkg.	29.6	18.7
1" cube	5.6	3.5
(Boar's Head)	10.0	7.0
(Crowley/Axelrod), 2 tbsp. or 1.1 oz.	10.0	6.0
(Friendship Light), 2 tbsp.	5.0	3.0
(Friendship Reduced Fat), 2 tbsp.	2.5	1.5
(Philadelphia Brand)	10.0	6.0
(Philadelphia Brand Free)	0	0
(Philadelphia Brand Neufchâtel)	6.0	4.0
(Weight Watchers Light), 2 tbsp.	2.5	1.5
w/chives *(Philadelphia Brand)*	9.0	6.0
w/pimientos *(Philadelphia Brand)*	9.0	6.0
cream, soft, 2 tbsp.:		
(Friendship)	10.0	6.0
(Philadelphia Brand)	10.0	7.0
(Philadelphia Brand Free)	0	0
(Philadelphia Brand Light)	5.0	3.5
spreadable *(Heluva Good)*	10.0	6.0
w/chives and onion *(Philadelphia Brand)*	10.0	7.0
w/herb and garlic *(Philadelphia Brand)*	10.0	7.0
w/olive and pimiento *(Philadelphia Brand)*	9.0	6.0
w/pineapple *(Philadelphia Brand)*	9.0	6.0
w/smoked salmon *(Philadelphia Brand)*	9.0	6.0

	total fat (grams)	saturated fat (grams)
w/strawberries (*Philadelphia Brand*)	9.0	6.0
cream, whipped, 3 tbsp.:		
(*Breakstone's Temp-Tee*)	10.0	7.0
(*Philadelphia Brand*)	11.0	7.0
w/smoked salmon (*Philadelphia Brand*)	9.0	6.0
curd, washed, medium, sharp, or extra sharp		
(*Heluva* Good)	9.0	5.0
Edam:		
1 oz.	7.9	5.0
(*Boar's Head*)	7.0	5.0
(*Dorman Slice*), 1-oz. slice	7.0	4.5
(*Hoffman's*)	8.0	6.0
hickory smoked (*may-bud*)	8.0	5.0
farmer:		
(*Friendship*)	2.5	1.5
(*Hoffman's*)	8.0	6.0
(*Kraft*)	8.0	6.0
feta:		
(*Athenos* Traditional/Mild)	6.0	4.0
(*Churny*)	6.0	4.0
(*Feta Classika* Portions)	7.0	5.0
(*Krinos*)	8.0	5.0
w/basil and tomato (*Athenos*)	6.0	4.0
w/garlic and herb (*Athenos*)	7.0	4.5
peppercorn (*Athenos*)	6.0	4.0
fontina	8.8	5.4
fontina (*Classica*)	8.5	5.0
gjetost, goat's milk	8.4	5.4
goat:		
hard type	10.1	7.0
semi-soft type	8.5	5.9
soft type	6.0	4.1
gorgonzola (*Galbani*)	8.0	4.0
Gouda:		
1 oz.	7.8	5.0

	total fat (grams)	saturated fat (grams)
Cheese, Gouda *(cont.)*		
(*Boar's Head*)	9.0	5.0
(*Churny* Domestic)	8.0	6.0
(*Dorman* Slice), 1-oz. slice	8.0	5.0
(*Hoffman's*)	8.0	6.0
(*Kraft*)	9.0	6.0
(*may-bud*)	8.0	6.0
w/caraway seeds (*may-bud*)	8.0	5.0
Gruyère	9.2	5.4
havarti:		
(*Boar's Head*)	10.0	7.0
(*Dorman* Slice), 1-oz. slice	8.0	5.0
(*Hoffman's*)	11.0	7.0
(*Kraft*)	11.0	7.0
hot pepper (*Hoffman's*)	7.0	5.0
hot pepper, reduced fat (Alpine Lace)	6.0	4.0
hoop cheese (*Friendship*)	0	0
Italian, grated (*Kraft* ⅓ Less Fat), 2 tsp.	1.0	.5
Italian blend, grated (*Kraft*), 2 tsp.	1.5	1.0
Italico, semi soft (*Classica*)	10.0	3.0
(*Laughing Cow* Bonbel)	8.0	5.0
(*Laughing Cow* Wedge)	6.0	4.0
(*Laughing Cow* Mini Babybel), .75-oz. piece	6.0	4.0
Limburger	7.7	4.8
Limburger (*Kraft*)	8.0	5.0
marscapone, domestic (*Classica*)	12.0	8.0
marscapone, imported (*Galbani*)	14.0	9.0
Monterey jack:		
(*Dorman* Bar)	8.0	5.0
(*Dorman* Bar Reduced Fat)	4.5	3.0
(*Dorman* Slice), 1.2-oz. slice	10.0	6.0
(*Dorman* Slice), 1-oz. slice	8.0	5.0
(*Dorman* Slice Reduced Fat), 1.5-oz. slice	7.0	4.5
(*Heluva* Good)	8.0	6.0
(*Hoffman's*)	9.0	6.0

	total fat (grams)	saturated fat (grams)
(*Kraft*)	9.0	6.0
(*Kraft* ⅓ Less Fat)	5.0	3.5
(*Weight Watchers*)	5.0	3.0
reduced fat (*Alpine Lace*)	4.5	3.0
reduced fat (*Alpine Lace* Slices), 1-oz. slice	5.0	3.0
shredded (*Heluva* Good), 1 oz. or ¼ cup	8.0	5.0
shredded (*Kraft*), 1 oz. or ¼ cup	9.0	6.0
w/jalapeño (*Heluva* Good)	8.0	6.0
w/jalapeños (*Hoffman's* Pepper Jack)	8.0	6.0
w/jalapeños (*Kraft*)	9.0	6.0
w/jalapeños (*Kraft* ⅓ Less Fat)	5.0	3.5
w/vegetables (*Hoffman's* Garden Jack)	8.0	6.0
Monterey jack and cheddar (*Hoffman's* Super Jack)	9.0	6.0
Monterey jack and cheddar, shredded (*Dorman* Reduced Fat), 1 oz., about ⅓ cup	5.0	3.0
mozzarella:		
whole milk	6.1	3.7
whole milk (*DiGiorno*)	6.0	4.0
whole milk (*Heluva* Good Chunk)	6.0	4.0
whole milk (*Polly-O*)	6.0	3.0
whole milk, low moisture	7.0	4.4
whole milk, low moisture (*Boar's Head*)	7.0	4.0
whole milk, low moisture, shredded (*Kraft*), 1 oz. or ¼ cup	7.0	5.0
part skim	4.5	2.9
part skim (*Heluva* Good), 1 oz. or ¼ cup shredded	5.0	3.0
part skim (*Polly-O*)	5.0	3.0
part skim, low moisture	4.9	3.1
part skim, low moisture (*Dorman* Slice), 1-oz. slice	5.0	3.0
part skim, low moisture (*Kraft*)	5.0	4.0
part skim, low moisture, shredded (*Kraft*), 1 oz. or ¼ cup	6.0	4.0

	total fat (grams)	saturated fat (grams)

Cheese, mozzarella *(cont.)*

part skim, low moisture, shredded (*Kraft* ⅓
  Less Fat), 1 oz. or ¼ cup .... 5.0 .... 3.0
part skim, low moisture, finely shredded (*Kraft*),
  1 oz. or ¼ cup .... 4.5 .... 3.0
part skim, reduced sodium (*Alpine Lace*) ..... 5.0 .... 3.0
light (*Polly-O* Lite) .... 3.0 .... 2.0
string, part skim, low moisture (*Kraft*),
  1 stick .... 6.0 .... 3.5
Muenster:
  1 oz. .... 8.5 .... 5.4
  (*Boar's Head/Boar's Head* Low Sodium) ...... 8.0 .... 5.0
  (*Dorman* Sandwich Slice), 1-oz. slice .... 8.0 .... 5.0
  (*Dorman* Slice), 1.5-oz. slice .... 13.0 .... 8.0
  (*Dorman* Slice Reduced Fat), 1.5-oz. slice .... 8.0 .... 4.5
  (*Heluva* Good) .... 8.0 .... 6.0
  (*Hoffman's*) .... 9.0 .... 6.0
  (*Kraft*) .... 9.0 .... 6.0
  reduced sodium (*Alpine Lace*) .... 9.0 .... 5.0
Neufchâtel .... 6.6 .... 4.2
Neufchâtel, 3-oz. pkg. .... 19.9 .... 12.6
w/onion (*Hoffman's* Chees'N Onion) .... 7.0 .... 5.0
Parmesan:
  hard .... 7.3 .... 4.7
  grated, 1 tbsp. .... 1.5 .... 1.0
  grated (*Kraft* 100%), 2 tsp. .... 1.5 .... 1.0
  grated (*Progresso*), 1 tbsp. .... 2.0 .... 1.0
  grated or shredded (*Classica*), 1 tbsp. .... 1.0 .... 1.0
  shredded (*DiGiorno*), 2 tsp. .... 1.5 .... 1.0
  shredded (*Kraft* 100%), 2 tsp. .... 1.5 .... 1.0
pimiento, processed .... 8.9 .... 5.6
pimiento, processed, 1" cube .... 5.5 .... 3.4
pizza cheese, shredded:
  cheddar, mild, and low moisture whole milk
    mozzarella (*Kraft*), 1 oz. or ¼ cup ..... 7.0 .... 5.0

	total fat (grams)	saturated fat (grams)
four cheese (*Kraft*), 1 oz. or ¼ cup	7.0	4.5
mozzarella, low moisture and cheddar (*Kraft*), 1 oz. or ¼ cup	8.0	5.0
mozzarella, low moisture and provolone with smoke flavor (*Kraft*), 1 oz. or ¼ cup	7.0	4.5
Port du Salut	8.0	4.7
provolone:		
1 oz.	7.6	4.8
(*Boar's Head*)	8.0	4.5
(*Dorman* Slices), 1-oz. slice	8.0	4.5
(*Dorman* Slices Reduced Fat), 1.5-oz. slice	7.0	4.0
mild (*DiGiorno*)	7.0	5.0
smoke flavor (*Kraft*)	7.0	5.0
smoked, reduced fat (*Alpine Lace*)	5.0	3.0
ricotta:		
(*Breakstone's*), 1 oz. or ¼ cup	8.0	5.0
whole milk	3.7	2.4
whole milk, ½ cup	16.1	10.3
whole milk (*Polly-O*)	4.0	0
part skim	2.2	1.4
part skim, ½ cup	9.8	6.1
part skim (*Polly-O*)	3.0	0
light (*Polly-O* Lite)	2.0	0
Romano:		
hard	7.6	n.a.
grated (*DiGiorno*), 1 tbsp.	1.5	1.0
grated (*Kraft* 100%), 2 tsp.	1.5	1.0
grated (*Progresso*), 1 tbsp.	2.0	1.0
grated, dry or fresh (*Classica* Pecorino), 1 tbsp.	1.5	.5
shredded (*Classica* Pecorino), 1 tbsp.	2.0	1.5
Roquefort, sheep's milk	8.7	5.5
w/salami (*Hoffman's* Chees'N Salami)	7.0	5.0
sharp, super, processed (*Hoffman*)	9.0	6.0

	total fat (grams)	saturated fat (grams)

Cheese *(cont.)*
Swiss:

(*Boar's Head* Domestic)	8.0	4.5
(*Boar's Head* Imported Gold Label Premium)	8.0	5.0
(*Boar's Head* No Salt)	8.0	5.0
(*Dorman* Bar Very Low Sodium)	8.0	5.0
(*Dorman* Sandwich Slice), 1-oz. slice	8.0	4.5
(*Dorman* Slice), 1.2-oz. slice	9.0	6.0
(*Dorman* Slice Low Sodium), 1.2-oz. slice	10.0	6.0
(*Dorman* Slice Reduced Fat), 1.2-oz. slice	5.0	3.5
(*Heluva* Good)	8.0	5.0
(*Kraft*)	9.0	6.0
baby (*Boar's Head*)	9.0	6.0
baby (*Kraft*)	9.0	6.0
natural	7.8	5.0
natural, 1" cube	4.1	2.7
processed	7.1	4.6
processed, 1" cube	4.5	2.9
reduced fat (*Alpine Lace*)	6.0	4.0
shredded (*Kraft*), 1 oz. or ¼ cup	9.0	6.0
smoked, and cheddar (*Hoffman's*)	8.0	6.0
w/caraway seeds (*Hoffman's* Swisson Rye)	7.0	5.0
Taleggio (*Tal-Fino*)	9.0	4.0
Tilsit, whole milk	7.4	4.8

Cheese, fat-free or nondairy:

(*Smart Beat* Low Sodium Nondairy), ⅔-oz. slice	2.0	<1.0
(*Smart Beat* Fat Free Nondairy), ⅔-oz. slice	0	0
all varieties:		
(*Alpine Lace*), 1 oz.	0	0
(*Kraft Healthy Favorites*), ¼ cup	0	0
(*Weight Watchers* Fat Free), .75 oz.	0	0
nondairy (*AlmondRella*), 1 oz.	3.0	.5
nondairy (*TofuRella*), 1 oz.	5.0	1.0
nondairy (*VeganRella*), 1 oz.	3.0	0
nondairy (*Zero-FatRella*), 1 oz.	0	0

	total fat (grams)	saturated fat (grams)
cheddar, imitation, shredded (*Georgio's*), 1 oz., ¼ cup	7.0	1.0
cottage, nonfat, plain or fruit:		
(*Crowley/Axelrod* Nonfat)	0	0
(*Friendship* Nonfat)	0	0
(*Knudsen Free*)	0	0
(*Light n' Lively Free*)	0	0
"cream cheese" (*Better than Cream Cheese*), 1 oz.	8.0	2.0
"cream cheese," garlic and herb (*Soyakaas* Tofu), 2 tbsp.	9.0	1.5
Jamaican jack, nondairy (*HempRella*), 1 oz.	3.0	0
mozzarella, imitation, shredded (*Georgio's*), 1 oz., ¼ cup	7.0	1.0
mozzarella or ricotta (*Polly-O* Free), 1 oz.	0	0
Cheese and bacon dip (*Nalley*), 2 tbsp.	11.0	2.5
Cheese bread, see "Bread, frozen or refrigerated"		
Cheese dip, 2 tbsp.:		
and bacon, see "Cheese and bacon dip"		
blue cheese (*Kraft* Premium)	4.0	2.5
cheddar, mild (*Frito-Lay*)	3.0	1.0
cheddar w/jalapeño:		
(*Breakstone's*)	4.0	3.0
(*Doritos*)	3.0	1.0
(*Heluva* Good Light)	2.0	1.5
yogurt (*Crowley's*)	2.5	1.5
cheddar and mustard pretzel (*Heluva* Good)	6.0	3.0
cheese w/jalapeño (*Kraft* Premium)	5.0	3.0
hot (*Price's* Fiesta)	7.0	3.0
nacho:		
(*Knudsen*)	4.0	3.0
(*Kraft* Premium)	5.0	3.0
(*Nalley*)	12.0	1.5
salsa:		
(*Chi-Chi's* Fiesta)	3.0	1.0

	total fat (grams)	saturated fat (grams)
Cheese dip, salsa *(cont.)*		
(*Doritos* Cheese N' Salsa)	2.0	.5
(*Eagle*)	3.0	1.0
(*Heluva* Good Cheese 'N Salsa)	5.5	5.0
(*Old El Paso* Cheese 'n Salsa)	3.0	1.0
(*Tostitos* Conqueso)	2.0	.5
Cheese dip mix, nacho (*Knorr*), ⅟₁₆ pkg.	0	0
Cheese food (see also "Cheese," "Cheese product," and "Cheese spread"), 1 oz., except as noted:		
(*Hoffman's Munst-ett*)	8.0	5.0
American, processed:		
cold pack	7.0	4.4
(*Golden Image*), ¾ oz.	5.0	1.5
(*Harvest Moon*), slice, ⅔ oz.	6.0	4.0
(*Heluva* Good Singles), .75-oz. slice	5.0	3.0
(*Kraft*)	9.0	6.0
(*Kraft* Singles), ⅔ oz.	4.5	3.0
(*Kraft* Singles ⅓ Less Fat), ¾ oz.	3.0	2.0
(*Kraft Free* Singles), ⅔ oz.	0	0
(*Light 'n Lively* 50% Less Fat), ¾ oz.	2.5	1.5
(*Lunchwagon*), ¾ oz.	5.0	1.0
(*Old English*)	9.0	6.0
(*Schwan's*), 1 slice, .7 oz.	6.0	4.0
shredded (*Harvest Moon*), ¼ cup	9.0	2.0
shredded (*Kraft*), ¼ cup	9.0	6.0
cheddar (*Kraft* Singles ⅓ Less Fat), ¾ oz.	3.0	2.0
cheddar, sharp/extra sharp (*Cracker Barrel*), 2 tbsp.	8.0	5.0
cheddar, sharp, plain or port wine (*Heluva* Good), 1 oz. or 2 tbsp.	7.0	3.0
cheddar, sharp, w/bacon, horseradish, or jalapeño (*Heluva* Good), 1 oz. or 2 tbsp.	7.0	3.0
cheddar, shredded (*Harvest Moon*), ¼ cup	9.0	2.0
garlic (*Hoffman's* Chees'N Garlic)	7.0	5.0
garlic (*Kraft*)	7.0	5.0

	total fat (grams)	saturated fat (grams)
grated (*Kraft*), 1 tbsp.	1.5	1.0
hot pepper (*Hoffman*)	7.0	5.0
jalapeño pepper (*Kraft*)	7.0	5.0
Mexican (*Hoffman's*)	8.0	6.0
Mexican w/jalapeños (*Kraft* Singles), ¾ oz.	5.0	3.5
Monterey (*Kraft* Singles), ¾ oz.	5.0	3.5
mozzarella, shredded (*Harvest Moon*), ¼ cup	8.0	1.5
pepper and pickle (*Hoffman's* Sweet Pepper'n Pickle)	8.0	5.0
pepperoni (*Hoffman's* Chees'n Pepperoni)	7.0	5.0
pimiento (*Hoffman's* Chees'n Pimento)	8.0	5.0
pimiento (*Kraft*), ¾ oz.	5.0	3.5
pizza, w/sausage and pepper (*Hoffman's* Instant Pizza)	7.0	5.0
port wine (*WisPride* Cup), 1.1 oz., 2 tbsp.	7.0	4.0
port wine (*WisPride* Cup Light), 1.1 oz., 2 tbsp.	3.0	2.0
sharp (*Kraft*), ¾ oz.	6.0	4.0
Swiss, processed	6.8	n.a.
Swiss, processed (*Kraft*), ¾ oz.	5.0	3.5
Swiss, processed (*Kraft* Singles ⅓ Less Fat), ¾ oz.	2.5	1.5
taco (*Hoffman's Tacos Cheez*)	7.0	5.0
(*Velveeta*), all flavors, ¼ cup	9.0	6.0
(*Velveeta Light*)	3.0	2.0
Cheese log, sharp cheddar, w/almonds (*WisPride*), 1.1 oz., 2 tbsp.	8.0	4.0
Cheese nuggets, mozzarella, frozen:		
(*Banquet*), 1.25 oz.	6.0	2.5
(*Schwan's*), 1.1 oz.	7.0	4.0
Cheese product (see also "Cheese food" and "Cheese spread"):		
(*Cheez Whiz Light*), 2 tbsp.	3.0	2.0
(*Kraft Free*), all varieties, ¾ oz.	0	0
(*Velveeta Light*), 1 oz.	3.0	2.0

	total fat (grams)	saturated fat (grams)

Cheese product *(cont.)*

American:

(*Harvest Moon*), ⅔ oz. 3.0 . . . . 2.0

(*Kraft* Deluxe 25% Less Fat), ¾ oz. . . . . 5.0 . . . . 3.0

(*Kraft* Singles ⅓ Less Fat), ¾ oz. . . . . 3.0 . . . . 2.0

(*Light n' Lively* 50% Less Fat), ¾ oz. . . . . 2.5 . . . . 1.5

cheddar:

(*Kraft* Singles ⅓ Less Fat), ¾ oz. . . . . 3.0 . . . . 2.0

(*Spreadery*), 2 tbsp. . . . . 4.5 . . . . 3.0

Neufchâtel:

w/garden vegetables (*Spreadery*), 2 tbsp. . . . . . 6.0 . . . . 4.0

ranch or garlic & herb (*Spreadery*), 2 tbsp. . . . 7.0 . . . . 5.0

pimiento (*Spreadery*), 2 tbsp. . . . . 8.0 . . . . 5.0

Swiss (*Kraft* Singles ⅓ Less Fat), ¾ oz. . . . . 2.5 . . . . 1.5

Cheese, freeze-dried, powdered cheddar

(*AlpineAire*), ½ cup sauce* . . . . 14.0 . . . . n.a.

Cheese nut casserole, freeze-dried*

(*AlpineAire*), 1⅓ cups . . . . 16.0 . . . . n.a.

Cheese omelette, see "Egg breakfast, freeze-dried"

Cheese salsa, see "Salsa dip"

Cheese sauce, refrigerated, four, w/white wine

(*Contadina*), ½ cup . . . . 28.0 . . . . 14.0

Cheese sauce mix:

½ cup* . . . . 8.6 . . . . 4.7

(*Durkee* Pouches), ¼ pkg. . . . . 1.5 . . . . 1.0

(*French's*), ¼ pkg. 5 0

four (*Knorr* Pasta Sauces), ⅙ pkg. 2.0 5

nacho (*Durkee* Pouches), ⅕ pkg. 2.0 0

Cheese sausage, see "Sausage"

Cheese snack, 1 piece, except as noted:

cheddar curds (*Heluva* Good), 1 oz. . . . . 9.0 . . . . 5.0

(*Handi-Snacks* Cheez'n Breadsticks) . . . . 7.0 . . . . 4.0

(*Handi-Snacks* Cheez'n Crackers) . . . . 8.0 . . . . 4.5

(*Handi-Snacks* Cheez'n Pretzels) . . . . 6.0 . . . . 4.0

mozzarella (*Handi-Snacks* String Cheese) . . . . . 6.0 . . . . 4.0

	total fat (grams)	saturated fat (grams)
Cheese spread (see also "Cheese," "Cheese food," and "Cheese, fat-free or nondairy"), 2 tbsp., except as noted:		
(*Cheez Whiz Light*)	3.0	2.0
(*Cheez Whiz Zap-A-Pack*)	8.0	5.0
(*Harvest Moon*), ¾ oz.	4.5	3.0
(*Old English*)	8.0	5.0
(*Squeeze-A-Snack*)	8.0	5.0
(*Velveeta*), all flavors, 1 oz.	6.0	4.0
all varieties (*Easy Cheese*)	7.0	4.0
all varieties, except jalapeño (*Cheez Whiz*)	7.0	5.0
American, processed, 1 oz.	6.0	3.8
w/bacon (*Kraft*)	8.0	5.0
cheddar (*Gracias*), ¼ cup	8.0	3.0
cheddar, all varieties (*Spreadery*)	4.5	3.0
cream cheese and smoked salmon (*Vita*), 2 oz., ¼ cup	17.0	11.0
garlic and herbs, soft (*Rondele*)	9.0	6.0
garlic and herbs, soft (*Rondele* Light)	4.0	2.5
jalapeño (*Cheez Whiz*)	8.0	5.0
jalapeño (*Kraft*), 1 oz.	6.0	4.0
(*Kraft Roka* Brand Blue)	7.0	4.5
limburger (*Mohawk Valley*)	7.0	4.5
nacho or nacho w/jalapeño (*Gracias*), ¼ cup	6.0	2.0
Neufchâtel:		
w/garden vegetables (*Spreadery*)	6.0	4.0
w/garlic & herb or ranch (*Spreadery*)	7.0	5.0
olive and pimiento (*Kraft*)	6.0	4.0
pimiento:		
(*Kraft*)	6.0	4.0
(*Price's*)	7.0	3.0
(*Price's* Light)	3.5	1.0
(*Spreadery*)	8.0	5.0
pineapple (*Kraft*)	5.0	3.5
w/salsa (*Cheez Whiz Zap-A-Pack*)	8.0	5.0
slices (*Velveeta*), ¾ oz.	4.5	3.0

	total fat (grams)	saturated fat (grams)
Cheese sprinkles (*Smart Seas*), ½ tsp.	0	0
Cheese sticks, breaded, frozen, 4 pieces, except as noted:		
cheddar (*Farm Rich*)	16.0	5.0
mozzarella (*Farm Rich*)	16.0	4.0
mozzarella (*Schwan's*), 1 oz., 2 pieces	6.0	3.0
provolone (*Farm Rich*)	14.0	7.0
Cheeseburger, see "Beef sandwich"		
Cheesecake, see "Cake, frozen"		
Cheesecake mix, see "Pie mix"		
Cherimoya:		
1 medium, 1.9 lb.	2.2	n.a.
trimmed, 1 oz.	.1	0
Cherry:		
fresh:		
sour, red, w/pits, 4 oz.	.3	.1
sour, red, pitted, ½ cup	.2	.1
sweet, w/pits, 4 oz.	1.0	.3
sweet, 10 medium or ½ cup pitted	.7	.2
canned, in syrup, ½ cup:		
dark, in heavy syrup (*Del Monte*)	0	0
dark, sweet (*Wilderness*)	0	0
dessert (*Wilderness*)	0	0
Royal Anne (*Wilderness*)	0	0
canned, in water (*Wilderness* Tart Red), ½ cup	0	0
dried (*Sonoma*), 1.4 oz., ¼ cup	0	0
frozen, dark sweet or red tart (*Stilwell*), 1 cup	0	0
Cherry, maraschino, in jars, w/liquid, 1 oz.	.1	0
Cherry juice or drink, all blends, all brands, 8 fl. oz.	0	0
Cherry pastry filling (*Solo*), 2 tbsp.	0	0
Chervil, dried, 1 tbsp.	.1	0
Chestnut, European:		
raw, in shell, 1 lb.	7.6	1.4
boiled or steamed, shelled, peeled, 1 oz.	.4	.1

	total fat (grams)	saturated fat (grams)
dried, shelled, peeled, 1 oz.	1.1	.2
roasted, shelled, peeled, 1 oz.	.6	.1
roasted, shelled, peeled, 1 cup, about 17 kernels	3.2	.6
Chestnut, Oriental:		
Chinese:		
raw, in shell, 1 lb.	4.2	.6
boiled or steamed, shelled, 1 oz.	.2	<.1
dried, 1 oz.	.5	.1
roasted, shelled, 1 oz.	.3	.1
Japanese:		
raw, in shell, 1 lb.	1.6	.2
boiled or steamed, shelled, 1 oz.	.1	<.1
dried, 1 oz.	.4	.1
roasted, shelled, 1 oz.	.2	<.1
Chia seeds, dried:		
1 oz.	7.5	3.0
(*Arrowhead Mills*), 3 tbsp.	7.0	2.0
Chicken, retail (see also "Chicken, frozen or refrigerated"):		
broiler or fryer, roasted:		
½ chicken, w/skin, 10.5 oz. (15.8 oz. w/bone)	40.7	11.3
meat, w/skin, 4 oz.	15.4	4.3
meat only, 4 oz.	8.4	2.3
meat only, chopped or diced, 1 cup	10.4	2.9
skin only, 1 oz.	11.5	3.2
dark meat, w/skin, 4 oz.	17.9	5.0
dark meat only, 4 oz.	11.0	3.0
dark meat only, chopped or diced, 1 cup	13.6	3.7
light meat, w/skin, 4 oz.	12.3	3.5
light meat only, 4 oz.	5.1	1.4
light meat only, chopped or diced, 1 cup	6.3	1.8
breast, w/skin, ½ breast, 3.5 oz. (8.5 oz. w/bone)	7.6	2.2
breast, skinned, ½ breast, 3 oz. (8.5 oz. w/bone and skin)	3.1	.9

	total fat (grams)	saturated fat (grams)
Chicken, broiler or fryer, roasted *(cont.)*		
breast, meat only, 4 oz.	4.0	1.1
drumstick, w/skin, 1.8 oz. (2.9 oz. w/bone)	5.8	1.6
drumstick, skinned, 1.6 oz. (2.9 oz. w/bone and skin)	2.5	.7
leg, w/skin, 4 oz. (5.7 oz. w/bone)	15.4	4.2
leg, skinned, 3.4 oz. (5.7 oz. w/bone and skin)	8.0	2.2
thigh, w/skin, 2.2 oz. (2.9 oz. w/bone)	9.6	2.7
thigh, skinned, 1.8 oz. (2.9 oz. w/bone and skin)	5.7	1.6
wing, w/skin, 1.2 oz. (2.3. w/bone)	6.6	1.9
wing, skinned, .7 oz. (2.3 oz. w/bone and skin)	1.7	.5
broiler or fryer, stewed:		
½ chicken, w/skin, 11.8 oz. (1.1 lbs. w/bone)	42.0	11.7
meat, w/skin, 4 oz.	14.2	4.0
meat only, 4 oz.	7.6	2.1
meat only, chopped or diced, 1 cup	9.4	2.6
dark meat, w/skin, 4 oz.	16.6	4.6
dark meat only, 4 oz.	10.2	2.8
dark meat only, chopped or diced, 1 cup	12.6	3.4
light meat, w/skin, 4 oz.	11.3	3.2
light meat only, 4 oz.	4.5	1.3
light meat only, chopped or diced, 1 cup	5.6	1.6
breast, w/skin, ½ breast, 3.9 oz. (9.5 oz. w/bone)	8.2	2.3
breast, skinned, ½ breast, 3.4 oz. (9.5 oz. w/bone and skin)	2.9	.8
drumstick, w/skin, .2 oz. (3.1 oz. w/bone)	6.1	1.7
drumstick, skinned, 1.6 oz. (3.1 oz. w/bone and skin)	2.6	.7
leg, w/skin, 4.4 oz. (6.3 oz. w/bone)	16.2	4.5
leg, skinned, 3.6 oz. (6.3 oz. w/bone and skin)	8.1	2.2

	total fat (grams)	saturated fat (grams)
thigh, w/skin, 2.4 oz. (3.2 oz. w/bone)	10.0	2.8
thigh, skinned, 1.9 oz (3.2 oz. w/bone and skin)	5.4	1.5
wing, w/skin, 1.4 oz. (2.7 oz. w/bone)	6.7	1.9
wing, skinned, .8 oz. (2.7 oz. w/bone and skin)	1.7	.5
capon, roasted:		
½ chicken, w/skin, 1.4 lbs. (2 lbs. w/bone)	74.2	20.8
meat w/skin, 4 oz.	13.2	3.7
roaster, roasted:		
½ chicken, w/skin, 1 lb. (1.5 lbs. w/bone)	64.3	17.9
meat, w/skin, 4 oz.	15.2	4.2
meat only, 4 oz.	7.5	2.1
meat only, chopped or diced, 1 cup	9.3	2.5
dark meat only, 4 oz.	9.9	2.8
dark meat only, chopped or diced, 1 cup	12.3	3.4
light meat only, 4 oz.	4.6	1.2
light meat only, chopped or diced, 1 cup	5.7	1.5
Chicken, canned:		
(*Hormel*), 2 oz.	3.0	1.0
(*Swanson*), ¼ cup	1.0	.5
breast (*Hormel/Hormel* No Salt), 2 oz.	1.5	.5
Chicken, ground:		
(*Longacre*), 1 oz. raw	4.0	n.a.
(*Perdue*), 4 oz. raw	13.0	4.0
(*Perdue*), 3 oz. cooked	11.0	3.5
burgers (*Perdue*), 1 burger, 4 oz. raw, 3 oz. cooked	11.0	3.5
Patties (*Perdue*), 1 patty, 4 oz. raw, 3 oz. cooked	11.0	3.5
Chicken, freeze-dried:		
diced (*AlpineAire*), ⅓ cup*	1.0	n.a.
Chicken, frozen or refrigerated:		
raw:		
(*Pilgrim's Pride* Family Pack), 4 oz.	17.0	3.0
breast, split (*Pilgrim's Pride*), 6.3-oz. piece	23.0	2.0

	total fat (grams)	saturated fat (grams)
Chicken, frozen or refrigerated, raw *(cont.)*		
breast, boneless (*Perdue/Perdue Fit 'N Easy/ Perdue* Family Pack), 4 oz.	3.0	1.0
breast, boneless (*Perdue Oven Stuffer*), 4 oz.	2.5	.5
breast, boneless, thin sliced (*Perdue Oven Stuffer*), 1 slice, 3 oz.	1.5	.5
breast, boneless, skinless (*Pilgrim's Pride*), 5-oz. piece	3.0	0
breast tenders (*Perdue Fit 'N Easy*), 4 oz.	1.0	0
drumstick (*Pilgrim's Pride*), 4.2 oz., 2 pieces	11.0	3.0
leg, whole (*Pilgrim's Pride*), 7.1-oz. piece	34.0	9.0
patty, fajita (*Pilgrim's Pride*), 3-oz. piece	4.0	0
pieces, selected (*Pilgrim's Pride*), 4 oz.	18.0	3.0
tenderloins (*Perdue Fit 'N Easy*), 4 oz.	1.0	.5
thighs, bone-in (*Pilgrim's Pride*), 3.5-oz. piece	18.0	5.0
thighs, boneless, skinless (*Pilgrim's Pride*), 5.9 oz., 2 pieces	18.0	4.0
wings, whole (*Pilgrim's Pride*), 5 oz., 4 pieces	21.0	5.0
wings, split (*Pilgrim's Pride* Drummettes), 4.3 oz., 7 pieces	18.0	4.0
barbecued (*Empire* Kosher), 5 oz. edible	17.0	4.5
barbecued (*Hebrew National/Falls*), 3 oz. edible	8.0	n.a.
fried:		
breast, battered, breaded (*Empire* Kosher), 3 oz.	8.0	2.0
cutlets, battered, breaded (*Empire* Kosher), 3.3-oz. cutlet	9.0	1.5
drum and thigh (*Empire* Kosher), 3 oz. w/out bone	16.0	4.0
ground, see "Chicken, ground"		
nuggets, see "Chicken entree, frozen"		
roasted, 3 oz., except as noted:		
whole or split, dark meat (*Perdue*)	15.0	4.5

	total fat (grams)	saturated fat (grams)
whole or split, white meat (*Perdue*)	10.0	3.0
whole, dark meat (*Perdue Oven Stuffer*)	14.0	4.0
whole, white meat (*Perdue Oven Stuffer*)	8.0	2.5
breast (*Longacre* Gourmet), 1 oz.	1.0	n.a.
breast (*Longacre* Premium), 1 oz.	3.0	n.a.
breast, boneless (*Perdue Oven Stuffer*)	1.5	.5
breast, boneless (*Perdue/Perdue Fit 'N Easy/ Perdue* Family Pack)	2.5	1.0
breast, boneless, thin sliced (*Perdue Oven Stuffer*), 2-oz. slice	1.0	.0
breast, whole (*Perdue/Perdue* Family)	9.0	2.5
breast, whole (*Perdue Oven Stuffer* Roaster)	7.0	2.0
breast, split (*Perdue/Perdue Family*), 1 breast, about 7 oz.	19.0	6.0
breast, split, skinless (*Perdue*), 1 breast, about 6 oz.	8.0	2.5
breast, split (*Perdue* Breast & Thigh Combo), 3.5 oz., ½ breast	2.5	1.0
breast quarters (*Perdue*), 3 oz.	11.0	3.5
breast, tenders (*Perdue Fit 'N Easy*)	.5	0
drumstick (*Perdue Oven Stuffer*), 1 piece, about 3.5 oz.	10.0	3.0
drumstick (*Perdue/Perdue* Value Pack/Family), 1 drumstick, about 2 oz.	6.0	2.0
drumsticks, skinless (*Perdue*), 3.5 oz., 2 drumsticks	6.0	1.5
leg (*Perdue/Perdue* Value Pack/*Family*), 1 leg, about 5.5 oz.	26.0	7.0
thigh (*Perdue*), 1 thigh, about 2.5 oz.	10.0	3.0
thigh (*Perdue/Perdue* Value Pack/Family)	18.0	5.0
thigh (*Perdue* Breast & Thigh Combo), 3.5 oz., 2 thighs	11.0	3.0
thigh, boneless (*Perdue/Perdue Fit 'N Easy*), 2 thighs, about 3.5 oz.	10.0	3.0

	total fat (grams)	saturated fat (grams)

Chicken, frozen or refrigerated, roasted *(cont.)*

thigh, boneless (*Perdue Oven Stuffer*), 1 thigh,
about 3.5 oz. .... 9.0 .... 2.5

thigh, boneless/skinless (*Perdue,* Roaster) 3.3-
oz. thigh .... 8.0 .... 2.5

thigh, boneless/skinless (*Perdue*), 3.5 oz.,
2 thighs .... 11.0 .... 3.0

thigh, skinless (*Perdue* Broiler), 1 thigh,
about 2.5 oz. .... 9.0 .... 2.5

wing (*Perdue/Perdue* Value Pack/Family),
2 wings .... 15.0 .... 4.5

wing drummettes (*Perdue*), 2 wings,
about 2.5 oz. .... 11.0 .... 3.5

wingettes (*Perdue*), 3 wings, about 3 oz. ..... 14.0 .... 4.0

wingettes (*Perdue Oven Stuffer*), 3 pieces,
about 3.5 oz. .... 15.0 .... 4.5

"Chicken," vegetarian, canned:

diced (*Worthington Chik*), 1.9 oz., ¼ cup 3.5 5

fried (*Worthington FriChik*), 3.2 oz., 2 pieces .... 8.0 .... 1.0

fried, and gravy (*Loma Linda Chik'n*), 5.2 oz.,
2 pieces .... 31.0 .... 4.5

sliced (*Worthington Chik*), 3.2 oz., 3 slices ...... 6.0 .... 1.0

"Chicken," vegetarian, frozen:

(*Worthington Chic-ketts*), 1.9 oz., 2 slices, ⅜" .... 7.0 .... 1.0

diced (*Worthington Chik*), 1.9 oz., ¼ cup .... 4.5 .... 1.0

fried (*Loma Linda Chik'n*), 2-oz. piece .... 15.0 .... 2.0

nuggets (*Loma Linda Chik*), 3 oz., 5 pieces ..... 16.0 .... 2.5

patties (*Morningstar Farms Chik*), 2.5-oz. patty ... 10.0 .... 1.5

patties (*Worthington CrispyChik*), 2.5-oz. patty ... 9.0 .... 1.5

pie (*Worthington*), 8-oz. pie .... 27.0 .... 6.0

sliced (*Worthington*), 2 oz., 2 slices .... 4.5 .... 1.0

sticks (*Worthington ChikStiks*), 1.7-oz. piece ..... 8.0 .... 2.0

"Chicken," vegetarian, mix, dry (*Loma Linda*
Supreme), ⅓ cup 1.0 0

	total fat (grams)	saturated fat (grams)

Chicken bologna:

(*Empire* Kosher), 3 slices, 1.8 oz.	7.0	2.0
(*Perdue*), 2 slices, 2 oz.	9.0	2.5

Chicken burger, see "Chicken, ground"

Chicken coating mix, see "Chicken
    seasoning/sauce mix"

Chicken dinner, frozen:

barbecue (*Banquet*), 9 oz.	12.0	2.5
w/barbecue sauce (*Healthy Choice*), 12.75 oz.	6.0	2.0
boneless (*Swanson Hungry-Man*), 17.2 oz.	28.0	11.0
breast tenders, Southern fried (*Banquet*), 8.75 oz.	30.0	8.0
w/broccoli Alfredo (*Healthy Choice*), 12.1 oz.	7.0	3.0
Burgundy (*Armour Classics Lite*), 10 oz.	5.0	1.5
chow mein (*Banquet*), 9 oz.	7.0	2.0
chow mein (*Chun King*), 13 oz.	14.0	5.0
Dijon (*Healthy Choice*), 11 oz.	3.0	1.0
and dumplings (*Banquet*), 10 oz.	8.0	2.5
fried:		
(*Banquet*), 9 oz.	27.0	9.0
(*Banquet Extra Helping*), 18 oz.	39.0	9.0
(*Morton*), 9 oz.	25.0	8.0
dark meat (*Swanson*), 9.7 oz.	28.0	11.0
dark meat (*Swanson* Budget), 9.5 oz.	22.0	8.0
Southern (*Banquet Extra Helping*), 17.5 oz. . . .	37.0	9.0
white meat (*Banquet Extra Helping*), 18 oz. . . .	41.0	9.0
white meat, mostly (*Swanson Hungry-Man*), 15.5 oz.	40.0	14.0
glazed (*Armour Classics*), 10.75 oz.	14.0	4.0
herb roasted (*Healthy Choice*), 11.5 oz.	7.0	3.0
herbed, w/fettuccine (*The Budget Gourmet* Light & Healthy), 11 oz.	8.0	3.0
honey mustard breast (*The Budget Gourmet* Light & Healthy), 11 oz.	6.0	1.5
imperial (*Chun King*), 13 oz.	10.0	3.0

	total fat (grams)	saturated fat (grams)

Chicken dinner *(cont.)*

mesquite:

    (*Armour Classics*), 9.5 oz. .... 13.0 .... 4.0

    (*Healthy Choice*), 10.5 oz. .... 4.0 .... 1.0

    barbecue sauce (*The Budget Gourmet* Light & Healthy), 11 oz. .... 6.0 .... 2.0

and noodles (*Armour Classics*), 11 oz. .... 9.0 .... 5.0

nuggets (*Swanson*), 9.5 oz. .... 24.0 .... 11.0

Oriental (*Banquet*), 9 oz. .... 9.0 .... 2.5

Oriental (*Healthy Choice*), 11.25 oz. .... 1.0 .... <1.0

Parmesan (*Banquet*), 9.5 oz. .... 15.0 .... 4.0

parmigiana:

    (*Armour Classics*), 10.75 oz. .... 18.0 .... 6.0

    (*Banquet Extra Helping*), 19 oz. .... 33.0 .... 8.0

    (*The Budget Gourmet* Light & Healthy), 11 oz. .. 10.0 .... 3.0

    (*Healthy Choice*), 11.5 oz. .... 6.0 .... 3.0

    (*Swanson*), 11.5 oz. .... 19.0 .... 7.0

roast breast, w/herb gravy (*The Budget Gourmet* Light & Healthy), 11 oz. .... 7.0 .... 2.0

salsa (*Healthy Choice*), 11.25 oz. .... 2.0 .... 1.0

southwestern style (*Healthy Choice*), 12.5 oz. .... 5.0 .... 2.0

sweet and sour (*Armour Classics Lite*), 11 oz. 1.0 0

sweet and sour (*Healthy Choice*), 10 oz. .... 4.0 .... 1.0

teriyaki (*Healthy Choice*), 12.25 oz. .... 4.0 .... 1.0

teriyaki, breast, w/Oriental vegetables (*The Budget Gourmet* Light & Healthy), 11 oz. .... 6.0 .... 1.0

vegetables, Italian style, and (*The Budget Gourmet* Light & Healthy), 11 oz. .... 7.0 .... 2.0

walnut (*Chun King*), 13 oz. .... 19.0 .... 5.0

w/wine and mushrooms (*Armour Classics*), 10 oz. .... 11.0 .... 5.0

Chicken entree, canned or packaged, 1 bowl or cup:

(*Hormel Top Shelf* Chix Acapulco/Fiesta) .... 16.0 .... 8.0

a la king (*Hormel Top Shelf*) .... 12.0 .... 5.0

a la king (*Swanson*) .... 21.0 .... 7.0

	total fat (grams)	saturated fat (grams)
breast, glazed (*Hormel Top Shelf*)	5.0	1.5
cacciatore (*Hormel Top Shelf*)	2.5	1.0
and dumpling (*Dinty Moore* Microwave Cup)	6.0	1.5
and noodles, see "Noodle and chicken entree"		
w/mashed potatoes (*Dinty Moore American*		
Classics)	4.0	1.5
stew (*Dinty Moore*)	11.0	3.0
stew (*Dinty Moore* Microwave Cup)	8.0	2.0
stew (*Swanson*)	8.0	3.0
Chicken entree, freeze-dried*, 1 cup, except as noted:		
a la king and noodles (*Mountain House*)	10.0	3.0
almond (*AlpineAire*), 1¼ cups	7.0	n.a.
honey-lime, w/rice (*Mountain House*)	4.0	1.0
noodles and (*Mountain House*)	3.0	1.0
Polynesian, w/rice (*Mountain House*)	4.0	1.0
primavera (*AlpineAire*), 1½ cups	2.0	n.a.
rice and (*Mountain House*)	10.0	2.0
rice, brown, and, w/vegetables (*AlpineAire*),		
1½ cups	4.0	n.a.
rotelle (*AlpineAire*), 1⅓ cups	3.0	n.a.
Sierra (*AlpineAire*), 1⅓ cups	2.0	n.a.
stew (*Mountain House*)	9.0	2.0
teriyaki, w/rice (*Mountain House*)	2.0	1.0
Chicken entree, frozen (see also "Chicken, frozen or		
refrigerated"):		
a la king (*Banquet Hot Sandwich Toppers*), 4.5 oz.	4.0	1.5
a la king (*Stouffer's*), 9.5 oz.	10.0	3.0
a l'orange (*Healthy Choice*), 9 oz.	2.0	<1.0
a l'orange (*Lean Cuisine*), 9 oz.	2.5	.5
Alfredo (*Stouffer's Lunch Express*), 9⅝ oz.	17.0	6.0
au gratin (*The Budget Gourmet* Light & Healthy),		
9.1 oz.	8.0	5.0
baked (*Stouffer's* Homestyle), 8⅞ oz.	12.0	3.0
baked, w/whipped potato (*Lean Cuisine* Cafe		
Classics), 8 oz.	5.0	.5

	total fat (grams)	saturated fat (grams)

Chicken entree, frozen *(cont.)*

in barbecue sauce, glazed (*Weight Watchers*),
7.4 oz. .... 3.5 .... 1.0
in barbecue sauce, honey (*Lean Cuisine*), 8¾ oz. ... 4.5 .... 1.0
breast:
    breaded (*Pilgrim's Pride*), 4-oz. piece .... 11.0 .... 2.0
    breaded (*Schwan's*), 3.1-oz. piece .... 7.0 .... 1.5
    breaded cutlet, pasta marinara and (*Celentano*),
     10 oz. .... 19.0 .... 4.0
    for fajitas (*Schwan's*), ½ cup .... 3.0 .... 1.0
    fillet (*Pilgrim's Pride*), 2 pieces .... 14.0 .... 3.0
    fried (*Banquet*), 1 piece .... 26.0 .... 13.0
    glazed (*Healthy Choice*), 8.5 oz. .... 3.0 .... 1.0
    nuggets (*Pilgrim's Pride* Ring Things),
     4 pieces .... 18.0 .... 4.0
    strips (*Pilgrim's Pride*), 4 strips .... 13.0 .... 2.0
    stuffed (*Schwan's*), 1 piece, 6.0 oz. .... 14.0 .... 6.0
    tenderloin, Southern style (*Schwan's*),
     2 tenders .... 9.0 .... 1.5
    tenders (*Banquet*), 4.5 oz. .... 18.0 .... 4.0
calypso (*Lean Cuisine* Cafe Classics), 8.5 oz. ..... 6.0 .... 2.0
carbonara (*Lean Cuisine* Cafe Classics), 9 oz. .... 8.0 .... 2.0
casserole (*Schwan's*), 1 cup .... 17.0 .... 5.0
chow mein:
    (*Healthy Choice*), 9 oz. .... 5.0 .... 2.0
    (*Weight Watchers Smart Ones*), 9 oz. 2.0 5
    w/rice (*Lean Cuisine*), 9 oz. .... 5.0 .... 1.0
    w/rice (*Stouffer's Lunch Express*), 10⅝ oz. ... 4.0 .... 1.0
chunks, fried (*Country Skillet*), 3 oz. .... 17.0 .... 3.0
cordon bleu (*Schwan's*), 1 piece, 4.9 oz. .... 13.0 .... 4.0
cordon bleu (*Weight Watchers*), 9 oz. .... 6.0 .... 2.0
creamed (*Stouffer's*), 6.5 oz. .... 20.0 .... 7.0
creamy, and broccoli (*Stouffer's*), 8⅞ oz. .... 15.0 .... 5.0
drummies (*Schwan's*), 3 pieces, 2.8 oz. .... 17.0 .... 4.0

	total fat (grams)	saturated fat (grams)
and dumplings (*Banquet* Family), 1 cup	15.0	5.0
enchilada, see "Enchilada" entree		
escalloped, and noodles (*Stouffer's*), 10 oz.	29.0	6.0
fettuccine, see "Fettuccine entree"		
w/fettuccine (*The Budget Gourmet*), 10 oz.	19.0	10.0
fiesta (*Weight Watchers Smart Ones*), 8.5 oz.	2.0	.5
fiesta, w/rice and vegetables (*Lean Cuisine*), 8.5 oz.	5.0	1.0
fillet, breaded, and potato rounds (*Stouffer's* Homestyle), 6⅝ oz.	18.0	3.0
fillet, Southern style (*Schwan's*), 3.5-oz. fillet	15.0	4.0
French recipe (*The Budget Gourmet* Light & Healthy), 10 oz.	8.0	3.0
fried:		
(*Kid Cuisine*), 10.1 oz.	20.0	6.0
(*Stouffer's* Homestyle), 7⅛ oz.	16.0	4.0
hot and spicy (*Banquet*), 3 oz.	18.0	5.0
hot and spicy (*Banquet* Snackin), 4 pieces	16.0	4.0
original or Southern (*Banquet*), 3 oz.	18.0	5.0
w/potatoes (*Swanson*), 7 oz.	21.0	8.0
skinless (*Banquet*), 3 oz.	13.0	3.0
thighs and wings (*Banquet*), 3 oz.	18.0	5.0
white portions (*Swanson*), 10.3 oz.	26.0	11.0
glazed, w/vegetable rice (*Lean Cuisine*), 8.5 oz.	6.0	1.0
grilled, and angel hair pasta (*Stouffer's* Lunch Express), 9⅞ oz.	13.0	3.0
grilled, salsa (*Lean Cuisine* Cafe Classics), 8⅞ oz.	6.0	1.5
herb roasted (*Lean Cuisine* Cafe Classics), 8 oz.	5.0	1.0
honey mustard:		
(*Healthy Choice*), 9.5 oz.	3.0	1.0
(*Weight Watchers Smart Ones*), 8.5 oz.	2.0	.5
w/vegetable rice (*Lean Cuisine*), 7.5 oz.	4.5	1.0
Italiano, w/fettuccini (*Lean Cuisine*), 9 oz.	6.0	1.5
Kiev (*Schwan's*), 1 piece	21.0	9.0

	total fat (grams)	saturated fat (grams)

Chicken entree, frozen *(cont.)*

legs, Buffalo (*Pilgrim's Pride*), 2 pieces	6.0	2.0
w/linguine (*Stouffer's Lunch Express*), 9⅝ oz.	11.0	2.0
mandarin (*The Budget Gourmet* Light & Healthy), 10 oz.	5.0	1.0
mandarin (*Healthy Choice*), 10 oz.	2.0	1.0
mandarin (*Lean Cuisine Lunch Express*), 9¾ oz.	6.0	<1.0
Marco Polo (*Schwan's*), 1 piece, 4.9 oz.	12.0	4.0
Marsala (*Weight Watchers Smart Ones*), 9 oz.	2.0	.5
Marsala, and vegetables (*Lean Cuisine*), 8⅛ oz.	4.0	1.0
Mediterranean (*Lean Cuisine* Cafe Classics), 10⅛ oz.	4.0	1.0
Mexican style, and rice (*Stouffer's Lunch Express*), 9⅛ oz.	8.0	1.0
Mirabella (*Weight Watchers Smart Ones*), 9 oz.	2.0	.5
Monterey (*Stouffer's* Homestyle), 9⅜ oz.	20.0	9.0
and noodles (*The Budget Gourmet*), 10 oz.	23.0	12.0
and noodles (*Stouffer's* Homestyle), 10 oz.	14.0	5.0
noodles and, see "Noodle dishes" and "Noodle entree"		
nuggets (see also "breast," above):		
(*Banquet*), 9 pieces	15.0	3.0
(*Banquet* Meals), 6.75 oz.	21.0	5.0
(*Country Skillet*), 3 oz.	18.0	4.0
(*Empire* Kosher Plain), 5 pieces, 3 oz.	9.0	1.5
(*Kid Cuisine*), 8.5 oz.	13.0	3.0
(*Morton*), 7 oz.	17.0	4.0
(*Pilgrim's Pride* 10.5 oz./23 oz.), 4 pieces	16.0	3.0
(*Pilgrim's Pride* 9 oz.), 6 pieces	16.0	3.0
(*Schwan's*), 6 pieces	15.0	3.0
(*Swanson*), 9.5 oz.	21.0	7.0
breaded, battered (*Empire* Kosher), 3.1 oz., 5 pieces	13.0	2.5
chicken and cheddar (*Banquet*), 2.5 oz.	19.0	6.0
Southern fried (*Banquet*), 9 pieces	15.0	3.0

	total fat (grams)	saturated fat (grams)
Southern fried (*Banquet* Micro), 6 pieces	20.0	4.0
sweet and sour (*Banquet* Micro), 6 pieces	18.0	4.0
orange glazed breast (*The Budget Gourmet* Light & Healthy), 9 oz.	2.0	1.0
Oriental:		
(*The Budget Gourmet* Light & Healthy), 9 oz.	6.0	2.0
(*Stouffer's Lunch Express*), 9¾ oz.	9.0	1.5
w/peanut sauce (*Healthy Choice*), 9.5 oz.	5.0	1.0
w/vegetables and vermicelli (*Lean Cuisine*), 9 oz.	6.0	1.0
Parmesan (*Banquet* Family), 1 patty	13.0	5.0
Parmesan and pasta (*Lean Cuisine*), 10⅞ oz.	5.0	1.5
parmigiana (*Stouffer's* Homestyle), 10⅞ oz.	10.0	2.0
parmigiana (*Weight Watchers*), 9.1 oz.	6.0	3.0
patties:		
(*Banquet*), 1 patty	12.0	2.5
(*Country Skillet*), 2.5 oz.	12.0	2.5
(*Pilgrim's Pride*), 2.5-oz. patty	12.0	3.0
(*Pilgrim's Pride*), 3-oz. patty	14.0	3.0
breaded (*Morton*), 6.75 oz.	15.0	3.0
breaded (*Schwan's*), 3-oz. patty	14.0	3.0
Southern fried (*Banquet*), 2.5 oz.	12.0	3.0
Southern fried (*Country Skillet*), 2.5 oz.	12.0	2.5
in peanut sauce (*Lean Cuisine*), 9 oz.	6.0	1.0
piccata (*Lean Cuisine* Cafe Classics), 9 oz.	6.0	1.5
piccata, lemon herb (*Weight Watchers Smart Ones*), 8.5 oz.	2.0	.5
pie:		
(*Banquet*), 7 oz.	18.0	7.0
(*Banquet* Family), 8 oz.	30.0	12.0
(*Banquet* Supreme), 7 oz.	15.0	5.0
(*Empire* Kosher), 8.2 oz.	21.0	5.0
(*Lean Cuisine*), 9.5 oz.	10.0	2.5
(*Morton*), 7 oz.	18.0	7.0

	total fat (grams)	saturated fat (grams)
Chicken entree, frozen, pie *(cont.)*		
(*Stouffer's*), 10 oz.	33.0	8.0
(*Stouffer's*), ½ of 16-oz. pkg.	30.0	10.0
(*Swanson*), 7-oz. pie	22.0	8.0
vegetarian, see "Chicken vegetarian"		
pie, hand-held, see "Chicken sandwich"		
popcorn (*Schwan's*), 3 oz.	16.0	3.0
popcorn, hot (*Banquet*), 3 oz.	19.0	4.0
rice and, see "Rice entrees"		
roasted, glazed (*Weight Watchers Smart Ones*), 8.9 oz.	5.0	2.5
sandwich, see "Chicken sandwich"		
Southern fried (*Weight Watchers*), 8 oz.	11.0	4.5
sticks (*Empire* Kosher Stix), 4 pieces, 3.1 oz.	9.0	2.0
stir-fry (*Pilgrim's Pride*), 1 cup	4.0	0
stir-fry, w/pasta (*Healthy Choice*), 12 oz.	5.0	1.0
sweet and sour (*The Budget Gourmet*), 10 oz.	5.0	1.0
sweet and sour, w/rice (*Lean Cuisine*), 10⅜ oz.	2.5	1.0
tenderloins (*Pilgrim's Pride*), 2 pieces	10.0	1.0
Tex-Mex (*Weight Watchers Smart Ones*), 8.3 oz.	4.0	1.5
and vegetables:		
(*Healthy Choice*), 11.5 oz.	3.0	1.0
(*Lean Cuisine*), 10.5 oz.	5.0	1.0
w/rice (*Stouffer's Lunch Express*), 9⅞ oz.	11.0	3.0
vegetables and, see "Vegetable entree"		
wings:		
barbecue (*Banquet Game Time*), 4 pieces	12.0	4.0
barbecue (*Schwan's*), 6 pieces	14.0	4.0
Buffalo (*Pilgrim's Pride*), 3 pieces	15.0	4.0
hot (*Schwan's Hot Wings*), 6 pieces	14.0	3.0
hot and spicy (*Banquet Game Time*), 4 pieces	16.0	5.0
Chicken entree, refrigerated (see also "Chicken, frozen or refrigerated"):		
barbecued:		
whole, dark meat (*Perdue*), 3 oz.	10.0	3.0

	total fat (grams)	saturated fat (grams)
whole, white meat (*Perdue*), 3 oz.	3.5	1.0
breast (*Perdue*), 5.5-oz. piece	8.0	2.5
drumstick (*Perdue*), about 2 pieces	4.0	1.0
smokey (*Longacre*), 4 oz.	7.0	n.a.
thigh (*Perdue*), about 1 piece	12.0	3.5
wings (*Perdue Done It!*), 3 oz.	12.0	3.0
bleu cheese, Italian (*Chicken By George*), 5 oz.	8.0	n.a.
breast cutlet (*Perdue Done It!*), 3.5 oz.	13.0	4.0
breast nugget (*Perdue Done It!*), 3 oz.	12.0	3.0
breast nugget, w/cheese (*Perdue Done It!*), 3 oz.	15.0	4.0
breast tenders (*Perdue Done It!*), 3 oz.	7.0	2.5
cacciatore (*Longacre*), 4 oz.	3.0	n.a.
Cajun (*Chicken By George*), 5 oz.	8.0	1.0
Caribbean grill (*Chicken By George*), 5 oz.	6.0	n.a.
lemon herb (*Chicken By George*), 5 oz.	6.0	1.0
lemon oregano (*Chicken By George*), 5 oz.	4.0	n.a.
mesquite barbecue (*Chicken By George*), 5 oz.	6.0	1.0
mustard dill (*Chicken By George*), 5 oz.	7.0	n.a.
roasted:		
(*Chicken By George*), 5 oz.	4.0	n.a.
whole, dark meat (*Perdue*), 3 oz.	11.0	3.0
whole, white meat (*Perdue*), 3 oz.	7.0	2.0
breast (*Perdue*), 5-oz. piece	6.0	2.0
drumstick (*Perdue*), 2.5 oz., about 2 drums	4.0	1.0
thigh (*Perdue*), about 1 piece	12.0	3.5
wings, hot and spicy (*Perdue Done It!*), 3 oz.	12.0	3.0
shaped, nugget, all shapes (*Perdue Done It! Fun Shapes*), 3 oz.	12.0	3.0
shaped, on a stick (*Perdue Done It! Fun Shapes*), 3.5 oz.	13.0	3.0
sweet and sour (*Longacre*), 4 oz.	<1.0	n.a.
Szechuan, w/peanuts (*Longacre*), 4 oz.	4.0	n.a.

	total fat (grams)	saturated fat (grams)
Chicken entree, refrigerated, roasted *(cont.)*		
teriyaki (*Chicken By George*), 5 oz.	5.0	1.0
tomato herb w/basil (*Chicken By George*), 5 oz.	7.0	n.a.
Chicken fat:		
1 oz.	14.0	n.a.
rendered (*Empire* Kosher), 1 tbsp.	13.0	4.0
Chicken frankfurter (see also "Chicken sausage"):		
(*Empire* Kosher), 2-oz. link	7.0	2.0
(*Longacre*), 2-oz. link	11.0	n.a.
(*Longacre*), 1.6-oz. link	9.0	n.a.
(*Perdue*), 2-oz. link	11.0	3.5
turkey and chicken, see "Turkey frankfurter"		
Chicken giblets, simmered:		
broiler-fryer, 4 oz.	5.4	1.7
broiler-fryer, chopped or diced, 1 cup	6.9	2.2
roaster, 4 oz.	5.9	1.9
roaster, chopped or diced, 1 cup	7.6	2.4
Chicken gizzard, broiler-fryer, simmered,		
1 medium, .8 oz.	.8	.2
Chicken gravy:		
canned, ¼ cup	3.4	.8
canned (*Franco-American*), 2 oz., ¼ cup	4.0	1.0
Chicken gravy mix:		
(*Durkee/French's*), ¼ pkg.	.5	0
(*Pillsbury*), 2 tsp.	0	0
(*Weight Watchers*), ¼ pkg.	0	0
roasted chicken (*Knorr Gravy Classics*), ⅛ pkg.	1.0	0
vegetarian (*Loma Linda Gravy Quik*), 1 tbsp.	0	0
Chicken heart, see "Heart"		
Chicken hors d'oeuvre, frozen:		
a la king (*Pepperidge Farm* Kit), 1 filled shell	26.0	10.0
Monterey, filling (*Pepperidge Farm* Kit),		
7 filled sheets	28.0	8.0
Chicken liver, see "Liver" and "Liver pâté"		

	total fat (grams)	saturated fat (grams)

Chicken luncheon meat:

breast, oven roasted:

(*Boar's Head* Golden), 2 oz.	1.0	0
(*Healthy Choice*), 2 oz.	2.0	<1.0
(*Hebrew National* Sliced), 1.8 oz., 5 slices	.5	0
(*Hillshire Farm*), 1 slice	<1.0	n.a.
(*Louis Rich* White), 1-oz. slice	2.5	.5
(*Louis Rich* Deli-Thin), 4 slices, 1.8 oz.	1.5	.5
(*Louis Rich* Deluxe), 1-oz. slice	1.0	0
(*Oscar Mayer Healthy Favorites*), 1.8 oz., 4 slices	0	0

breast, honey glaze (*Oscar Mayer Deli-Thin*),

4 slices, 1.8 oz.	1.0	0

breast, skinless (*Healthy Choice* Deli Meats),

1 oz.	<1.0	<1.0

breast, smoked:

(*Healthy Choice*), 2 oz.	2.0	<1.0
(*Hillshire Farm Deli Select*), 1 slice	<1.0	n.a.
(*Hillshire Farm Flavor Pack*), .75 oz. slice	<1.0	n.a.
hickory (*Boar's Head*), 2 oz.	1.0	0
hickory (*Louis Rich*), 1-oz. slice	1.0	0
roll (*Longacre* Sliced), .8-oz. slice	4.0	n.a.
roll (*Wampler-Longacre*), 1 oz.	5.0	n.a.

Chicken marinade, see "Chicken seasoning/sauce mix"

Chicken pie, see "Chicken entree, frozen"

Chicken salad:

(*Longacre*), 1 oz.	3.0	n.a.
(*Longacre* Lite), 1 oz.	2.0	n.a.

Chicken sandwich, frozen:

(*Hormel Quick Meal*), 1 piece	12.0	3.0
(*Kid Cuisine*), 8.25 oz.	14.0	3.0
(*Schwan's*), 3.3-oz. piece	6.0	1.0
broccoli, cheddar (*Weight Watchers*), 5 oz.	6.0	2.5
w/cheese on French bread (*Schwan's*), 4.5 oz.	8.0	3.5

	total fat (grams)	saturated fat (grams)
Chicken sandwich, frozen *(cont.)*		
grilled (*Hormel Quick Meal*), 1 piece	9.0	3.0
grilled (*Weight Watchers*), 4 oz.	5.0	2.0
hand-held pie (*Mrs. Paterson's Aussie Pie*), 1 piece	25.0	8.0
Chicken sauce, see "Cooking sauce" and specific sauce listings		
Chicken sausage (see also "Chicken frankfurter" and "Vienna sausage"), 3.2-oz. link:		
and broccoli, w/cheese (*Bilinski's*)	3.5	1.5
and jalapeño pepper (*Bilinski's*)	4.0	1.0
and pesto (*Bilinski's*)	4.5	1.0
and spinach, with garlic and fennel (*Bilinski's*)	3.0	1.0
and sun-dried tomatoes (*Bilinski's*)	3.5	1.0
Chicken seasoning/sauce mix (see also specific listings):		
(*Blue Plate* Coating Mix), ¼ tsp.	0	0
(*Durkee/French's* Roasting Bag), ⅙ pkg.	0	0
(*Perc*), 1 tsp.	.2	0
(*Shake 'N Bake* Original), ⅛ pkg.	1.0	0
(*Shake 'N Bake* Hot and Spicy), ⅛ pkg.	1.0	0
barbecue (*Shake 'N Bake*), ⅛ pkg.	1.0	0
cacciatore or Mexican salsa (*Durkee* "Easy"), ⅒ pkg.	0	0
country (*Durkee* Roasting Bag), ⅙ pkg.	1.5	1.0
Creole (*McCormick*), ¼ pkg.	0	0
crispy (*Oven Fry*), ⅛ pkg.	1.0	0
curry, creamy (*McCormick*), ¼ pkg.	1.5	.5
Dijonne (*Knorr* Recipe Mix), ⅙ pkg.	1.0	1.0
fried (*Durkee* Spices), ¼ tsp.	0	0
herb and spice (*McCormick Rotisserie Recipe*), 2 tsp.	0	0
home style (*Oven Fry*), ⅛ pkg.	1.0	0

	total fat (grams)		saturated fat (grams)

hot and spicy (*McCormick Bag'n Season*),

⅙ pkg.	0	....	0
marinade (*Lawry's* Spices & Seasonings), 1 tsp.	0	....	0

marinade, mesquite or Southwestern style

(*McCormick*), ⅙ pkg.	0	....	0
mushroom (*Durkee* "Easy" Pouch), ⅑ pkg.	0	....	0
piccata, lemon and wine (*McCormick*), ¼ pkg.	0	....	0
sweet and sour (*Durkee* "Easy" Pouch), ⅑ pkg.	0	....	0

Chicken spread, canned:

1 tbsp.	1.5	....	n.a.
(*Libby Spreadables*), ⅓ cup	9.0	....	1.5
chunky (*Underwood*), 2 oz., ¼ cup	8.0	....	2.5

chunky, w/crackers (*Underwood Red Devil*

Snackers*), 1 pkg.	16.0	....	3.5
Chicken stock base (*Spice Island*), 2 tsp.	0	....	0

Chicken wing sauce, 2 tbsp.:

hot (*Chelten House*)	0	....	0
mild or hot (*Nance's*)	0	....	0

Chick-fil-A, 1 serving:

sandwiches:

chicken	9.0	....	2.0
chicken, chargrilled	3.0	....	1.0
chicken, chargrilled club (no dressing)	12.0	....	5.0
chicken, chargrilled, deluxe	3.0	....	1.0
chicken deluxe	9.0	....	2.0
chicken salad on whole wheat	5.0	....	2.0
Chick-n-Q	13.0	....	3.0

chicken dishes:

chicken salad jplate	5.0	....	0
Chick-fil-A Nuggets, 8-pack	14.0	....	3.0
Chick-n-Strips, 4 pieces	8.0	....	2.0
Chick-n-Strips Salad	9.0	....	2.0
garden salad, chargrilled	3.0	....	1.0
Grilled'n Lites, 2 skewers	2.0	....	0

	total fat (grams)	saturated fat (grams)
Chick-fil-A *(cont.)*		
side dishes:		
carrot and raisin salad	2.0	0
chicken soup, breast of, hearty	1.0	0
Chick-fil-A Waffle Fries, salted or unsalted	10.0	4.0
coleslaw	6.0	1.0
tossed salad, w/out dressing	0	0
desserts:		
cheesecake	21.0	9.0
cheesecake, w/blueberry topping	23.0	10.0
cheesecake, w/strawberry topping	23.0	10.0
fudge brownie w/nuts	16.0	3.0
Icedream, small cone	4.0	1.0
Icedream small cup	10.0	3.0
lemon pie	22.0	6.0
lemonade, small	0	0
Chickpeas:		
dry, 1 oz.	1.7	.2
dry (*Arrowhead Mills* Garbanzo), ¼ cup	2.0	0
dry, boiled, ½ cup	2.1	.2
canned, ½ cup:		
(*Allens*)	2.5	.5
(*Eden*)	1.5	0
(*Green Giant/Joan of Arc*)	1.5	0
(*Old El Paso* Garbanzo)	2.5	0
(*Progresso*)	2.5	0
(*Stokely*)	1.5	0
w/tamari (*Eden*)	1.0	0
Chicory, witloof:		
untrimmed, 1 lb.	.4	.1
1 head, 5–7" long, 2.1 oz.	.1	<.1
Chicory greens:		
untrimmed, 1 lb.	1.1	.3
trimmed, chopped, ½ cup	.3	.1
Chicory root, 1 medium, 2.6 oz.	.1	<.1

	total fat (grams)	saturated fat (grams)

Chili, canned:

(*Chi-Chi's* San Antonio), 1 cup	19.0	1.0

w/beans:

(*Hormel*), 1 cup	17.0	7.0
(*Hormel*), 7.5-oz. can	11.0	5.0
(*Hormel* Micro Cup), 7.3-oz. cup	11.0	5.0
(*Hormel* Micro Cup), 10.5-oz. cup	17.0	7.0
(*Libby's*), 1 cup	27.0	13.0
(*Libby's Diner*), 7.75 oz.	22.0	8.0
(*Nalley*), 7.5 oz.	8.0	4.0
(*Nalley* Real Hearty)	14.0	6.0
(*Old El Paso*), 1 cup	7.0	1.5
(*Van Camp's*), 1 cup	21.0	8.0
(*Wolf*), 1 cup	18.0	7.0
and cheddar cheese (*Nalley*), 7.5 oz.	12.0	6.0
chunky (*Hormel*), 1 cup	16.0	6.0
and frankfurters (*Nalley Chili Dog Chili*), 7.5 oz.	12.0	5.0
hot (*Hormel*), 1 cup	17.0	7.0
hot (*Hormel*), 7.5-oz. can	11.0	5.0
hot (*Hormel* Micro Cup), 1 cup	11.0	5.0
hot (*Nalley*), 7.5 oz.	8.0	4.0
and jalapeño (*Nalley*), 7.5 oz.	8.0	4.0
jalapeño style (*Wolf*), 1 cup	18.0	7.0
thick (*Nalley*), 7.5 oz.	9.0	4.0

w/out beans:

(*Hormel*), 1 cup	30.0	13.0
(*Hormel,* 7.5-oz. can	30.0	14.0
(*Hormel* Micro Cup), 1 cup	17.0	8.0
(*Libby's*), 1 cup	37.0	17.0
(*Nalley Big Chuck*), 7.5 oz.	14.0	7.0
(*Wolf*), 1 cup	30.0	12.0
hot (*Hormel*), 1 cup	30.0	13.0
jalapeño style (*Wolf*), 1 cup	30.0	12.0
and onion (*Nalley* Walla Walla), 7.5 oz.	15.0	7.0

	total fat (grams)	saturated fat (grams)
Chili, canned *(cont.)*		
w/macaroni (*Hormel* Chili Mac), 7.5-oz. can	9.0	4.0
w/macaroni (*Hormel* Micro Cup Chili Mac), 1 cup	9.0	4.0
turkey, w/or w/out beans (*Hormel*), 1 cup	3.0	1.0
vegetarian (see also specific listings):		
(*Natural Touch*), 1 cup	12.0	2.0
(*Worthington*), 1 cup	15.0	2.5
all varieties (*Health Valley* Fat Free), ½ cup	0	0
Chili, frozen:		
(*Stouffer's* Entree), 8¾ oz.	10.0	4.0
three bean, w/rice (*Lean Cuisine* Entree), 9 oz.	6.0	2.0
vegetarian, w/meatless meats (*Bodin's*), 8 oz.	1.5	0
vegetarian (*Tabatchnick*), 7.5 oz.	6.0	1.0
Chili, mix see also "Chili seasoning mix":		
(*Aunt Patsy's Pantry* Cowgirl), 1 cup	.5	0
(*Knorr* Four Bean), 1 pkg.	1.5	0
(*Tabasco* 7 Spice Recipe), regular or spicy, ½ cup	.7	.1
w/black beans (*Aunt Patsy's Pantry*), 1 cup	.5	0
w/black beans (*Buckeye*), ¼ pkg.	1.0	0
chicken (*Aunt Patsy's Pantry*), 1 cup	.5	0
chicken, white (*Buckeye*), ⅕ pkg.	1.0	0
lentil (*Aunt Patsy's Pantry*), 1 cup	1.0	0
lentil (*Buckeye* Rip Roar'n), ⅛ pkg.	1.0	0
spicy three-bean or vegetarian (*Spice Islands*), 1 pkg.	1.5	0
vegetarian (*Fantastic Foods*), about ⅛ cup	0	0
Chili beans, canned, ½ cup:		
all varieties (*Brooks*)	.5	0
all varieties, except Mexican (*Green Giant/Joan of Arc*)	1.0	0
Mexican (*Green Giant/Joan of Arc*)	1.5	0
Mexican style (*Van Camp's*)	2.0	.5
chili caliente dip mix (*Knorr*), ⅟₂₀ pkg.	0	0

	total fat (grams)	saturated fat (grams)

Chili entree, freeze-dried*

macaroni, w/beef (*Mountain House* Chili Mac), 1 cup	6.0	2.0
meatless (*AlpineAire* Mountain Chili), 1½ cups	2.0	n.a.
sauce, w/beans and beef (*Mountain House*), 1 cup	4.0	2.0

Chili entree, frozen, see "Chili, frozen"

Chili pepper, see "Pepper, chili"

Chili powder (see also "Chili seasoning mix"):

1 tbsp.	1.3	0
1 tsp.	.4	0
(*Spice Islands*), ¼ tsp.	0	0
all varieties (*Durkee*), ¼ tsp.	0	0

Chili sauce:

(*Del Monte*), 1 tbsp.	0	0
(*Heinz*), 1 tbsp.	0	0
(*Nance's*), 2 tbsp.	0	0
(*Wolf*), 1 tbsp.	1.0	0
red (*Las Palmas*), ¼ cup	.5	0

Chili seasoning mix (see also "Chili, mix"):

(*Durkee*), ⅕ pkg.	0	0
(*Durkee* Pot-O-Chili), ⅛ pkg.	0	0
(*French's Chili-O* Original), ⅕ pkg.	0	0
(*Lawry's* Spices & Seasonings), 1 tbsp.	.5	0
(*Lawry's* Tex-Mex Spices & Seasonings), 2 tbsp.	1.5	0
(*McCormick*), ⅛ pkg.	.5	0
(*Old El Paso*), 1 tbsp.	.5	0
mild (*Durkee*), ⅕ pkg.	.5	0
mild (*French's Chili-O*), ⅕ pkg.	.5	0
onion (*French's Chili-O*), ⅕ pkg.	0	0
Texas red (*Durkee*), ⅓ pkg.	1.0	0
Texas style (*French's Chili-O*), ⅕ pkg.	1.0	0

Chilies, see "Pepper, chili"

Chimichanga, frozen:

beef (*Old El Paso*), 1 piece	20.0	5.0
beef or chicken (*Schwan's*), 1 piece, 4 oz.	10.0	2.0

	total fat (grams)	saturated fat (grams)
Chimichanga, frozen *(cont.)*		
chicken (*Old El Paso*), 1 piece	16.0	4.0
Chimichanga dinner, frozen		
(*Banquet* Meals), 9.5 oz.	23.0	7.0
Chinese parsley, see "Coriander"		
chinese yam, see "Yam bean tuber"		
Chitterlings, pork:		
raw, 1 oz.	6.5	2.3
simmered, 4 oz.	32.6	11.5
Chives:		
fresh, 1 oz.	.2	<.1
fresh-cut, raw (*Frieda's*), 3.5 oz.	.3	n.a.
freeze-dried, ¼ cup	<.1	0
Chocolate, see "Candy"		
Chocolate, baking (see also "Cocoa"):		
(*Nestlé Choco-Bake*), .5 oz.	8.0	5.0
bar:		
bittersweet (*Ghirardelli*), 1.5 oz.	15.0	8.0
semisweet (*Baker's*), 1-oz. square	9.0	5.0
semisweet or sweet dark (*Ghirardelli*),		
1.5 oz.	14.0	8.0
semisweet or sweet dark (*Nestlé*), .5 oz.	4.0	2.5
sweet (*German's*), .5 oz., 2 squares	3.5	2.0
unsweetened (*Baker's*), 1-oz. square	14.0	9.0
unsweetened (*Ghirardelli*), 1.5 oz.	23.0	13.0
unsweetened (*Nestlé*), .5 oz.	7.0	2.0
white (*Baker's*), 1-oz. square	9.0	6.0
white (*Nestlé* Premier), .5 oz.	5.0	3.0
chips, chunks or morsels:		
cookie (*Guittard* Super), 10 pieces, about		
.5 oz.	4.5	2.5
milk (*Ghirardelli*), .5 oz., 2 tbsp.	4.0	2.0
milk (*Guittard* Maxi), 12 pieces, about .5 oz.	4.5	2.5
milk (*Nestlé* Morsels), 1 tbsp.	4.0	2.0
milk, real (*Baker's*), .5 oz., about 27 chips	4.0	2.0

	total fat (grams)	saturated fat (grams)
mint (*Andes* Creme de Menthe), 1.4 oz., 2 tbsp.	13.0	12.0
mint (*Nestlé* Morsels), 1 tbsp.	4.0	2.0
semisweet (*Ghirardelli*), .5 oz., 2 tbsp.	4.0	2.5
semisweet (*Guittard*), 30 pieces, about .5 oz.	4.0	2.5
semisweet (*Nestlé* Morsels), 1 tbsp.	4.0	2.0
semisweet, mini (*Nestlé* Morsels), 1 tbsp.	4.0	2.0
semisweet, flavored (*Baker's*), .5 oz., about 27 chips	3.0	3.0
semisweet, real (*Baker's*), .5 oz., about 27 chips	3.5	2.0
white, vanilla (*Ghirardelli*), .5 oz., 2 tbsp.	4.0	3.0
white, vanilla (*Guittard* Choc-Au-Lait), 30 pieces, about .5 oz.	5.0	4.0
Chocolate flavor drink (see also "chocolate milk"):		
canned, all flavors:		
(*Nestlé Sweet Success*), 10 fl. oz.	3.0	1.0
(*Sego* Very), 1 can	1.5	0
(*Sego* Lite Very), 1 can	3.0	n.a.
canned, milk, creamy (*Carnation* Instant Breakfast), 10 fl. oz.	2.5	1.0
refrigerated, milk, creamy (*Carnation*), 8 fl. oz.	3.0	2.0
Chocolate flavor drink mix (see also "Cocoa, hot, mix"), 1 pkt., except as noted:		
all flavors, except chocolate chip (*Nestlé Sweet Success*)	1.5	1.0
chocolate (*Nestlé Quik*), 2 tbsp.	.5	.5
chocolate (*Nestlé Quik* No Sugar Added), 2 tbsp.	1.0	.5
chocolate chip (*Nestlé Sweet Success*)	2.0	1.5
creamy milk (*Carnation* Instant Breakfast)	1.0	.5
regular or malt (*Pillsbury* Instant Breakfast)	0	0
malt (*Carnation* Instant Breakfast)	1.5	.5
malt (*Carnation* Instant Breakfast No Sugar)	1.5	1.0

	total fat (grams)	saturated fat (grams)

Chocolate flavor drink mix *(cont.)*
shake (*Weight Watchers*), .75 oz. 1.0 0
Chocolate milk (see also "Chocolate shake"), 8 fl.oz.:
(*Crowley*) . . . . 8.0 . . . . 5.0
(*Nestlé Quik*) . . . . 9.0 . . . . 5.0
lowfat (*Nestlé Quik*) . . . . 5.0 . . . . 3.0
lowfat, 1% (*Crowley*) . . . . 2.5 . . . . 2.0
lowfat, 2% (*Hershey's*) . . . . 4.5 . . . . 2.5
Chocolate pastry (see also specific listings),
    milk or dark (*Pepperidge Farm* Clouds),
    4.3 oz., 2 pieces . . . . 38.0 . . . . 15.0
Chocolate shake (*Nestlé Killer Shakes*), 1 carton . . . . 17.0 . . . . 10.0
Chocolate syrup (see also "Chocolate topping"):
    1 fl. oz., 2 tbsp. 3 2
    (*Hershey's* Syrup), 2 tbsp. 0 0
Chocolate topping, 2 tbsp.:
    (*Barbara's Chocolate Mountain* Sauce) . . . . 4.0 . . . . 3.0
    (*Hershey's* Chocolate Shoppe) . . . . 4.5 . . . . 2.0
    all varieties (*Smucker's Magic Shell*) . . . . 16.0 . . . . 6.0
    chocolate (*Kraft*) 0 0
    dark chocolate fudge (*Mrs. Richardson's*) . . . . 6.0 . . . . 5.0
    fudge (*Smucker's*) 1.5 5
    fudge, hot:
        (*Kraft*) . . . . 4.0 . . . . 2.0
        (*Mrs. Richardson's*) . . . . 6.0 . . . . 6.0
        (*Mrs. Richardson's* Fat Free) 0 0
        (*Smucker's*) . . . . 4.0 . . . . 1.0
        (*Smucker's* Light Fat Free) 0 0
Chops, vegetarian, see "Vegetarian dishes, canned"
Chorizo sausage:
    beef and pork, 1 oz. . . . . 10.9 . . . . n.a.
    (*Hillshire Farm*), 2 oz. . . . . 17.0 . . . . n.a.
    (*Hillshire Farm* Lower Fat), 2 oz. . . . . 11.0 . . . . n.a.
Chow mein, see "Beef entree" and "Chicken entree"
Chow mein noodles, see "Noodle, Chinese"

	total fat (grams)	saturated fat (grams)
Chow mein seasoning mix (*Kikkoman*), 1⅛ oz.	.8	n.a.
Chowder, see "Soup"		
Chrysanthemum garland:		
raw, 1" pieces, ½ cup	<.1	0
boiled, drained, 1" pieces, ½ cup	.1	0
Chub, see "Cisco, smoked"		
Churro, frozen (*Tio Pepe's*), 1 piece	5.0	1.5
Chutney, mango (*Genuine Sun Brand* Major Grey's),		
1 tbsp.	0	0
Cilantro, see "Coriander"		
Cinnamon:		
1 oz.	.9	.2
ground, 1 tbsp.	.2	<.1
Cinnamon sugar (*Durkee* Spices), ¼ tsp.	0	0
Cisco, meat only:		
raw, 4 oz.	2.2	.5
smoked, 4 oz.	13.5	2.0
Citrus drink, all varieties (*Ocean Spray Refreshers*),		
8 fl. oz.	0	0
Clam, meat only:		
fresh, mixed species:		
raw, 1 lb.	4.4	.4
raw, 9 large or 20 small, about 6.3 oz.	1.8	.2
boiled, poached, or steamed, 4 oz.	2.2	n.a.
Clam, canned:		
drained, 1 cup	3.1	.3
minced (*Progresso*), ¼ cup	0	0
minced or chopped, in juice (*Doxsee*), ¼ cup	0	0
Clam chowder, see "Soup"		
Clam dip, 2 tbsp.:		
(*Heluva* Good New England).	5.0	3.0
(*Kraft*)	4.0	3.0
(*Kraft* Premium)	4.0	2.5
(*Nalley*)	10.0	1.5

	total fat (grams)	saturated fat (grams)

Clam dip *(cont.)*
Chesapeake (*Breakstone's*) . . . . 4.0 . . . . 2.5
Clam entree, frozen, fried:
  (*Gorton's*), 3 oz., about 15 pieces . . . . 17.0 . . . . 4.0
  (*Mrs. Paul's*), 3 oz., about 28 pieces w/½ tsp.
    relish mix . . . . 16.0 . . . . 3.0
  breaded strips (*Schwan's*), 4 oz. . . . . 14.0 . . . . 1.5
Clam juice:
  1 cup 1 0
  (*Bookbinder's*), 1 can, 10.5 oz. 0 0
  (*Doxsee*), 1 tbsp. 0 0
Clam sauce, canned, ½ cup:
  red (*Progresso*) 3.0 5
  white:
    (*Progresso*) . . . . 9.0 . . . . 1.5
    (*Progresso* Authentic) . . . . 7.0 . . . . 1.9
    creamy (*Progresso*) . . . . 6.0 . . . . 1.5
    w/Romano cheese (*Bookbinder's*) . . . . 30.0 . . . . 5.0
Clover sprouts (*Jonathan's Sprouts*), 3 oz., 1 cup 5 0
Cloves, ground:
  1 tbsp. 1.3 3
  1 tsp. 4 1
Coating mix, see "Seasoning and coating mix" and
  specific listings
Cobbler, apple or blueberry, deep dish (*Awrey's*),
  ⅛ pkg. . . . . 14.0 . . . . 3.0
Cobbler, freeze-dried, apple-blueberry (*AlpineAire*),
  ½ cup . . . . 2.0 . . . . n.a.
Cobbler, frozen or refrigerated, 4 oz., ⅛ pkg.,
  except as noted:
  apple:
    (*Pet-Ritz*), ⅙ pkg. . . . . 12.0 . . . . 5.0
    (*Stilwell*) . . . . 9.0 . . . . 4.0
    (*Stilwell* Lite) . . . . 4.5 . . . . 1.0
    crumb (*Pet-Ritz*), ⅙ pkg. . . . . 9.0 . . . . 4.0

	total fat (grams)	saturated fat (grams)
apricot (*Stilwell*)	9.0	4.0
berry (*Stilwell* Festival)	9.0	4.0
berry (*Stilwell* Festival Lite)	4.5	1.0
blackberry:		
(*Stilwell*)	9.0	4.0
(*Stilwell* Lite)	4.5	1.0
(*Pet-Ritz*), ⅙ pkg.	11.0	4.0
crumb (*Pet-Ritz*), ⅙ pkg.	8.0	3.0
blueberry (*Pet-Ritz*), ⅙ pkg.	11.0	5.0
cherry:		
(*Pet-Ritz*), ⅙ pkg.	11.0	4.0
(*Stilwell*)	9.0	4.0
(*Stilwell* Lite)	4.5	1.0
crumb (*Pet-Ritz*), ⅙ pkg.	6.0	2.5
peach:		
(*Pet-Ritz*), ⅙ pkg.	9.0	3.0
(*Stilwell*)	9.0	4.0
(*Stilwell* Lite)	4.5	1.0
crumb (*Pet-Ritz*), ⅙ pkg.	7.0	3.0
strawberry (*Pet-Ritz*), ⅙ pkg.	9.0	3.0
strawberry (*Stilwell*)	9.0	4.0
Cocktail sauce (see also "Tartar sauce"), ¼ cup, except as noted:		
(*Del Monte* Seafood)	0	0
(*Gold's*), 1 tsp.	0	0
(*Heinz*)	0	0
(*Heluva* Good)	0	0
(*Kraft Sauceworks*)	.5	0
(*Nalley*)	0	0
regular or hot (*Dockside/Chelten House*), 1 tbsp.	0	0
regular or hot and spicy (*Bookbinder's*)	1.5	0
Cocoa, dry:		
(*Nestlé* Baking), 1 tbsp.	1.0	0
(*Weight Watchers*), .7 oz.	0	0
unsweetened (*Ghirardelli*), 1 heaping tbsp.	3.0	1.5

	total fat (grams)	saturated fat (grams)

Cocoa, dry *(cont.)*
sweet, chocolate and *(Ghirardelli)*, 2½ tbsp. ..... 1.5 .... 1.0
Cocoa hot mix (see also "Chocolate flavor drink mix"):
(Carnation No Sugar Added), 3 tbsp. 0 0
(Carnation 70 Calorie/Fat Free), 1 pkt. 0 0
chocolate:
French creme *(Nestlé* European Style), 3 tbsp. .. 1.0 .... 1.0
Irish creme *(Nestlé* European Style), 3 tbsp. .. 1.5 .... 1.5
milk or rich, w/ or w/out marshmallows
(Carnation) 3 tbsp. 1.0 0
rich, w/ or w/out marshmallows *(Nestlé)*,
1 pkt. 1.0 5
Swiss truffle *(Nestlé* European Style), 3 tbsp. .. 1.5 .... 1.0
Cocoa butter oil, 1 tbsp. .... 13.6 .... 8.1
Coconut:
in shell, 1 lb. .... 79.0 .... 70.0
shelled, 1 oz. .... 9.5 .... 8.4
shelled, shredded or grated, 1 cup not packed ... 26.8 .... 23.8
Coconut, dried, 2 tbsp., except as noted:
(Angel Flake Bag) .... 4.5 .... 4.0
(Angel Flake Can) .... 5.0 .... 4.5
(Baker's Premium Shred) .... 4.0 .... 4.0
(Durkee Famous) .... 6.0 .... 6.0
sweetened:
flaked, canned, ¼ cup .... 6.1 .... 5.4
flaked, packaged, 1 oz. .... 9.1 .... 8.1
shredded, 1 oz. .... 10.1 .... 8.9
cookie shred, ¼ cup .... 8.3 .... 7.3
toasted, 1 oz. .... 13.4 .... 11.8
Coconut bar, see "Fruit bars"
Coconut cream:
canned, sweetened, ¼ cup .... 13.1 .... 11.6
drink mix *(Coca Casa)*, 3 tbsp. .... 3.0 .... 3.0
Coconut milk, canned, 1 tbsp. .... 3.6 .... 3.2

	total fat (grams)	saturated fat (grams)
Coconut nectar (*R.W. Knudsen* Tropical Blends), 8 fl. oz.	5.0	n.a.
Coconut oil, 1 tbsp.	13.6	11.8
Cod, meat only, 4 oz. except as noted:		
Atlantic:		
raw	.8	.2
baked, broiled, or microwaved	1.0	.2
dried, salted, 1 oz.	.7	.1
Pacific, raw	.7	.1
Pacific, baked, broiled, or microwaved	.9	.1
Cod, canned, Atlantic, w/liquid, 11-oz. can	2.7	.5
Cod, frozen:		
fillets (*Schwan's*), 4 oz.	.5	0
Pacific, loins (*Peter Pan*), 4 oz., about 1 fillet	.5	0
Cod entree, frozen:		
battered (*Schwan's Battercrisp*), 2-oz. piece	7.0	1.0
lightly breaded (*Van de Kamp's*), 1 fillet	10.0	1.5
Cod liver oil, 1 tbsp.	13.6	3.1
Coffee:		
brewed, 6 fl. oz.	0	0
freeze-dried, all varieties (*Taster's Choice*), 1 cup	<1.0	0
instant, regular, 1 oz. powder	.1	<.1
Coffee, flavored, mix (see also "Cappuccino, iced"), 1 cup*, except as noted:		
all varieties (*Taster's Choice*), 1 tsp.	0	0
amaretto (*General Foods International Coffee*)	3.0	.5
cappuccino:		
(*Nescafé* Instant Authentic Unsweetened), 1 pkt.	2.5	.5
(*Nescafé* Instant Authentic Sweetened), 1 pkt.	1.5	.5
cinnamon (*Maxwell House*)	1.5	0
coffee (*Maxwell House*)	1.0	0
Italian (*General Foods International Coffee*)	1.5	.5
mocha (*Nescafé* Instant Authentic), 1 pkt.	2.0	.5

	total fat (grams)	saturated fat (grams)

Coffee, flavored, mix, cappuccino *(cont.)*

mocha, regular or decaffeinated

(*Maxwell House*) .... 2.5 .... 1.0

orange (*General Foods International Coffee*) ... 2.0 5

orange (*General Foods International Coffee Sugar Free*) 1.5 5

vanilla, regular or decaffeinated (*Maxwell House*) 1.0 0

chocolate, Viennese (*General Foods International Coffee*) .... 2.0 .... 1.0

Français (*General Foods International Coffee*) ..... 3.5 .... 1.0

French vanilla:

(*General Foods International Coffee*) 2.5 5

(*General Foods International Coffee Sugar Free*) 2.0 5

hazelnut Belgian (*General Foods International Coffee*) 2.0 5

Kahlua Cafe (*General Foods International Coffee*) 2.0 5

Suisse mocha:

(*General Foods International Coffee*) 2.5 5

(*General Foods International Coffee Sugar Free*) 2.0 5

decaffeinated (*General Foods International Coffee*) 3.0 5

decaffeinated (*General Foods International Coffee Sugar Free*) 1.5 5

Vienna:

(*General Foods International Coffee*) 2.5 5

(*General Foods International Coffee Sugar Free*) 1.5 5

Coffee flavored drink mix (*Carnation Instant Breakfast*), 1 pkt. 5 0

Coffee substitute, cereal grain (*Natural Touch Kaffree Roma*), 1 tsp. 0 0

	total fat (grams)	saturated fat (grams)

Coffee whitener, see "Creamer"

Cold cuts, see "Luncheon meat" and specific listings

Collard greens:

fresh:

raw, untrimmed, 1 lb.	.6	0
raw, chopped, ½ cup	<.1	0
boiled, drained, chopped, ½ cup	.5	0
canned (*Allens/Sunshine*), ½ cup	.5	0
frozen (*McKenzie's*), 1 cup	0	0

Cookie:

all varieties:

(*Archway* Fat Free), 1 oz.	0	0
(*Barbara's* Mini Fat Free), 1.1 oz., 6 pieces	0	0
(*Health Valley* Fat Free), 1 oz.	0	0

almond:

(*Archway* Crescents), .8 oz., 2 pieces	3.5	.5
(*Stella D'Oro* Breakfast Treats), 1 piece	4.0	n.a.
(*Stella D'Oro* Chinese Dessert), 1 piece	9.0	n.a.
(*Sunshine* Almond Crescents), 1.1 oz., 4 pieces	6.0	1.5
toast (*Stella D'Oro* Mandel), 1 piece	1.0	n.a.

animal crackers:

(*Barnum's Animals*), 1.1 oz., 12 pieces	4.0	.5
(*Sunshine*), 2-oz. pkg.	7.0	1.5
(*Tom's*), 1 oz.	3.0	1.0
candied (*Grandma's*), 5 pieces	6.0	4.0
cinnamon or vanilla (*Barbara's*), 1 oz., 8 pieces	5.0	2.5

anise:

(*Stella D'Oro* Anisette Sponge), 1 piece	1.0	n.a.
(*Stella D'Oro* Anisette Toast), 1 piece	1.0	n.a.
(*Stella D'Oro* Anisette Toast Jumbo), 1 piece	1.0	n.a.

apple:

(*Sunshine* Golden Fruit), .7-oz. piece	1.5	0

	total fat (grams)	saturated fat (grams)

Cookie, apple *(cont.)*

bar (*Newtons* Fat Free), 1 oz., 2 pieces	0	0
bar, Dutch (*Stella D'Oro*), 1 piece	3.0	n.a.
filled (*Little Debbie Apple Delights*), 1 pkg.	5.0	2.0
pastry (*Stella D'Oro* Low Sodium), 1 piece	2.5	n.a.
apple cinnamon (*Stella D'Oro* Fat Free Fruit Delight), 1 piece	0	0
apple cinnamon (*Tastykake* Bar), 1.5-oz. piece	7.0	1.5
apple and raisin (*Archway*), 1.1-oz. piece	4.5	1.0
apple and raisin (*Smart Snackers*), .75 oz.	2.0	.5
apricot filled (*Archway*), 1-oz. piece	4.0	1.0
apricot raspberry (*Pepperidge Farm*), 1.1 oz., 3 pieces	6.0	2.0
(*Archway* Bells and Stars), 3 pieces, about 1 oz.	7.0	1.5
(*Archway* Holiday Pak), 1.1 oz., 3 pieces	8.0	1.5
(*Archway* New Orleans Cake), 1-oz. piece	4.0	1.0
(*Archway* Old Fashioned Windmill), .75-oz. piece	4.0	.5
(*Archway* Party Treats), 1.1 oz., 3 pieces	7.0	2.0
(*Archway* Select Assortment), 3 pieces, about 1 oz.	6.0	1.5
(*Archway* Wedding Cakes), 1.1 oz., 3 pieces	8.0	1.5
arrowroot biscuit (*Nabisco National*), .2-oz. piece	.5	0
arrowroot biscuit (*Peek Freans*), 1.4 oz., 5 pieces	5.1	n.a.
biscotti:		
almond (*Pepperidge Farm*), 1.3-oz. piece	6.0	1.5
almond (*Pepperidge Farm* Caruso), .7-oz. piece	3.5	1.0
anise (*Pepperidge Farm* La Scala), .7-oz. piece	3.0	1.0
anise (*Pepperidge Farm*), 1.3-oz. piece	5.0	2.0
chocolate hazelnut (*Pepperidge Farm*), .7-oz. piece	5.0	1.0

	total fat (grams)	saturated fat (grams)
chocolate hazelnut (*Pepperidge Farm*), 1.3-oz. piece	9.0	2.0
cinnamon chip (*Pepperidge Farm*), .7-oz. piece	3.5	1.0
cinnamon chip (*Pepperidge Farm*) 1.3-oz. piece	6.0	2.0
cranberry pistachio (*Pepperidge Farm* Tosca), .7-oz. piece	3.0	1.0
cranberry pistachio (*Pepperidge Farm*), 1.3-oz. piece	6.0	2.0
biscotti, chocolate dipped:		
almond (*Pepperidge Farm* Figaro), .8-oz. piece	4.0	2.0
almond (*Pepperidge Farm*), 1.5-oz. piece	10.0	3.5
orange (*Pepperidge Farm*), .8-oz. piece	4.5	1.5
orange (*Pepperidge Farm*), 1.3-oz. piece	8.0	3.0
biscottini cashews (*Stella D'Oro*), 1 piece	5.5	n.a.
blueberry filled (*Archway*), 1-oz. piece	4.0	1.0
brown edge wafer (*Nabisco*), 1 oz., 5 pieces	6.0	1.5
brownie, large (*Pepperidge Farm*), 1.8 oz., 2 pieces	13.0	3.5
brownie chocolate nut (*Pepperidge Farm* Old Fashioned), 1.1 oz., 3 pieces	9.0	3.0
bourbon creme (*Peek Freans*), 1.4 oz., 3 pieces	8.0	n.a.
bran crunch (*Peek Freans*), 1.4 oz., 4 pieces	7.3	n.a.
butter/butter flavor:		
(*Peek Freans Petit Beurre*), 1.4 oz., 6 pieces	5.0	n.a.
(*Pepperidge Farm* Chessmen), 9 oz., 3 pieces	5.0	3.0
(*Pepperidge Farm* Médaillon au Beurre), 1.2 oz., 4 pieces	5.0	3.0
(*Sunshine* Mini Butter Enrobed), 1.1 oz., 15 pieces	8.0	4.5
assortment (*Pepperidge Farm* Toy Chest), .9 oz., 3 pieces	5.0	3.0

	total fat (grams)	saturated fat (grams)

Cookie *(cont.)*

butter pecan bites (*Barbara's* Small Indulgences),
1 oz., 6 pieces .... 8.0 .... 8.0

caramel (*Dare* Golden), 1 piece .... 3.0 .... 2.0

caramel cookie bar:

(*Little Debbie*), 1 pkg. .... 8.0 .... 1.5

(*Twix* Family), 1-oz. piece .... 7.0 .... 2.5

(*Twix* Fun Size), .6-oz. piece .... 4.0 .... 1.5

(*Twix* King Size), .9-oz. piece .... 6.0 .... 2.0

(*Twix* Singles), 2 oz., 2 pieces .... 14.0 .... 5.0

caramel pecan (*Pepperidge Farm* Soft Baked),
.9-oz. piece .... 7.0 .... 1.5

carrot cake (*Archway*), 1-oz. piece .... 5.0 .... 1.0

cherry cobbler (*Pepperidge Farm*), .6-oz piece .... 2.5 .... 1.0

cherry filled (*Archway*), 1-oz. piece .... 4.0 .... 1.0

cherry nougat (*Archway*), 1 oz., 3 pieces .... 9.0 .... 1.5

chocolate:

(*Archway* Dutch Cocoa), 1-oz. piece .... 4.0 .... 1.0

(*Pepperidge Farm* Goldfish), 1.5-oz. pouch ... 7.0 .... 2.5

(*Pepperidge Farm* Goldfish), 1.1 oz., 30 pieces .. 5.0 .... 1.5

(*Stella D'Oro* Castelets), 1 piece .... 3.0 .... n.a.

(*Stella D'Oro* Margherite), 1 piece .... 3.0 .... n.a.

(*Sunshine Tru Blu*), .6-oz. piece 3.5 5

bits (*Grandma's*), 9 pieces .... 8.0 .... 2.0

brownie (*Entenmann's* Fat Free), .8 oz.,
2 pieces 0 0

covered cracker (*Ritz*), 1 oz., 3 pieces .... 9.0 .... 5.0

dark (*Peek Freans*), 1.4 oz., 3 pieces .... 10.1 .... n.a.

fudge (*Dare*), 1 piece .... 4.2 .... 2.3

fudge brownie (*Eagle* Gourmet), 1 piece ...... 16.0 .... 5.0

fudge w/mint (*Grasshopper*), 1.1 oz., 4 pieces .. 7.0 .... 5.0

galore (*Dare*), 1 piece .... 4.0 .... 2.6

milk (*Peek Freans*), 1.4 oz., 3 pieces .... 10.4 .... n.a.

milk (*Pepperidge Farm* Bordeaux), 1.1 oz.,
3 pieces .... 9.0 .... 3.5

	total fat (grams)	saturated fat (grams)
milk, fudge (*Dare*), 1 piece	4.6	2.2
milk, toffee, mini (*Pepperidge Farm*), 2 oz.,		
9 pieces	14.0	5.0
w/nuts (*Pepperidge Farm Geneva*), 1.1 oz.,		
3 pieces	9.0	3.5
orange (*Pepperidge Farm* Chocolat a l'Orange),		
1.1 oz., 2 pieces	6.0	2.2
w/raisins (*Dare Sun-Maid*), 1 piece	3.0	.7
snaps (*Nabisco*), 1.1 oz., 7 pieces	5.0	2.0
wafers (*Nabisco Famous*), 1.1 oz., 5 pieces ...	4.0	1.5
chocolate chip/chunk:		
(*Archway* Bag), 1 oz., 3 pieces	7.0	2.0
(*Archway* Ice Box), 1-oz. piece	6.0	2.5
(*Archway* Super Pak), 1-oz. piece	6.0	1.5
(*Archway* Supreme), 1-oz. piece	4.5	1.5
(*Barbara's*), 1.3 oz., 2 pieces	7.0	1.5
(*Chips Ahoy!*), 1.1 oz., 3 pieces	8.0	2.5
(*Chips Ahoy! Reduced Fat*), 1.1 oz., 3 pieces ..	6.0	1.5
(*Dare*), 1 piece	3.3	1.1
(*Dare Breaktime*), 1 piece	1.7	.4
(*Drake's*), 1 oz., 2 pieces	7.0	2.5
(*Eagle*), 1 piece	8.0	2.5
(*Entenmann's*), 1.1 oz., 3 pieces	7.0	2.0
(*Famous Amos*), 1 oz., 3 pieces	6.0	n.a.
(*Grandma's* Big), 1.4-oz. piece	9.0	2.5
(*Grandma's* Rich N' Chewy), 1 pkg.	11.0	4.0
(*Keebler Chips Deluxe*), .5 oz, 1 piece	4.5	1.5
(*Keebler Chocolate Lovers Chip Deluxe*), .6 oz.,		
1 piece	5.0	2.5
(*Keebler* Soft Batch), .6 oz., 1 piece	3.5	1.0
(*Pepperidge Farm* Large), 1.8 oz., 2 pieces ...	11.0	3.5
(*Pepperidge Farm* Old Fashioned), 1 oz.,		
3 pieces	7.0	2.5
(*Pepperidge Farm Goldfish*), 1.1 oz., 19 pieces ..	7.0	2.5
(*Pepperidge Farm Nantucket*), .9-oz. piece	7.0	3.0

	total fat (grams)	saturated fat (grams)

Cookie, chocolate chip/chunk *(cont.)*

(*Schwan's*), 1-oz. piece	5.0	....	1.5
(*Smart Snackers*), 1.1 oz.	3.5	....	1.0
(*Snackwell's* Reduced Fat), .6-oz. piece	3.5	....	1.5
(*Sunshine Chip A Roos*), 1.3 oz., 3 pieces	10.0	....	3.5
(*Sunshine Classics*), .7-oz. piece	5.0	....	3.0
(*Tastykake* Bar), 1.5-oz. piece	8.0	....	2.0
(*Tastykake* Soft & Chewy), 2.8 oz., 2 pieces ..	14.0	....	4.0
chewy (*Chips Ahoy!*), 1.3 oz., 3 pieces	8.0	....	2.5
chocolate (*Barbara's*), 1.3 oz., 2 pieces	7.0	....	1.5
chocolate (*Pepperidge Farm* Soft Baked), .9-oz. piece	6.0	....	2.0
chocolate (*Tastykake* Soft & Chewy), 2.8 oz., 2 pieces	13.0	....	4.0
chocolate, large (*Pepperidge Farm*), 1.8 oz., 2 pieces	12.0	....	3.5
chocolate, walnuts (*Pepperidge Farm Beacon Hill*), .9-oz. piece	7.0	....	2.0
chunk (*Pepperidge Farm* Soft Baked), .9-oz. piece	6.0	....	2.5
chunky (*Chips Ahoy!*), .6-oz. piece	4.0	....	3.0
crisps (*Barbara's* Small Indulgences), 1 oz., 6 pieces	7.0	....	4.0
drop (*Archway*), 1-oz. piece	10.0	....	3.0
fudge (*Grandma's* Big), 1.4-oz. piece	6.0	....	2.0
macadamias (*Pepperidge Farm Sausalito*), .9-oz. piece	7.0	....	2.0
macadamias (*Pepperidge Farm* Soft Baked), .9-oz. piece	6.0	....	2.5
mini (*Chips Ahoy!* Bite Size), 1.1 oz. 14 pieces	7.0	....	2.5
mini (*Pepperidge Farm*), 2 oz., 9 pieces	14.0	....	5.0
mini (*Sunshine*), 1.1 oz., 5 pieces	8.0	....	3.0
pecan (*Famous Amos*), 1 oz., 3 pieces	8.0	....	n.a.

	total fat (grams)	saturated fat (grams)
pecan (*Pepperidge Farm* Chesapeake), .9-oz. piece	8.0	1.5
w/pecans (*Sunshine Classics*), .7-oz. piece	7.0	2.0
snaps (*Nabisco*), 1.1 oz., 7 pieces	5.0	1.5
sprinkled (*Chips Ahoy!*), 1.3 oz., 3 pieces	8.0	2.5
striped (*Chips Ahoy!*), .6-oz. piece	4.0	1.5
toffee (*Pepperidge Farm Charleston*), .9-oz. piece	7.0	2.5
and toffee (*Archway*), 1-oz. piece	7.0	1.5
w/walnuts (*Sunshine Classics*), .7-oz. piece	6.0	2.5
white chunk (*Pepperidge Farm Tahoe*), .9-oz. piece	7.0	3.0
chocolate sandwich:		
(*Elfin Delights*), .9-oz., 2 pieces	2.5	.5
(*E. L. Fudge*), 1.2 oz., 3 pieces	8.0	2.0
(*Famous Amos*), 3 pieces	8.0	2.0
(*Grandma's*), 3 pieces	5.0	1.5
(*Pepperidge Farm Brussels*), 1.1 oz., 3 pieces	7.0	3.0
(*Pepperidge Farm Lido*), .6-oz. piece	4.5	1.5
(*Pepperidge Farm Milano*), 1.2 oz., 3 pieces	10.0	3.5
(*Smart Snackers*), 1.1 oz.	3.5	1.0
creme (*Oreo*), 1.2 oz., 3 pieces	7.0	1.5
creme (*Oreo* Reduced Fat), 1.2 oz., 3 pieces	5.0	1.0
creme (*Oreo Double Stuf*), 1 oz., 2 pieces	7.0	1.5
creme (*Snackwell's* Reduced Fat), .9-oz., 2 pieces	2.5	.5
creme (*Sunshine Hydrox*), 1.1 oz., 3 pieces	7.0	2.0
creme (*Sunshine Hydrox* Reduced Fat), 1.1 oz., 3 pieces	4.0	1.0
creme, fudge (*Elfin Delights*), 1.2 oz., 3 pieces	3.5	1.0
creme, fudge or white fudge covered (*Oreo*), .75-oz. piece	6.0	1.5
double chocolate (*Pepperidge Farm Milano*), 1 oz., 2 pieces	8.0	3.0

	total fat (grams)	saturated fat (grams)

Cookie, chocolate sandwich *(cont.)*

hazelnut (*Pepperidge Farm Milano*), .9 oz.,
2 pieces .... 7.0 .... 2.0
mint (*Pepperidge Farm Brussels*), 1.3 oz.,
3 pieces .... 10.0 .... 3.5
mint (*Pepperidge Farm Milano*), .9-oz.,
2 pieces .... 8.0 .... 3.5
orange (*Pepperidge Farm Milano*), .9 oz.,
2 pieces .... 8.0 .... 2.5
cinnamon apple (*Archway*), 1-oz. piece 3.5 5
cinnamon chip (*Pepperidge Farm* Large), 1.8 oz.,
2 pieces .... 10.0 .... 2.5
cinnamon danish (*Dare*), 1 piece 1.8 4
coconut:
(*Dare* Breaktime), 1 piece 1.4 5
(*Drake's*), 1 oz., 2 pieces .... 6.0 .... 4.0
chocolate drop (*Keebler*), .6-oz. piece .... 5.0 .... 2.0
creme (*Dare*), 1 piece ...,............ 4.8 .... 1.6
macaroon (*Archway*), .8-oz. piece .... 5.0 .... 4.0
coffee cake crunch (*Barbara's* Small Indulgences),
1 oz., 6 pieces .... 6.0 .., 6.0
coffee creme (*Peek Freans*), 1.4 oz., 3 pieces .... 9.1 .... n.a.
cranberry (*Sunshine* Golden Fruit Low Fat), .7-oz.
piece 1.0 0
cranberry bar (*Newtons* Fat Free), 1 oz.,
2 pieces 0 0
creme sandwich (see also specific cookie listings),
all varieties (*Barbara's Cookies & Creme*),
.9-oz., 2 pieces .... 5.0 .... 4.0
Danish, imported (*Nabisco*), 1.2 oz., 5 pieces .... 8.0 .... 2.0
(*Dare* Harvest From the Rain Forest), 1 piece .... 4.0 .... 1.0
egg biscuit (see also "kitchel," below):
(*Stella D'Oro* Low Sodium), 3 pieces .... 3.0 .... n.a.
(*Stella D'Oro* Jumbo), 1 piece .... 1.0 .... n.a.
Roman (*Stella D'Oro*), 1 piece .... 5.0 .... n.a.
sugared (*Stella D'Oro*), 1 piece .... 1.0 .... n.a.

	total fat (grams)	saturated fat (grams)
fig bar:		
(*Fig Newtons*), 1.1 oz., 2 pieces	2.5	1.0
(*Little Debbie Figaroo*), 1.5 oz.	4.0	.5
(*Smart Snackers*), .7 oz.	0	0
(*Sunshine*), 2 pieces, 1 oz.	2.5	.5
(*Tom's*), 1.75 oz. piece	0	0
French creme (*Dare*), 1 piece	4.7	2.0
fruit (see also individual fruit cookies):		
bar, chewy (*Newtons* Fat Free), 1 oz., 2 pieces	0	0
cake (*Archway*), 1.1 oz., 3 piece	7.0	1.5
creme (*Peek Freans*), 1.4 oz., 3 pieces	8.6	n.a.
shortcake (*Peek Freans*), 1.4 oz., 3 pieces	8.5	n.a.
slices (*Stella D'Oro*), 1 piece	2.0	n.a.
slices (*Stella D'Oro* Fat Free), 1 piece	0	0
fruit and honey bar (*Archway*), 1-oz. piece	4.0	.5
fudge (see also "chocolate," above):		
(*Stella D'Oro* Swiss), 1 piece	3.0	n.a.
(*Tastykake* Bar), 1.5-oz. piece	7.0	2.0
brownie w/chocolate chips (*Eagle*), 1 piece	11.0	4.0
caramel peanut bar (*Heyday*), .8-oz. piece	5.0	1.0
deep night (*Stella D'Oro*), 1 piece	4.0	n.a.
nut bar (*Archway*), 1-oz. piece	4.5	1.0
nutty (*Grandma's* Big), 1.4-oz. piece	8.0	1.5
stripe creme pie (*Eagle*), 1 piece	12.0	4.0
fudge or devil's food cakes (*Snackwell's* Fat Free), 1 piece	0	0
garden creme (*Peek Freans*), 1.4 oz., 3 pieces	9.8	n.a.
ginger:		
(*Dare* Breaktime), 1 piece	1.1	.2
(*Drake's*), 1 oz., 2 pieces	3.0	1.0
(*Eagle* Gourmet), 1 piece	3.5	1.0
(*Little Debbie*), ¾ oz.	3.0	.5
(*Pepperidge Farm* Gingerman), 1 oz., 4 pieces	3.5	1.0
crisps (*Peek Freans*), 1.4 oz., 5 pieces	4.5	n.a.

	total fat (grams)	saturated fat (grams)

Cookie, ginger *(cont.)*

snaps (*Archway*), 1.1 oz., 5 pieces	5.0	1.0
snaps (*Nabisco* Old Fashioned), 1 oz., 4 pieces ..	2.5	.5
snaps (*Sunshine*), 1 oz., 7 pieces	4.5	1.0

gingerbread, iced:

(*Archway*), 1.1 oz., 3 pieces	5.0	1.0
(*Sunshine*), 1.4 oz., 5 pieces	6.0	.3

golden bar (*Stella D'Oro*), 1 piece .... 4.0 .... n.a.

graham cracker:

(*Bugs Bunny*), 1.1 oz., 10 pieces	5.0	1.0
(*Keebler Selects* Original), 1 oz., 8 pieces	3.0	1.0
(*Nabisco* Original), 1 oz., 8 pieces	3.0	.5
(*Pepperidge Farm Goldfish*), 1.1 oz., 19 pieces ..	7.0	2.5
(*Sunshine Grahamy Bears*), 1.1 oz., 10 pieces ..	5.0	1.0
amaranth (*Health Valley*), 1 oz., 6 pieces	3.0	0
apple cinnamon (*Keebler Selects*), 1 oz., 8 pieces	3.0	1.0
chocolate (*Bugs Bunny*), 1.1 oz., 13 pieces ...	5.0	1.0
chocolate (*Keebler Selects*), 1.1 oz., 8 pieces ...	5.0	1.5
chocolate (*Nabisco*), 1.1 oz., 3 pieces	8.0	5.0
chocolate (*Teddy Grahams* Snacks), 1.1 oz., 24 pieces	5.0	1.0
cinnamon (*Bugs Bunny*), 1.1 oz., 13 pieces ...	4.5	.5
cinnamon (*Honey Maid*), 1.2 oz., 10 pieces ...	3.0	.5
cinnamon (*Snackwell's* Fat Free), 1.1 oz., 30 pieces	0	0
cinnamon (*Sunshine*), 1.1 oz., 2 pieces	6.0	1.5
cinnamon (*Pepperidge Farm Goldfish*), 1.1 oz., 19 pieces	7.0	2.5
cinnamon crisp (*Keebler Selects*), 1.1 oz., 8 pieces	5.0	1.0
cinnamon crisp (*Keebler Selects* Low Fat), 1.1 oz., 9 pieces	1.5	.5
cinnamon or honey (*Teddy Grahams* Snacks), 1.1 oz., 24 pieces	4.0	1.0

	total fat (grams)	saturated fat (grams)
fudge covered (*Nabisco* Family Favorites), 1 oz., 3 pieces	7.0	1.5
fudge-dipped (*Sunshine*), 1.2 oz., 4 pieces	9.0	6.0
honey (*Honey Maid*), 1 oz., 8 pieces	3.0	.5
honey (*Keebler Selects*), 1.1 oz., 8 pieces	6.0	1.5
honey (*Keebler Selects* Low Fat), 1.1 oz., 9 pieces	1.5	.5
honey (*Sunshine*), 1 oz., 2 pieces	4.0	1.0
honey, w/amaranth (*New Morning*), 1 piece	1.5	0
oat or rice bran (*Health Valley*), 1 oz., 6 pieces	3.0	0
peanut butter (*Frito-Lay*), 1 pkg.	9.0	2.5
vanilla (*Frito-Lay*), 1 pkg.	11.0	2.5
w/vanilla frosting (*Betty Crocker*), 1 oz.	4.5	1.5
whole wheat (*New Morning*), 1.1 oz., 2 pieces	3.0	0
hazelnut (*Pepperidge Farm* Old Fashioned), 1.1 oz., 3 pieces	8.0	2.0
hermits (*Archway* Cookie Jar), 1-oz. piece	3.0	.5
holiday tub (*Tastykake*), 1.1 oz., 4 pieces	8.0	1.5
kichel, egg (*Stella D'Oro* Low Sodium), 21 pieces	9.0	n.a.
lemon:		
(*Archway* Frosty), 1-oz. piece	5.0	1.0
(*Drake's*), 1 oz., 2 pieces	5.0	1.5
(*Sunshine* Lemon Coolers), 1.1 oz., 5 pieces	6.0	1.5
(*Sunshine* Tru Blu), 1 piece	3.5	.5
almond delights (*Barbara's* Small Indulgences), 1 oz., 6 pieces	6.0	6.0
bits (*Grandma's*), 9 pieces	6.0	2.5
creme (*Dare*), 1 piece	4.1	1.1
creme sandwich (*Eagle*), 6 pieces	11.0	2.5
drop (*Archway*), 1-oz. piece	3.5	.5
nut, mini (*Pepperidge Farm*), 2 oz., 9 pieces	18.0	9.0

	total fat (grams)	saturated fat (grams)

Cookie, lemon *(cont.)*

nut crunch (*Pepperidge Farm*), 1.1 oz., 3 pieces	9.0	2.0
macadamia coconut (*Eagle* Gourmet), 1 piece	16.0	5.0
maple leaf creme (*Dare*), 1 piece	3.6	.9
maple walnut fudge (*Dare*), 1 piece	4.6	3.0

marshmallow:

(*Mallomars*), .9 oz., 2 pieces	5.0	3.0
(*Pinwheels*), 1.1-oz. piece	5.0	2.5
(*Sunshine* Mallo Puff), 1 piece	2.0	1.5
cake (*Dare Belmont Mallow*), 1 piece	2.8	2.0
fudge cake (*Nabisco* Twirls), 1.1-oz. piece	6.0	1.5
fudge puff (*Nabisco* Puffs), .75-oz. piece	4.0	1.0

mint:

(*Dare* Midnight Mint), 1 piece	4.0	2.3
(*Sunshine* Enrobed Mint Patties), .85 oz., 2 pieces	7.0	3.5
sandwich (*Mystic Mint*), .6-oz. piece	4.0	1.0

molasses:

(*Archway*), 1-oz. piece	3.5	.5
(*Archway* Old Fashioned), 1-oz. piece	3.0	1.0
(*Grandma's* Big), 1.4-oz. piece	4.0	1.0
dark (*Archway*), 1-oz. piece	3.5	.5
crisps (*Pepperidge Farm* Old Fashioned), 1.1 oz., 5 pieces	6.0	1.5
iced (*Archway*), 1-oz. piece	4.0	1.0
iced (*Archway* Super Pak), 1-oz. piece	3.5	1.0
soft drop (*Archway*), 1-oz. piece	3.5	1.0
mud pie (*Archway*), 1-oz. piece	4.0	1.0
nutty nougat (*Archway*), 1.1 oz., 3 pieces	10.0	2.0

oatmeal:

(*Archway*), 1 piece, about 1 oz.	3.0	1.0
(*Archway Ruth's Golden*), 1-oz. piece	5.0	1.0
(*Dare* Breaktime), 1 piece	1.3	.2
(*Dare Oats Up!*), 1 piece	2.9	.5

	total fat (grams)	saturated fat (grams)
(*Drake's*), 1 oz., 2 pieces	5.0	1.5
(*Nabisco* Family Favorites), .6-oz. piece	3.0	.5
(*Peek Freans* Traditional), 1.4 oz., 2 pieces	6.2	n.a.
(*Pepperidge Farm* Irish), 1 oz., 3 pieces	6.0	1.5
(*Pepperidge Farm* Large), 1.8 oz., 2 pieces	9.0	2.0
(*Ruth's*), 1-oz. piece	4.5	1.0
(*Sunshine* Country Style), 1.2 oz., 3 pieces	7.0	1.5
butterscotch (*Pepperidge Farm* Old Fashioned), 1.2 oz., 3 pieces	9.0	3.0
iced (*Archway*), 1-oz. piece	5.0	1.0
iced (*Sunshine*), .9 oz., 2 pieces	5.0	1.0
apple filled (*Archway*), 1-oz. piece	3.0	.5
apple spice (*Grandma's* Big), 1.4-oz. piece	6.0	1.5
w/chocolate chips (*Sunshine*), 1.3 oz., 3 pieces	8.0	3.0
chocolate chip or raisin (*Entenmann's* Fat Free), 2 pieces	0	0
creme pie (*Eagle*), 1 piece	12.0	3.0
date filled (*Archway*), 1-oz. piece	4.0	1.0
iced (*Eagle*), 1 piece	5.0	1.0
pecan (*Archway*), 1-oz. piece	5.0	1.5
sandwich, coconut (*Famous Amos*), 3 pieces	7.0	2.0
sandwich, peanut butter or vanilla (*Famous Amos*), 3 pieces	7.0	1.5
oatmeal raisin (see also "raisin oatmeal," below):		
(*Archway*), 1-oz. piece	4.0	1.0
(*Barbara's*), 1.3 oz., 2 pieces	7.0	.5
(*Dare*), 1 piece	2.7	.7
(*Eagle* Gourmet), 1 piece	17.0	4.0
(*Pepperidge Farm* Old Fashioned), 1.2 oz., 3 pieces	6.0	1.5
(*Pepperidge Farm* Santa Fe), .9 oz-piece	4.5	1.0
(*Pepperidge Farm* Soft Baked), .9-oz. piece	4.0	1.0
(*Smart Snackers*), 1.1 oz.	2.0	0
(*Snackwell's* Reduced Fat), .9 oz., 2 pieces	2.5	0

	total fat (grams)	saturated fat (grams)

Cookie, oatmeal raisin *(cont.)*

(*Tastykake* Bar), 1.5-oz. piece	7.0	1.5
(*Tastykake* Soft & Chewy), 2.8 oz., 2 pieces	14.0	2.5
bran (*Archway*), 1-oz. piece	3.5	1.0
cinnamon (*Famous Amos*), 1 oz., 3 pieces	6.0	n.a.
mini (*Pepperidge Farm*), 2 oz., 9 pieces	10.0	2.5
peach tart (*Pepperidge Farm*), 1.1 oz., 2 pieces	3.0	1.0

peach-apricot:

(*Stella D'Oro* Fruit Delight), 1 piece	0	0
(*Stella D'Oro* Sodium Free), 1 piece	3.0	n.a.
peanut jumble (*Archway*), 1-oz. piece	7.0	1.5

peanut butter:

(*Archway*), 1-oz. piece	7.0	1.5
(*Archway* Ol' Fashion), 1-oz. piece	6.0	1.0
(*Dare* Delites), 1 piece	4.0	2.4
(*Drake's*), 1 oz., 2 pieces	6.0	1.0
(*Grandma's* Big), 1.4-oz. piece	9.0	2.0
bar (*Eagle*), 1 piece	10.0	3.0
bar (*Grandma's*), 1 pkg.	9.0	2.5
bar, chunky (*Tastykake*), 1.5-oz. piece	11.0	3.0
bits (*Grandma's*), 9 pieces	6.0	1.5
chip (*Dare*), 1 piece	2.9	.7
and chips (*Archway*), 1-oz. piece	7.0	1.5
chocolate chip (*Eagle* Gourmet), 1 piece	20.0	6.0
chocolate chip (*Grandma's* Big), 1.4-oz. piece	10.0	3.0
creme patties (*Nutter Butter*), 1.1 oz., 5 pieces	9.0	1.5
milk, mini (*Pepperidge Farm*), 2 oz., 9 pieces	15.0	7.0
wafer (*Sunshine*), 1.1 oz., 4 pieces	9.0	2.0

peanut butter sandwich:

(*Grandma's*), 5 pieces	9.0	2.0
(*Nutter Butter*), 1 oz., 2 pieces	6.0	1.0
(*Nutter Butter* Bites), 1.1 oz., 10 pieces	7.0	1.5
and graham (*Eagle*), 6 pieces	10.0	2.5

pecan:

(*Archway* Ice Box), 1-oz. piece	7.0	1.5

	total fat (grams)	saturated fat (grams)
(*Pecan Sandies*), .6 oz., 1 piece	5.0	1.0
(*Pecan Sandies* Low Fat), .5-oz. piece	3.0	.5
crunch (*Archway*), 1.1 oz., 6 pieces	8.0	2.0
ice box (*Archway*), 1-oz. piece	8.0	1.5
mini (*Pepperidge Farm* Scotties), 2 oz., 9 pieces	17.0	7.0
(*Peek Freans* Delectable), 1.4 oz., 2 pieces	8.1	n.a.
(*Peek Freans* Nice), 1.4 oz., 5 pieces	6.6	n.a.
(*Peek Freans* Sweetmeal), 1.4 oz., 5 pieces	8.5	n.a.
(*Pepperidge Farm* Biarritz), 1.1 oz., 6 pieces	8.0	4.0
(*Pepperidge Farm* Espirit Blanc), .6-oz. piece	4.5	2.5
(*Pepperidge Farm* Espirit Noir), .6-oz. piece	5.0	3.5
pfeffernusse, see "spice," below		
pound cake cookie (*Aunt Bea's*), .9-oz. piece	4.0	1.0
prune pastry (*Stella D'Oro* Sodium Free), 1 piece	3.0	n.a.
raisin (*Sunshine* Golden Fruit), .7-oz. piece	1.5	0
raisin oatmeal (*Archway* Bag), 1 oz., 3 pieces	6.0	1.5
raisin oatmeal (*Dare Sun-Maid*), 1 piece	2.5	.5
raspberry:		
(*Stella D'Oro* Fat Free Fruit Delight), 1 piece	0	0
bar (*Newtons* Fat Free), 1 oz., 2 pieces	0	0
filled (*Archway*), 1-oz. piece	4.0	1.0
filled (*Pepperidge Farm* Linzer), .8-oz. piece	4.0	1.0
filled (*Smart Snackers*), .7 oz.	0	0
filled, hazelnut (*Pepperidge Farm* Chantilly), .8-oz. piece	3.0	.5
shortcake (*Tom's*), 2 oz.	1.5	.5
rocky road (*Archway*), 1-oz. piece	4.5	1.0
sandwich, see specific cookie listings		
sesame (*Stella D'Oro* Regina), 1 piece	2.0	n.a.
shortbread:		
(*Lorna Doone*), 1 oz., 4 pieces	7.0	1.0
(*Pepperidge Farm* Highland), 1 oz., 2 pieces	7.0	5.0

	total fat (grams)	saturated fat (grams)

Cookie, shortbread *(cont.)*

(*Pepperidge Farm* Old Fashioned), .9 oz.,
    2 pieces .... 7.0 .... 2.5
almond, mini (*Pepperidge Farm*), 2 oz.,
    9 pieces .... 17.0 .... 7.0
butter (*Dare*), 1 piece .... 3.7 .... 1.5
w/chocolate (*Keebler Sweet Spots*), 1 pkg. .... 6.0 .... 3.0
fudge coated (*Keebler Fudge 'n Caramel*),
    .8 oz., 2 pieces .... 6.0 .... 4.0
fudge striped (*Nabisco Family Favorites*), 1.1
    oz., 3 pieces .... 8.0 .... 1.5
fudge striped (*Sunshine*), 1.1 oz., 3 pieces ... 9.0 .... 5.0
pecan (*Pecan Passion*), .6-oz. piece .... 5.0 .... 1.0
pecan (*Pepperidge Farm* Old Fashioned), .9 oz.,
    2 pieces .... 9.0 .... 2.5
shortcake (*Peek Freans*), 1.4 oz., 3 pieces .... 9.6 .... n.a.
spice:
    (*Archway* Pfeffernusse), 1.3 oz., 2 pieces 1.0 0
    drops (*Stella D'Oro* Pfeffernusse), 1 piece .... 1.0 .... n.a.
    (*Stella D'Oro Angel Bars*), 1 piece .... 5.0 .... n.a.
    (*Stella D'Oro Angel Wings*), 1 piece .... 5.0 .... n.a.
    (*Stella D'Oro Angelica Goodies*), 1 piece ..... 4.0 .... n.a.
    (*Stella D'Oro Anginette*), 1 piece .... 1.0 .... n.a.
    (*Stella D'Oro Como Delights*), 1 piece .... 7.0 .... n.a.
strawberry:
    (*Pepperidge Farm*), 1.1 oz., 3 pieces .... 5.0 .... 2.0
    bar (*Newtons* Fat Free), 1 oz., 2 pieces 0 0
    filled (*Archway*), .9-oz. piece .... 3.5 .... 1.0
    filled (*Archway*), 1-oz. piece .... 4.0 .... 1.0
sugar:
    (*Archway*), 1-oz. piece .... 4.0 .... 1.0
    (*Biscos* Waffle Cremes), 1.2 oz., 4 pieces .... 9.0 .... 2.0
    (*Dare*), 1 piece 1.4 2
    (*Pepperidge Farm*), 1.1 oz., 3 pieces .... 6.0 .... 1.5
    (*Pepperidge Farm* Large), 1.8 oz., 2 pieces ... 10.0 .... 2.5

	total fat (grams)	saturated fat (grams)
soft (*Archway*), 1-oz. piece	4.0	1.0
wafer (*Biscos*), 1 oz., 8 pieces	6.0	1.5
wafer, chocolate (*Sunshine*), .9 oz., 3 pieces	7.0	2.0
wafer, vanilla (*Sunshine*), .9 oz., 3 pieces	6.0	1.5
wafer, vanilla (*Tastykake*), 1.1 oz., 5 pieces	10.0	2.0
tea biscuit:		
(*Dare* Social Tea), 1 piece	1.0	.2
(*Social* Tea), 1 oz., 6 pieces	4.0	.5
rich (*Peek Freans*), 1.4 oz., 5 pieces	6.2	n.a.
toffee (*Toffee Sandies*), .9 oz., 2 pieces	7.0	2.0
vanilla:		
(*Pepperidge Farm* Bordeaux), 1 oz., 4 pieces	5.0	2.5
(*Pepperidge Farm* Goldfish), 1.5-oz. pouch	10.0	3.5
(*Pepperidge Farm* Goldfish), 1.1 oz., 19 pieces	7.0	2.5
(*Stella D'Oro* Margherite), 1 piece	3.0	n.a.
(*Sunshine* Dixie Vanilla), .9 oz., 2 pieces	4.5	1.0
(*Sunshine Tru Blue*), .6-oz. piece	3.5	.5
bits (*Grandma's*), 9 pieces	7.0	1.5
chocolate-laced (*Pepperidge Farm* Pirouettes), 1.2 oz., 5 pieces	10.0	2.5
chocolate nut coated (*Pepperidge Farm* Geneva), 1.1 oz., 3 pieces	9.0	3.5
raspberry tart (*Pepperidge Farm* Wholesome Choice), 1.1 oz., 2 pieces	3.0	1.0
wafer (*Archway*), 1.1 oz., 5 pieces	4.0	1.0
wafer (*Keebler*), 1.1 oz., 8 pieces	7.0	2.0
(*Keebler* Lowfat), 1.1 oz., 8 pieces	3.5	.5
wafer (*Nilla*), 1.1 oz., 8 pieces	5.0	1.0
vanilla sandwich:		
(*Cameo* Creme), 1 oz., 2 pieces	5.0	1.0
(*Cookie Break*), 1.1 oz., 3 pieces	6.0	1.5
(*Eagle* Creme), 6 pieces	11.0	2.5
(*Elfin Delights*), .9 oz., 2 pieces	2.5	.5
(*Grandma's*), 5 pieces	9.0	2.5
(*Keebler* French Creme), .6-oz. piece	3.5	1.0

	total fat (grams)	saturated fat (grams)

Cookie, vanilla sandwich *(cont.)*

    (*Nabisco* Family Favorites), 1.2 oz., 3 pieces .. 8.0 .... 1.5

    (*Peek Freans* French), 1.4 oz., 3 pieces ...... 10.3 .... n.a.

    (*Smart Snackers*), 1.1 oz. .... 3.0 .... 1.0

    (*Snackwell's* Reduced Fat), .9 oz., 2 pieces ... 2.5 5

    (*Sunshine Vienna Fingers*), 1 oz., 2 pieces .... 6.0 .... 1.5

    (*Sunshine Vienna Fingers* Reduced Fat), 1 oz.,

        2 pieces 3.5 5

    wafer (see also specific cookie listings):

    (*Dare*), 1 piece 6 2

    (*Sunshine*), 1.1 oz., 7 pieces .... 7.0 .... 1.5

    fudge coated (*Keebler* Fudge Sticks), 1 oz.,

        3 pieces .... 8.0 .... 4.5

    sandwich, strawberry or vanilla (*Grandma's*),

        1 pkg. .... 8.0 .... 2.0

    walnut, black, ice box (*Archway*), .8-oz. piece .... 6.0 .... 1.5

Cookie crumbs, see "Pie crust or shell"

Cookie, frozen or refrigerated, dough:

    candy (*Pillsbury*), 1 oz. .... 6.0 .... 2.0

    chocolate chip (*Mrs. Goodcookie*), .9 oz.,

        2 pieces .... 6.0 .... 2.0

    chocolate chip or chocolate chocolate chip

        (*Pillsbury*), 1 oz. .... 6.0 .... 1.5

    dinosaurs (*Pillsbury*), 1 oz., 2 pieces .... 5.0 .... 1.5

    holiday (*Pillsbury*), 1 oz., 2 pieces .... 7.0 .... 2.0

    oatmeal chocolate chip (*Pillsbury*), 1 oz. .... 6.0 .... 1.5

    peanut butter (*Pillsbury*), 1 oz. .... 5.0 .... 1.0

    sugar (*Pillsbury*), 1.1 oz., 2 pieces .... 5.0 .... 1.5

    teddy bears (*Pillsbury*), 1 oz., 2 pieces .... 5.0 .... 1.0

Cookie, mix, see "Brownie mix" and "Dessert bars"

Cooking sauce (see also specific sauce listings),

    in jars, ½ cup:

    broccoli, creamy (*Campbell's Simmer Chef*) .... 8.0 .... 3.0

    cacciatore (*Campbell's Simmer Chef*) .... 4.0 .... 1.0

    country French (*Ragu Chicken Tonight*) .... 10.0 .... 1.5

	total fat (grams)	saturated fat (grams)
dopiaza (*Patak's*)	6.0	0
honey mustard, golden (*Campbell's Simmer Chef*)	2.0	0
jalfrezi (*Patak's*)	10.0	3.0
mushroom, creamy (*Campbell's Simmer Chef*)	9.0	2.0
saag (*Patak's*)	11.0	1.0
stir-fry, see "Stir-fry sauce"		
Stroganoff, family style (*Campbell's Simmer Chef*)	7.0	5.0
sweet and sour (*Ragu Chicken Tonight*)	0	0
sweet and sour, Oriental (*Campbell's Simmer Chef*)	1.0	0
Cone, ice cream, see "Ice cream cone and cup"		
Coriander:		
fresh, untrimmed, 1 lb.	2.3	n.a.
fresh, trimmed, 9 plants, about .8 oz.	.1	0
dried, crumbled leaf, 1 tbsp.	.1	0
Coriander seeds, 1 tbsp.	.9	.1
Corkscrew pasta mix, w/creamy garlic (*Golden Grain Noodle Roni*), 1 cup∗	25.0	6.0
Corn, fresh:		
raw, in husks, 1 lb.	1.9	.3
raw, kernels from 3.2-oz. ear	1.1	.2
raw, cut kernels, ½ cup	.9	.1
boiled, drained, cut kernels, ½ cup	1.1	.2
Corn, canned, ½ cup, except as noted:		
kernel:		
(*Green Giant Niblets*), ⅓ cup	0	0
(*Seneca*)	0	0
(*Seneca* Natural Pack)	1.0	0
gold or white (*Stokely*)	1.0	0
golden (*Del Monte* Supersweet / Vacuum Pack)	1.0	0
sweet (*Green Giant*), ⅓ cup	1.0	0
sweet (*Green Giant* 50% Less Salt), ⅓ cup	0	0
vacuum-pack	.5	.1

	total fat (grams)	saturated fat (grams)
Corn, canned, kernel *(cont.)*		
white (*Del Monte*)	0	0
white, shoepeg (*Green Giant*), ⅓ cup	1.0	0
whole kernel, sweet (*Green Giant*)	1.0	0
whole kernel, sweet (*Green Giant 50% Less Salt*)	1.0	0
w/peppers (*Green Giant Mexicorn*), ⅓ cup	0	0
cream style:		
(*Green Giant*)	1.0	0
(*Seneca*)	0	0
(*Stokely*)	1.0	0
golden (*Del Monte*)	.5	0
white (*Del Monte*)	0	0
Corn, dried:		
toasted (*John Cope's*), ¼ cup	1.0	0
freeze-dried (*AlpineAire*), ½ cup*	1.0	0
freeze-dried (*Mountain House*), ½ cup*	1.0	0
Corn, frozen:		
on cob:		
(*Green Giant Nibblers*), 1 ear	.5	0
(*Green Giant Niblets*), 1 ear	1.5	0
(*John Cope's*), 1 ear	1.5	0
(*Ore-Ida*), 1 ear	2.5	0
(*Ore-Ida Mini Gold*), 1 ear	1.0	0
(*Schwan's*), 1 ear	2.0	1.0
extra sweet (*Green Giant*), 1 ear	2.0	0
kernel:		
(*Green Giant Harvest Fresh Niblets*), ⅔ cup	.5	0
(*Green Giant Niblets*), ⅔ cup	.5	0
(*Schwan's*), ⅔ cup	1.0	0
(*Stilwell*), ⅔ cup	1.0	0
white, extra sweet (*Green Giant*), ⅔ cup	.5	0
white (*John Cope's*), ⅓ cup	.5	0
white shoepeg (*Green Giant*), ½ cup	1.0	0

	total fat (grams)	saturated fat (grams)
white shoepeg (*Green Giant Harvest Fresh*), ½ cup	.5	0
cream style:		
(*Green Giant*), ½ cup	1.0	0
white (*John Cope's* Sweet n' Creamy), ⅓ cup	2.5	1.5
in butter sauce:		
(*Green Giant* One Serving), 4.5 oz.	2.0	1.0
(*Green Giant Niblets*), ⅔ cup	3.0	1.5
white shoepeg (*Green Giant*), ¾ cup	2.5	1.5
Corn, combinations, frozen, ⅔ cup:		
w/peas (*John Cope's* Vegetable Blend)	1.0	0
w/zucchini and pepper (*John Cope's* Fiesta)	1.0	0
Corn, whole grain:		
1 oz.	1.3	.2
1 cup	7.9	1.1
Corn bran, crude:		
1 oz.	.3	<.1
1 cup	.7	.1
Corn bread, see "Bread" and "Bread, mix"		
Corn chips, puffs, and similar snacks:		
(*Barbara's Pinta* Chips), 1 oz., 13 pieces	6.0	1.5
(*Brewer's Yeast Kettle Poppins*), 1 oz.	8.0	1.0
(*Eagle* Baked Shamu Shapes), 1 cup	10.0	2.0
(*Fritos* Original), 1 oz., 32 pieces	10.0	1.5
(*Fritos* Crisp N' Thin), 1 oz., 17 pieces	10.0	2.0
(*Fritos* Dip Size), 1 oz., 12 pieces	10.0	1.5
(*Fritos* Scoops), 1 oz., 10 pieces	9.0	1.5
(*Fritos* Wild N' Mild), 1 oz., 28 pieces	10.0	1.5
(*Garden of Eatin'* Cantina Chips), 1 oz.	5.0	.5
(*Garden of Eatin' Topopos* Cantina Chips), 1 oz.	5.0	.5
(*Kettle* Chips Light Salt /No Salt), 1 oz.	9.0	1.0
(*Planters*), 1 oz.	10.0	1.5
(*Tom's* Light Bugles), .75 oz.	2.0	0

	total fat (grams)	saturated fat (grams)

Corn chips, puffs, and similar snacks *(cont.)*

all varieties:

   (*Barbara's Amazing Bakes*), 1 oz.,

      24 pieces 1.0 0

   (*Kettle Chips Tia*), 1 oz. 6.0 5

   (*Sunchips*), 1 oz. . . . . 7.0 . . . . 1.0

bacon cheddar (*Tom's* Fries), 1 oz. . . . . 4.5 . . . . 1.5

baked (*Garden of Eatin' California Bakes*), 1 oz. . . . 1.0 0

baked, yogurt and green onion or hot and smoky

   (*Garden of Eatin' California Bakes*), 1 oz. . . . 2.0 0

barbecue (*Tom's Skinny Snacks*), .75 oz. . . . . 2.5 . . . . 1.0

barbecue or chili cheese (*Fritos*), 1 oz.,

   29 pieces . . . . 10.0 . . . . 1.5

blue corn:

   (*Barbara's*), 1 oz., 15 pieces . . . . 7.0 . . . . <1.0

   (*Barbara's Pinta Blues*), 1 oz., 14 pieces . . . . . 7.0 . . . . 1.5

   (*Garden of Eatin' Blue Chips*), 1 oz. 7.0 5

   herb and garlic (*Barbara's True Blues*), 1 oz. . . 9.0 . . . . n.a.

   hot (*Garden of Eatin' Red Hot Blues*), 1 oz. . . . 7.0 . . . . 1.0

   picante (*Barbara's Pinta Blues*), 1 oz.,

      13 pieces . . . . 7.0 . . . . 1.5

   and sesame seeds (*Garden of Eatin' Sesame*

      Blues), 1 oz. . . . . 8.0 . . . . 1.0

   and sunflower seeds (*Garden of Eatin' Sunny*

      Blues), 1 oz. . . . . 8.0 . . . . 1.0

cheese:

   (*Chee•tos* Crunchy/Flamin' Hot), 1 oz.,

      9 pieces . . . . 9.0 . . . . 2.0

   (*Chee•tos* Wild Fangs), 1 oz., 9 pieces . . . . 10.0 . . . . 1.5

   (*Health Valley* Cheddar Lites), 1.1 oz.,

      1½ cups . . . . 2.0 . . . . 1.0

   (*Husman's*), 1 pkg., 1½ cups . . . . 8.0 . . . . 1.5

   (*Planters* Cheez Balls), 1 oz. . . . . 10.0 . . . . 2.0

   (*Planters* Cheez Puffs), 1 oz. . . . . 10.0 . . . . 2.5

   (*Snyder of Berlin*), 1 oz. . . . . 6.0 . . . . 1.0

   (*Tom's* Light Bugles), .75 oz. 2.0 5

	total fat (grams)	saturated fat (grams)
all varieties (*Health Valley* Fat Free Puffs), 1 oz.	0	0
baked (*Tom's* Baked Cheezers), 1 oz.	6.0	1.0
balls (*Eagle Cheegles*), 2½ cups	10.0	2.0
balls (*Eagle Cheegles* Reduced Fat), 2½ cups	6.0	1.5
balls, puffed (*Chee•tos*), 1 oz., 38 pieces	10.0	2.5
cheddar, New York, w/herb (*Kettle* Chips), 1 oz.	9.0	1.0
chili w/corn shell (*Combos*), 1.7-oz. bag	11.0	2.0
chili w/corn shell (*Combos*), 1 oz.	6.0	1.0
crunch (*Eagle Cheegles*), 1 cup	10.0	2.0
curls (*Chee•tos*), 1 oz., 15 pieces	9.0	2.5
green onion (*Health Valley* Cheddar Lites), 1.1 oz., 1½ cups	2.0	1.0
hot (*Tom's* Fries), 1 oz.	3.5	1.0
nacho (*Barbara's Pinta* Chips), 1 oz., 12 pieces	6.0	1.0
nacho (*Tom's* Skinny Snack), .75 oz.	2.0	.5
nacho w/tortilla shell (*Combos*), 1.7-oz. bag	11.0	2.0
nacho w/tortilla shell (*Combos*), 1 oz.	6.0	1.0
paws (*Chee•tos*), 1 oz., 20 pieces	10.0	2.5
puffs (*Barbara's*), 1 oz., ¾ cup	10.0	1.5
puffs (*Chee•tos*), 1 oz., 29 pieces	10.0	2.5
puffs, baked (*Barbara's*), 1 oz., 1½ cups	11.0	2.0
puffs, jalapeño (*Barbara's*), 1 oz., ¾ cup	9.0	1.5
puffs, jumbo (*Chee•tos*), 1 oz., 13 pieces	10.0	2.5
jalapeño jack (*Kettle* Chips), 1 oz.	9.0	1.0
mesquite barbecue (*Tom's* Fries), 1 oz.	2.0	.5
mini (*Garden of Eatin'*), 1 oz.	7.0	.5
onion flavor, see "Onion flavor snack"		
red corn (*Garden of Eatin' Red Chips*), 1 oz.	7.0	1.0
red corn, hot and spicy (*Garden of Eatin' Salsa Reds*), 1 oz.	7.0	1.0
salsa (*Barbara's Pinta* Chips), 1 oz., 12 pieces	6.0	1.0

	total fat (grams)	saturated fat (grams)

Corn chips, puffs, and similar snacks *(cont.)*

salsa w/mesquite (*Kettle* Chips), 1 oz.	8.0	1.0
tortilla chips:		
(*Chi-Chi's*), 1.1 oz., 11 pieces	8.0	1.0
(*Doritos* Original Thin), 1 oz., 9 pieces	7.0	1.0
(*Eagle* Restaurant Style Canola Oil), 1 oz., 13 pieces	6.0	.5
(*Eagle* Restaurant Style Rounds El Grande), 1 oz., 9 pieces	6.0	1.0
(*Garden of Eatin' Corntilla* Chips), 1 oz.	6.0	.5
(*Kettle Tias*), 1 oz.	6.0	.5
(*Old El Paso Nachips*), 1 oz., 9 pieces	8.0	1.5
(*Planters*), 1 oz.	7.0	3.0
(*Tostitos* Restaurant Style), 1 oz., 6 pieces	6.0	1.0
all varieties (*Eagle* Restaurant Style Canola Oil), 1 oz.	6.0	.5
all varieties (*Santitas*), 1 oz.	6.0	1.0
baked (*Tostitos* Original/Unsalted), 1 oz., 13 pieces	1.0	0
baked (*Tom's*), 1 oz.	0	0
black bean (*Garden of Eatin'*), 1 oz.	7.0	.5
black bean, w/jalapeño (*Garden of Eatin'* Chili Chips), 1 oz.	7.0	.5
blue corn (*Kettle Tias*), 1 oz.	6.0	.5
cheese, nacho (*Doritos* Cheesier), 1 oz., 15 pieces	7.0	1.0
cinnamon thins (*Tostitos*), 1 oz., 15 pieces	7.0	1.0
lime and chili (*Kettle Tias*), 1 oz.	6.0	.5
lime and chili (*Tostitos*), 1 oz., 6 pieces	7.0	1.0
nacho (*Tom's*), 1 oz.	0	0
nacho or ranch (*Eagle* Thins), 1 oz., 12 pieces	7.0	1.0
ranch (*Combos*), 1.7-oz. bag	12.0	2.5
ranch (*Combos*), 1 oz.	7.0	1.5
ranch, cool, baked (*Tostitos*), 1 oz., 11 pieces	3.0	.5
ranch, cooler (*Doritos*), 1 oz., 15 pieces	7.0	1.0

	total fat (grams)	saturated fat (grams)
salsa, zesty (*Doritos*), 1 oz., 15 pieces	7.0	1.5
salsa and cheese (*Doritos* Thins), 1 oz., 9 pieces	8.0	1.5
sea salt and vinegar (*Kettle* Chips), 1 oz.	8.0	1.0
sesame (*Hain*), 1 oz.	7.0	5.0
taco (*Doritos*), 1 oz., 15 pieces	7.0	1.5
toasted corn (*Doritos*), 1 oz., 18 pieces	6.0	1.0
tomato and basil (*Kettle Tias*), 1 oz.	6.0	.5
white corn (*Old El Paso*), 1 oz., 11 pieces	8.0	1.0
white corn, bite size (*Tostitos*), 1 oz., 24 pieces	8.0	1.0
white corn, round (*Tostitos*), 1 oz., 13 pieces	8.0	1.0
yellow (*Barbara's* Organic), 1 oz., 14 pieces	6.0	1.0
yellow (*Eagle* Restaurant Style), 1 oz., 13 pieces	7.0	1.0
yogurt and green onion (*Kettle* Chips), 1 oz.	8.0	1.0
Corn dog, see "Frankfurter, coated" and " 'Frankfurter,' vegetarian"		
Corn flake crumbs (*Kellogg's*), 1 oz.	0	0
Corn flour (see also "Cornmeal"), whole grain, 1 cup	4.5	.6
Corn grits, uncooked:		
1 oz.	.3	<.1
1 tbsp.	.1	<.1
all varieties (*Aunt Jemima*), 3 tbsp.	.5	0
hominy, all varieties (*Quaker*), ¼ cup	.5	0
white or yellow (*Arrowhead Mills*), ¼ cup	0	0
instant:		
original (*Quaker*), 1-oz. pkt.	0	0
w/bacon bits (*Quaker*), 1-oz. pkt.	5	0
w/butter (*Quaker*), 1-oz. pkt.	1.5	0
w/cheddar cheese (*Quaker*), 1-oz. pkt.	1.5	.5
quick (*Albers* Hominy), ¼ cup	.5	0
w/red gravy and ham flavor (*Quaker*), 1-oz. pkt.	.5	0
w/sausage bits (*Quaker*), 1-oz. pkt.	1.0	0

	total fat (grams)	saturated fat (grams)

Corn grits, uncooked, instant *(cont.)*

    zesty cheddar (*Quaker*), 1-oz. pkt. 1.5 5

Corn grits, cooked, 1 cup 5 1

Corn nuggets, breaded, frozen

    (*Quik-Krisp*), 6 pieces .... 8.0 .... 2.0

Corn nuts (*Frito-Lay*), ⅓ cup .... 5.0 .... 1.0

Corn oil:

    1 tbsp. .... 13.6 .... 1.7

    (*Hain*), 1 tbsp. .... 14.0 .... 2.0

    canola (*Crisco*), 1 tbsp. .... 14.0 .... 1.5

Corn pasta, see "Pasta"

Corn relish:

    (*Green Giant*), 1 tbsp. 0 0

    (*Nance's*), 2 tbsp. 0 0

    (*New Morning*), 1 tbsp. 0 0

Corn soufflé, frozen (*Stouffer's* Side Dish), ½ cup ... 7.0 .... 1.5

Cornbread, see "Bread, sweet, mix"

Corned beef, see "Beef, corned" and "Beef

    luncheon meat"

Cornish game hen:

    fresh, roasted:

        dark meat, w/skin (*Perdue*), 3 oz. .... 15.0 .... 5.0

        dark meat, split half (*Perdue*), about 6.5 oz. .. 15.0 .... 4.5

        white meat, w/skin (*Perdue*), 3 oz. .... 10.0 .... 3.0

        white meat, split half (*Perdue*), about 6.5 oz. .. 11.0 .... 3.5

    refrigerated, roasted:

        dark meat (*Perdue*), 3 oz. .... 9.0 .... 2.5

        white meat (*Perdue*), 3 oz. .... 7.0 .... 2.0

Cornmeal, ¼ cup, except as noted:

    blue (*Arrowhead Mills*) 1.5 0

    degermed 6 1

    high lysine (*Arrowhead Mills*) 1.0 0

    self-rising, bolted 1.1 2

    self-rising, bolted, w/wheat flour 1.2 2

    white or yellow (*Albers*), 1 oz. 0 0

	total fat (grams)	saturated fat (grams)
white or yellow (*Arrowhead Mills*)	1.0	0
Cornstarch, 1 tbsp.	0	0
Cottonseed flour:		
partially defatted, ¼ cup	1.5	.4
low-fat, 1 oz.	.4	.1
Cottonseed kernels, roasted, ¼ cup	13.5	3.6
Cottonseed meal, partially defatted, 1 oz.	1.4	.3
Cottonseed oil, 1 tbsp.	13.6	3.5
Country style gravy mix:		
(*Durkee/French's*), ⅛ pkg.	2.0	1.0
vegetarian (*Loma Linda Gravy Quik*), 1 tbsp.	.5	0
Couscous, ¼ cup, except as noted:		
dry:		
1 oz.	.2	<.1
(*Arrowhead Mills*)	0	0
(*Fantastic*)	0	0
(*Frieda's*)	0	0
whole wheat (*Fantastic Foods*)	1.0	0
cooked, 1 cup	.3	.1
Couscous mix:		
(*Casbah*), 2 oz.	1.3	n.a.
(*Near East*), 1¼ cup*	6.0	1.5
w/lentils (*Fantastic Foods Only A Pinch*), 2.3 oz.	1.0	0
pilaf (*Casbah*), 1 oz.	0	0
pilaf, savory (*Fantastic Foods* Quick Pilaf), ⅓ cup	1.0	0
spicy, w/raisins and almonds (*Knorr*), ¼ pkg.	1.0	0
whole wheat (*Casbah*), 2 oz.	1.4	n.a.
Cowpeas (see also "Blackeye peas"):		
fresh:		
raw, in pods, 1 lb.	.8	.2
raw and trimmed or boiled, drained, ½ cup	.3	.1
leafy tips, raw, chopped, ½ cup	<.1	<.1
young pods, w/seeds, boiled, drained, 4 oz.	.3	.1
dried, see "Cowpeas, mature"		

	total fat (grams)	saturated fat (grams)

Cowpeas *(cont.)*

canned, ½ cup:

    (*Allens/East Texas Fair*) 1.0 5

    w/jalapeños (*Home Folks*) 1.0 5

    w/snaps (*Allens/East Texas Fair*) 1.0 5

Cowpeas, mature (see also "Blackeye peas"):

raw, ½ cup 1.1 3

boiled, ½ cup 5 1

canned, ½ cup:

    (*Allens/East Texas Fair*) 1.0 5

    (*Green Giant/Joan of Arc*) 0 0

    w/bacon (*Allens/Trappey's*) 2.0 5

    w/bacon and jalapeños (*Allens/Trappey's*) 1.5 5

    w/pork (*East Texas Fair*) 1.5 5

Crab, meat only:

Alaska king:

    raw, 1 leg, 6.1 oz. (1 lb. whole leg) .... 1.0 .... n.a.

    raw, 4 oz. .... .7 .... n.a.

    boiled, poached, or steamed, 4 oz. .... 1.7 .... n.a.

blue, raw, .7 oz. (1.3 lbs. whole crab) .... .2 .... <.1

blue, boiled, poached, or steamed, 4 oz. 2.0 3

dungeness, raw, 5.75 oz. (1.5 lbs. whole crab) ... 1.6 2

dungeness, raw, 4 oz. .... .3 .... <.1

queen, raw, 4 oz. 1.4 2

Crab, canned, meat only:

blue, 4 oz. 1.4 3

blue, 1 cup, about 4.75 oz. 1.7 3

Crab, frozen:

(*Schwan's* Crab Rangoon), 5 oz., 7 pieces .... 22.0 .... 8.0

cake, deviled (*Mrs. Paul's*), 2.8-oz. piece w/1 tsp.

    relish mix .... 9.0 .... 3.0

cake, deviled, miniatures (*Mrs. Paul's*), 6 pieces

    1 tsp. relish mix .... 11.0 .... 3.0

"Crab," imitation (*Seablends* Classic/Standard), 3 oz.,

    about ½ cup 0 0

	total fat (grams)	saturated fat (grams)
Crabapple:		
fresh, untrimmed, 1 lb.	1.3	.2
fresh, trimmed, w/skin, sliced, ½ cup	.2	.1
canned, in heavy syrup (*Wilderness*), 1 piece	0	0
Cracker:		
all varieties:		
(*Hain* Fat Free), .5 oz.	0	0
(*Health Valley* Fat Free), .5 oz.	0	0
(*SnackWells* Fat Free), 1 oz.	0	0
arrowroot biscuit, see "Cookie"		
bacon flavor (*Nabisco*), 1.1 oz., 15 pieces	8.0	1.5
bacon-cheddar (*Frito-Lay*), 1 pkg.	10.0	3.0
butter flavor:		
(*Ritz* Original/Low Sodium), .6 oz., 5 pieces	4.0	.5
(*Ritz Bits*), 1.1 oz., 30 pieces	9.0	1.5
(*Sunshine Hi Ho*), 1.1 oz., 9 pieces	9.0	1.5
(*Town House* Classic/Reduced Sodium), .6 oz., 5 pieces	4.5	1.0
(*Town House* 50% Reduced Fat), .6 oz., 5 pieces	2.0	.5
crisp (*Toasteds Complements*), 1 oz., 9 pieces	7.0	1.5
thins (*Pepperidge Farm*), .5 oz., 4 pieces	3.0	1.0
cheese (see also "wheat," below):		
(*Cheese Nips*), 1.1 oz., 29 pieces	6.0	1.5
(*Cheez-It/Cheez-It* Low Sodium), 1.1 oz., 27 pieces	8.0	2.0
(*Cheez-It* Reduced Fat), 1.1 oz., 30 pieces	4.5	1.0
(*Hain*), 6 pieces	3.0	n.a.
(*Jarlsberg Cheese Crisps*), 1.1 oz., 10 pieces	7.0	3.0
(*Snackwell's* Reduced Fat), 1.1 oz., 30 pieces	2.0	.5
(*Tid-bits*), 1.1 oz., 32 pieces	8.0	1.5
(*Tom's* Cheese Bites), 1.25 oz.	4.5	1.5
cheddar (*Keebler Club*), .5 oz., 4 pieces	2.5	1.0
cheddar (*Munch'ems*), 1.1 oz., 28 pieces	6.0	1.0
cheddar (*Pepperidge Farm Goldfish*), 1-oz. pouch	5.0	1.5

	total fat (grams)	saturated fat (grams)

Cracker, cheese *(cont.)*

cheddar (*Pepperidge Farm Goldfish*), 1.1 oz.,
    55 pieces .... 6.0 .... 1.5

cheddar (*Snorkles*), 1.1 oz., 30 pieces .... 5.0 .... 1.5

cheddar, mild (*Sunshine Krispy*), .6 oz.,
    5 pieces 2.0 5

cheddar, white (*Cheez-It*), 1.1 oz., 26 pieces .. 9.0 .... 2.0

cheddar, zesty (*Pepperidge Farm Goldfish*), 1.3
    oz., ½ cup .... 10.0 .... 1.5

cheddar thins (*Better Cheddars*), 1.1 oz.,
    22 pieces .... 8.0 .... 2.0

cheddar thins (*Better Cheddars* Low Sodium),
    1.1 oz., 22 pieces .... 7.0 .... 1.5

cheddar thins (*Better Cheddars* Reduced Fat),
    1.1 oz., 24 pieces .... 6.0 .... 1.5

garlic (*Jarlsberg Cheese Crisps*), 1.1 oz.,
    11 pieces .... 7.0 .... 3.0

hot and spicy (*Cheez-It*), 1.1 oz., 26 pieces .. 8.0 .... 1.5

Parmesan (*Pepperidge Farm Goldfish*), 1.1 oz.,
    60 pieces .... 5.0 .... 1.5

snack (*Cheez-It* Party Mix), 1.1 oz., ½ cup ... 5.0 .... 1.0

Swiss (*Nabisco Swiss*), 1 oz., 15 pieces ..... 7.0 .... 1.5

three (*Pepperidge Farm* Snack Sticks), 1.1 oz.,
    9 pieces .... 5.0 .... 2.0

cheese sandwich (see also "toast sandwich" and
    "wheat," below):

(*Ritz*), 1.4-oz. pkg. .... 12.0 .... 3.0

(*Ritz Bits*), 1.1 oz., 14 pieces .... 10.0 .... 2.5

cheddar cheese (*Combos*), 1.7-oz. bag .... 13.0 .... 3.0

cheddar cheese (*Combos*), 1 oz. .... 8.0 .... 2.0

cheese on cheese (*Eagle*), 1.4 oz., 6 pieces ... 11.0 .... 3.0

crisp (*Tom's*), 1.4-oz. piece .... 7.0 .... 1.5

peanut butter (*Combos*), 1 oz. .... 8.0 .... 1.5

peanut butter (*Frito-Lay*), 1 pkg. .... 10.0 .... 2.0

peanut butter (*Handi-Snacks*), 1 piece .... 12.0 .... 3.0

	total fat (grams)	saturated fat (grams)
peanut butter (*Keebler* Cracker Packs), 1 pkg. ...	9.0	2.0
peanut butter (*Nabs*), 1.4 oz., 6 pieces	10.0	2.0
peanut butter (*Ritz Bits*), 1.1 oz., 13 pieces ...	8.0	1.5
peanut butter (*Tom's*), 1.4-oz. piece	7.0	1.5
peanut butter, grahamsticks (*Handi-Snacks*), 1 piece	10.0	2.5
peanut butter, honey roast (*Eagle*), 1.4 oz., 6 pieces	12.0	2.0
(*Chicken In A Biscuit*), 1.1 oz., 14 pieces	9.0	1.5
cracked pepper, see "soda or water" and "wheat," below		
crispbread, all varieties (*Wasa*), 1 piece	0	0
(*Dare Breton*), 1 piece	.9	.3
(*Dare Breton* 50% Less Salt), 1 piece	1.0	.4
(*Dare Breton* Light), 1 piece	.6	.3
(*Dare Cabaret*), 1 piece	1.1	.3
(*Dare Vivant*), 1 piece	1.0	.1
flatbread:		
all varieties, except sesame, plain, or pumpernickel (*New York*), 1 piece	1.0	0
sesame, plain, or pumpernickel (*New York*), 1 oz.	1.5	.5
whole wheat (*Garden of Eatin' Thin Tin*), 2-oz. piece	2.0	0
(*Frito-Lay* Original Snacks), 1 pkg.	12.0	2.5
garlic (*Keebler Club* Partners), .5 oz., 4 pieces ...	2.0	.5
graham, see "Cookies"		
(*Hain* Rich), 4 pieces	3.0	0
hot (*Frito-Lay* Snacks), 1 pkg.	9.0	2.0
jalapeño and cheddar (*Frito-Lay*), 1 pkg.	10.0	2.5
(*Keebler Club* Partners Original/Reduced Sodium), .5 oz., 4 pieces	3.0	1.0
matzo (*Manischewitz Premium Gold*), 1 oz., 1 sheet or 10 pieces	4.0	2.5
milk (*Royal Lunch*), .4-oz. piece	2.0	0

	total fat (grams)	saturated fat (grams)

Cracker, cheese sandwich *(cont.)*

mixed (*Red Oval Farms* Club), .9 oz., 3.5 pieces .. 4.6 .... n.a.

multigrain:

(*Harvest Crisps* 5 Grain), 1.1 oz., 13 pieces ...	3.5	....	.5
(*Sunshine Hi Ho*), 1.1 oz., 9 pieces	9.0	....	1.5
(*Wheat Thins*), 1.1 oz., 30 pieces	4.0	....	.5

oat (*Harvest Crisps*), 1.1 oz., 13 pieces .... 4.5 .... 1.0

oat (*Oat Thins*), 1.1 oz., 30 pieces .... 6.0 .... 1.0

onion (*Toasteds Complements*), 1 oz., 9 pieces ... 6.0 .... 1.0

pappadum, plain or garlic (*Patak's*), 1.1 oz.,
   3 pieces 5 0

peanut butter sandwich, see "Cheese sandwich" and
   "Toast sandwich"

pepper, cracked:

(*Sunshine Hi Ho*), 1.1 oz., 9 pieces	9.0	....	1.5
(*Sunshine Krispy*), .5 oz., 5 pieces	1.5	....	0

(*Pepperidge Farm Goldfish* Original), 1-oz. pouch ... 6.0 .... 2.0

(*Pepperidge Farm Goldfish Original*), 1.1 oz.,
   55 pieces .... 6.0 .... 2.0

pizza (*Pepperidge Farm Goldfish*), 1.1 oz.,
   55 pieces .... 6.0 .... 1.5

pretzel, see "Pretzel"

pumpernickel (*Pepperidge Farm* Snack Sticks),
   1.1 oz., 9 pieces 6.0 5

ranch (*Munch'ems*), 1.1 oz., 28 pieces .... 5.0 .... 1.0

rice, brown (*Eden*), 5 pieces 2.0 0

rye:

(*Rye-Krisp* Original), .5 oz., 2 pieces	0	....	0
seasoned (*Ry-Krisp*), .5 oz., 2 pieces	1.5	....	0
sesame (*Ry-Krisp*), .5 oz., 2 pieces	1.5	....	0
stoned (*Red Oval Farms*), .9 oz., 3.5 pieces ...	2.5	....	n.a.

saltine, .5 oz., 5 pieces, except as noted:

(*Premium* Original/Unsalted Tops)	1.5	....	0
(*Premium* Low Sodium)	1.0	....	0
(*Premium* Fat Free)	0	....	0

	total fat (grams)	saturated fat (grams)
(*Sunshine Hi-Ho* Original/Low Salt), 1.1 oz., 9 pieces	9.0	1.5
(*Sunshine Hi-Ho* Reduced Fat), 1.1 oz., 10 pieces	5.0	1.0
(*Sunshine Krispy/Krispy* Unsalted)	1.5	0
(*Sunshine Krispy* Fat Free)	0	0
(*Zesta* Original/Low Salt)	2.0	.5
(*Zesta* Fat Free)	0	0
mini (*Premium* Bits), 1.1 oz., 30 pieces	7.0	1.0
seasoned (*Munch'ems* Original), 1.1 oz., 28 pieces	5.0	1.0
sesame:		
(*American Heritage*), 1.1 oz., 9 pieces	9.0	1.5
(*Barbara's Wheatines*), .5 oz., 1 large square	1.0	0
(*Dare Breton*), 1 piece	1.1	.6
(*Hain*), 6 pieces	3.0	0
(*Pepperidge Farm*), .5 oz., 3 pieces	2.5	0
(*Pepperidge Farm* Snack Sticks), 1.1 oz., 9 pieces	6.0	.5
(*Toasteds Complements*), 1 oz., 9 pieces	6.0	1.0
and cheese (*Twigs* Snack Sticks), 1.1 oz., 15 pieces	7.0	1.5
and onion (*Red Oval Farms*), .9 oz., 3.5 pieces	4.0	n.a.
(*Sociables*), .5 oz., 7 pieces	4.0	.5
soda or water:		
(*Crown Pilot*), .6-oz. piece	1.5	0
(*Pepperidge Farm* Original Water), .5 oz., 5 pieces	1.0	.5
cracked pepper (*Pepperidge Farm*), .5 oz., 5 pieces	1.0	.5
cracked pepper (*Carr's*), .6 oz., 5 pieces	1.5	0
cracked pepper (*Snackwell's*), .5 oz., 7 pieces	0	0
poppy and sesame seed (*Carr's*), .5 oz., 4 pieces	4.0	.5

	total fat (grams)	saturated fat (grams)
Cracker, soda or water *(cont.)*		
sesame seed (*Carr's*), .6 oz., 5 pieces	1.5	0
soup and oyster:		
(*Campbell's*), .5 oz., 32 pieces	3.0	0
(*Oysterettes*), .5 oz., 19 pieces	2.5	.5
(*Pepperidge Farm* ABC), .7 oz., 20 pieces	4.0	.5
(*Premium*), .5 oz., 23 pieces	1.5	0
(*Sunshine Krispy*), .5 oz., 17 pieces	1.5	0
sour cream and onion (*Munch'ems*), 1.1 oz., 28 pieces	6.0	1.0
Southwestern style (*Munch'ems*), 1.1 oz., 28 pieces	4.0	1.0
toast, teething (*Zwieback*), 1 piece	1.0	0
toast sandwich:		
(*Tom's* Oven Toasted), 1.3 oz. piece	7.0	1.5
golden, and cheddar (*Frito-Lay*), 1 pkg.	13.0	4.0
peanut butter (*Eagle*), 1.4 oz., 6 pieces	10.0	2.5
peanut butter (*Frito-Lay*), 1 pkg.	9.0	1.5
peanut butter (*Nabs*), 1.4 oz., 6 pieces	10.0	2.0
peanut butter and cheese (*Planters*), 1 pkg.	10.0	2.0
(*Toasteds Complements* 50% Less Fat), 1 oz., 10 pieces	3.0	1.0
(*Uneeda* Biscuit), .5 oz., 2 pieces	1.5	0
vegetable:		
(*Garden Crisps*), 1.1 oz., 15 pieces	3.5	.5
(*Hain/Hain* No Salt Added), 6 pieces	3.0	0
(*Vegetable Thins*), 1.1 oz., 14 pieces	9.0	1.5
water, see "soda or water," above		
wheat:		
(*Barbara's Wheatines*), .5 oz., 1 large square	1.0	0
(*Snackwell's* Fat Free), .5 oz., 5 pieces	0	0
(*Sociables*), .5 oz., 7 pieces	4.0	.5
(*Toasteds Complements*), 1 oz., 9 pieces	6.0	1.5
(*Triscuit/Triscuit* Deli Style), 1.1 oz., 7 pieces	5.0	1.0

	total fat (grams)	saturated fat (grams)
(*Triscuit* Low Sodium), 1.1 oz., 7 pieces	6.0	1.0
(*Triscuit* Reduced Fat), 1.1 oz., 8 pieces	3.0	.5
(*Waverly*), .5 oz., 5 pieces	3.5	1.0
(*Wheat Krisp*), .6 oz., 2 pieces	1.5	0
(*Wheatables*), 1.1 oz., 26 pieces	7.0	2.0
(*Wheatsworth*), .6 oz., 5 pieces	3.5	.5
and bran (*American Heritage*), 1 oz., 9 pieces	7.0	1.5
w/bran or rye (*Triscuit*), 1.1 oz., 7 pieces	5.0	1.0
cheddar (*Eagle*), 1.4 oz., 6 pieces	10.0	3.0
cheddar (*Frito-Lay*), 1 pkg.	12.0	3.0
cheddar, white (*Wheatables*), 1.1 oz., 25 pieces	7.0	2.0
cheese (*Frito-Lay*), 1 pkg.	9.0	2.0
cracked (*Pepperidge Farm*), .5 oz., 2 pieces	2.5	1.0
cracked pepper (*Barbara's Wheatines*), .5 oz., 1 large square	1.0	1.0
French onion (*Wheatables*), 1.1 oz., 25 pieces	7.0	2.0
garden herb (*Triscuit*), 1 oz., 6 pieces	4.5	1.0
hearty (*Pepperidge Farm*), .6 oz., 3 pieces	3.5	0
ranch (*Wheatables*), 1.1 oz., 25 pieces	7.0	2.0
thins (*Wheat Thins* Original/Low Salt), 1 oz., 16 pieces	6.0	1.0
thins (*Wheat Thins* Reduced Fat), 1. oz., 18 pieces	4.0	.5
thins, mini (*Red Oval Farms*), .9 oz., 16 pieces	2.5	n.a.
thins, stoned (*Red Oval Farms*), .9 oz., 3.5 pieces	2.6	n.a.
whole (*Sunshine Hi Ho*), 1.1 oz., 9 pieces	8.0	1.5
whole (*Sunshine Krispy*), .5 oz., 5 pieces	1.5	0
zwieback toast (*Nabisco*), .3-oz. piece	1.0	0
Cracker crumbs:		
(*Premium* Fat Free), 1 oz., ¼ cup	0	0

	total fat (grams)	saturated fat (grams)
Cracker crumbs *(cont.)*		
(*Ritz*), 1 oz., ⅓ cup	7.0	1.0
Cranberry:		
raw, trimmed, whole or chopped, ½ cup	.1	0
canned, see "Cranberry sauce"		
dried (*Sonoma*), 1.4 oz., ⅓ cup	.5	0
Cranberry bean:		
raw, ½ cup	1.2	.3
boiled, ½ cup	.4	.1
canned, w/liquid, ½ cup	.4	.1
Cranberry juice, all blends:		
(*Ocean Spray*), 8 fl. oz.	0	0
(*R.W. Knudsen*), 8 fl. oz.	0	0
Cranberry relish, for chicken, orange		
or raspberry (*Cran•Fruit*), ¼ cup	0	0
Cranberry sauce:		
sweetened, 4 oz.	.2	0
whole or jelly (*Ocean Spray*), ½ cup	0	0
Crayfish, mixed species, meat only:		
raw, 1 oz., about 8 medium	.3	<.1
boiled or steamed, 4 oz.	1.5	.3
Cream, dairy:		
coffee milk (*Weeks*), 10 fl. oz.	3.0	2.0
half and half:		
1 oz.	3.3	2.0
¼ cup	7.0	4.3
1 tbsp.	1.7	1.1
(*Weeks*), 1 tbsp.	1.5	1.0
light, coffee or table:		
1 oz.	5.5	3.4
¼ cup	11.6	7.2
1 tbsp.	2.9	1.8
(*Weeks*), 1 tbsp.	3.0	2.0
medium, 25% fat:		
1 oz.	7.1	4.4

	total fat (grams)	saturated fat (grams)
¼ cup	15.0	9.3
1 tbsp.	3.8	2.3
sour, see "Cream, sour"		
whipping, light		
1 oz.	8.8	5.5
¼ cup, about ½ cup whipped	18.5	11.6
1 tbsp., about 2 tbsp. whipped	4.6	2.9
whipping, heavy:		
1 oz.	10.5	6.5
¼ cup, about ½ cup whipped	22.0	13.7
1 tbsp., about 2 tbsp. whipped	5.6	3.5
(*Weeks*), 1 tbsp.	6.0	3.5
whipped topping, see "Cream topping"		
Cream, sour (see also "Cream, sour, fat-free/nondairy"), 2 tbsp.:		
(*Breakstone's*)	5.0	4.0
(*Crowley/Axelrod*)	5.0	3.5
(*Friendship*)	5.0	3.5
(*Heluva* Good)	5.0	3.5
(*Knudsen Hampshire*)	6.0	4.0
(*Sealtest*)	5.0	3.5
half and half (*Breakstone's*)	3.5	2.5
light:		
(*Friendship*)	2.5	1.5
(*Heluva* Good)	2.5	1.5
(*Knudsen Light*)	2.5	2.0
(*Land O'Lakes*)	2.0	1.0
(*Sealtest Light*)	2.5	2.0
w/chives, light (*Land O'Lakes*)	2.0	1.0
"Cream," sour, fat-free/nondairy, 2 tbsp., except as noted:		
(*Breakstone's/Knudsen/Sealtest Free*)	0	0
(*Friendship* Nonfat)	0	0
(*Heluva* Fat Free)	0	0

	total fat (grams)	saturated fat (grams)
"Cream," sour, fat-free/nondairy (cont.)		
(Land O'Lakes No-Fat)	0	0
nondairy (Sour Supreme), 1 oz.	5.0	2.0
Cream of tartar, 1 tbsp.	0	0
Cream topping, whipped (see also "Cream"), 2 tbsp.:		
(Cool Whip Extra Creamy)	2.0	2.0
(Cool Whip Lite)	1.0	1.0
(Cool Whip Non-Dairy)	1.5	1.5
(Kraft)	1.5	1.0
(La Creme Lite)	1.0	1.0
(Pet Whip)	2.0	2.0
bowl (Rich's)	1.5	1.5
pressurized	1.4	.8
pressurized (Reddi Whip Light Cream)	2.0	1.0
pressurized (Rich's)	2.0	2.0
Cream topping mix, 2 tbsp.*:		
(D-Zerta)	1.0	.5
(Dream Whip)	1.0	1.0
Creamer, nondairy:		
fluid, 1 tbsp.:		
(Coffee-mate)	1.0	0
(Rich's Coffee Rich)	1.5	0
(Rich's Farm Rich, Quart)	1.5	0
fat free (Coffee-mate)	0	0
fat free (Rich's Farm Rich)	0	0
light (Coffee-mate)	.5	0
light (Rich's Coffee/Farm Rich)	1.0	0
powder:		
(Coffee-mate), 1 tbsp.	.5	.5
(Coffee-mate Lite/Fat Free), 1 tsp.	0	0
(Cremora), 1 tsp.	1.0	.5
(Cremora Fat Free), 1 tsp.	0	0
Creamer, flavored, nondairy:		
fluid, all flavors (Coffee-mate), 1 tbsp.	2.0	0
powder, all flavors (Coffee-mate), 1⅓ tbsp.	3.0	2.5

	total fat (grams)	saturated fat (grams)

Creme caramel, see "Pudding mix"

Crepes, refrigerated (*Frieda's*), .4-oz. piece .... 1.0 .... n.a.

Cress, garden:
    raw, untrimmed, 1 lb. 2.3 1
    raw, trimmed, ½ cup .... .2 .... <.1
    boiled, drained, ½ cup .... .4 .... <.1

Cress, water, see "Watercress"

Croaker, Atlantic, meat only, raw, 4 oz. .... 3.6 .... 1.2

Croissant:
    (*Pepperidge Farm* Petite), 1-oz. piece .... 8.0 .... 3.5
    (*Sara Lee* Original), 1 piece .... 8.0 .... 3.0
    butter:
        (*Awrey's*), 1-oz. piece .... 6.0 .... 3.0
        (*Awrey's*), 2-oz. piece .... 11.0 .... 5.0
        (*Awrey's*), 3-oz. piece .... 17.0 .... 8.0
        (*Pepperidge Farm*), 2-oz. piece .... 14.0 .... 7.0
        petite (*Pepperidge Farm*), 1.1-oz. piece ... 8.0 .... 3.5
    margarine (*Awrey's*), 1.25-oz. piece .... 7.0 .... 2.0
    margarine (*Awrey's*), 2.5-oz. piece .... 14.0 .... 3.0
    wheat (*Awrey's*), 2.5-oz. piece .... 14.0 .... 3.0

Croissant pizza, see "Pizza, croissant crust"

Croissant club sandwich, frozen (*Schwan's*),
    4-oz. piece .... 19.0 .... 11.0

Crookneck squash:
    fresh:
        raw, untrimmed, 1 lb. 1.1 2
        raw, ends trimmed, sliced, ½ cup .... .2 .... <.1
        boiled, drained, sliced, ½ cup 3 1
    canned, cut (*Allens/Sunshine*), ½ cup 0 0
    frozen:
        10-oz. pkg. 4 1
        boiled, drained, sliced, ½ cup .... .2 .... <.1

Croquette, vegetarian see "Vegetable dishes, frozen"

Croutons:
    Caesar (*Pepperidge Farm* Homestyle), ¼ oz.,
        6 pieces 1.5 0

	total fat (grams)	saturated fat (grams)

Croutons *(cont.)*

Caesar salad (*Brownberry*), ¼ oz., 2 tbsp.	1.5	0
cheddar cheese (*Brownberry*), ¼ oz., 2 tbsp.	1.5	0
cheddar and Romano (*Pepperidge Farm*), ¼ oz., 6 pieces	1.0	0
cheese garlic:		
(*Arnold/Brownberry*), ¼ oz., 2 tbsp.	1.0	0
(*Pepperidge Farm*), ¼ oz., 6 pieces	1.5	0
cracked pepper (*Pepperidge Farm*), ¼ oz., 6 pieces	1.5	0
herb, fine (*Arnold* Crispy), ¼ oz., 2 tbsp.	1.0	0
Italian:		
(*Arnold* Crispy), ¼ oz., 2 tbsp.	1.0	0
(*Pepperidge Farm* Zesty Homestyle), ¼ oz., 6 pieces	1.5	.5
(*Progresso*), ½ oz.	1.0	0
(*Kellogg's Croutettes*), 1 oz.	0	0
olive oil and garlic (*Pepperidge Farm*), ¼ oz., 6 pieces	1.0	0
onion and garlic:		
(*Arnold/Brownberry*), ¼ oz., 2 tbsp.	1.0	0
(*Pepperidge Farm*), ¼ oz., 6 pieces	1.0	0
ranch (*Arnold/Brownberry*), ¼ oz., 2 tbsp.	1.0	0
ranch (*Pepperidge Farm*), ¼ oz., 6 pieces	1.5	.5
seasoned (*Arnold/Brownberry*), ¼ oz., 2 tbsp.	1.0	0
seasoned (*Pepperidge Farm*), ¼ oz., 6 pieces	1.5	0
sourdough cheese (*Pepperidge Farm*), ¼ oz., 6 pieces	1.0	0
toasted (*Brownberry*), ¼ oz., 2 tbsp.	1.0	0
Cucumber, unpeeled:		
untrimmed, 1 lb.	.6	.1
1 medium, 8¼" long, 10.9 oz.	.4	.1
sliced, ½ cup	.1	<.1
Cucumber, pickled, see "Pickles"		
Cucumber dip, creamy (*Kraft* Premium), 2 tbsp.	4.0	3.0

	total fat (grams)	saturated fat (grams)
Cucumber salad (*Hebrew National/Rosoff/Schorr's*), 1 oz., about 3 slices	0	0
Cumin seeds:		
1 tbsp.	1.3	0
1 tsp.	.5	0
Cupcake, see "Cake, snack"		
Cupuassu oil, 1 tbsp.	13.6	7.2
Currant:		
black, ½ cup	.2	<.1
red or white, ½ cup	.1	<.1
dried, zante, ½ cup	.2	<.1
Curry powder:		
1 tbsp.	.9	0
1 tsp.	.3	0
(*Durkee/Spice Island*), ¼ tsp.	0	0
Curry sauce mix (*Knorr*), ⅕ pkg.	1.5	0
Cusk, meat only:		
raw, 4 oz.	.8	n.a.
baked, broiled, or microwaved, 4 oz.	1.0	n.a.
Custard apple, trimmed, 1 oz.	.2	0
Cutlet, vegetarian, see "Vegetarian dishes, canned"		
Cuttlefish, mixed species, meat only, raw, 4 oz.	.8	.1

D

	total fat (grams)	saturated fat (grams)
Daikon, see "Radish, Oriental"		
Daiquiri mixer:		
regular or strawberry (*Holland House*), 4 fl. oz. ...	0	 0
strawberry (*Mr. & Mrs. "T"*), 3.5 fl. oz.	0	 0
frozen, all flavors (*Bacardi*), 8 fl. oz.*	0	 0
Dairy Queen/Brazier, 1 serving:		
DQ Homestyle burgers:		
bacon cheeseburger, double	36.0	.... 18.0
burger, ultimate	43.0	.... 19.0
cheeseburger	17.0	.... 8.0
cheeseburger, double, regular or deluxe	31.0	.... 16.0
hamburger	12.0	.... 5.0
hamburger, double deluxe	22.0	.... 10.0
hot dogs:		
plain	14.0	.... 5.0
cheese dog	18.0	.... 8.0
chili dog	16.0	.... 6.0
chili 'n' cheese dog	21.0	.... 9.0
sandwiches:		
chicken breast fillet	20.0	.... 4.0
chicken breast fillet, w/cheese	25.0	.... 7.0

	total fat (grams)	saturated fat (grams)
chicken breast fillet, grilled	10.0	2.5
fish fillet	16.0	3.5
fish fillet, w/cheese	21.0	6.0
Chicken Strip Basket, w/BBQ sauce	37.0	9.0
Chicken Strip Basket, w/gravy	42.0	11.0
side dishes:		
french fries, small	10.0	2.0
french fries, regular	14.0	3.0
french fries, large	18.0	4.0
onion rings	12.0	2.5
ice cream and frozen desserts:		
banana split	11.0	<1.0
Blizzard:		
Heath, small	23.0	4.0
Heath, regular	36.0	5.0
strawberry, small	12.0	1.0
strawberry, regular	16.0	1.0
Breeze:		
Heath, small	12.0	3.0
Heath, regular	21.0	4.0
strawberry, small	<1.0	<1.0
strawberry, regular	1.0	<1.0
Buster Bar	29.0	8.0
cone:		
chocolate, small	7.0	<1.0
chocolate, regular	11.0	<1.0
chocolate dipped, small	16.0	3.0
vanilla, child's	4.0	<1.0
vanilla, small	7.0	1.0
vanilla, regular	10.0	1.0
Dilly bar	13.0	3.0
DQ frozen cake slice	18.0	4.0
DQ sandwich	4.0	1.0
DQ Big Scoop, chocolate or vanilla	14.0	1.0
Hot Fudge Brownie Delight	29.0	2.0

	total fat (grams)	saturated fat (grams)

Dairy Queen/Brazier, ice cream and frozen desserts *(cont.)*

malt, vanilla, small	14.0	2.0
Mr. Misty, small	0	0
Nutty Double Fudge	22.0	3.0
Peanut Buster parfait	32.0	9.0
shake, chocolate or vanilla, small	14.0	2.0
shake, vanilla, regular	16.0	2.0
sundae, chocolate, small	7.0	1.0
Waffle Cone Sundae, strawberry	12.0	3.0
yogurt cone or cup	<1.0	<1.0

Dandelion greens:

raw, trimmed, 1 oz., ½ cup chopped	.2	0
boiled, drained, chopped, ½ cup	.3	0

Danish pastry (see also "Cake"):

apple:

(*Awrey's* Round), 2.75-oz. piece	14.0	3.0
(*Awrey's* Round), 4.5-oz. piece	20.0	4.0
(*Awrey's* Square), 3-oz. piece	8.0	2.0
(*Hostess*), 3.8-oz. piece	22.0	10.0
mini (*Awrey's* Round), 1.7-oz. piece	8.0	2.0
apple fruit roll (*Hostess*), 2-oz. piece	4.0	2.0

cheese:

(*Awrey's* Round), 2.75-oz. piece	15.0	3.0
(*Awrey's* Round), 4.5-oz. piece	22.0	5.0
(*Awrey's* Square), 2.5-oz. piece	11.0	3.0
mini (*Awrey's* Round), 1.7-oz. piece	9.0	2.0
cinnamon raisin (*Awrey's* Square), 3-oz. piece	12.0	3.0
cinnamon raisin, mini (*Awrey's* Round), 1.7-oz. piece	8.0	2.0
cinnamon walnut (*Awrey's* Round), 2.75-oz. piece	18.0	3.0
pineapple, mini (*Awrey's* Round), 1.7-oz. piece	8.0	2.0
raspberry (*Awrey's* Square), 3-oz. piece	8.0	2.0
raspberry (*Hostess*), 1.2-oz. piece	2.5	1.0

	total fat (grams)	saturated fat (grams)
strawberry:		
(*Awrey's* Round), 2.75-oz. piece	14.0	3.0
(*Awrey's* Round), 4.5-oz. piece	20.0	4.0
mini (*Awrey's* Round), 1.7-oz. piece	8.0	2.0
Danish pastry, frozen and refrigerated:		
apple (*Pepperidge Farm*), 2.3-oz. piece	9.0	2.5
cheese (*Pepperidge Farm*), 2-oz. piece	10.0	3.0
cinnamon raisin (*Pepperidge Farm*), 2.3-oz. piece	12.0	2.5
cinnamon raisin or orange, iced (*Pillsbury*), 1 piece	7.0	2.0
raspberry (*Pepperidge Farm*), 2.3-oz. piece	9.0	2.5
Date, dried:		
(*Sonoma*), 1.4 oz., 5–6 pieces	0	0
pitted or chopped (*Del Monte*), 1.4 oz., ¼ cup	0	0
whole or chopped (*Dole*), ½ cup	0	0
Date nut pastry (*Awrey's*), 1 piece	10.0	2.0
Date pastry filling (*Solo*), 2 tbsp.	0	0
Demi-glacé mix (*Knorr* Classic Sauces), ⅕ pkg.	1.0	0
Denny's, 1 serving:		
breakfast:		
All-American Slam	84.0	35.0
applesauce, 2 oz.	0	0
bacon, 4 strips, 3 oz.	12.0	4.0
bagel	1.0	0
banana strawberry medley	0	0
Belgian waffle:		
plain	22.0	3.0
Senior Slam, w/out syrup	46.0	13.0
w/blueberry topping	22.0	3.0
w/strawberry topping	22.0	3.0
w/whipped topping	24.0	3.0
biscuit, unbuttered	9.0	2.0
biscuit, w/sausage gravy	30.0	9.0
blueberry muffin	14.0	n.a.
chicken fried steak and eggs, w/out bread	49.0	18.0

	total fat (grams)	saturated fat (grams)

Denny's, breakfast *(cont.)*

cinnamon roll	30.0	n.a.
cream cheese, 1 oz.	10.0	6.0
egg, 1	10.0	4.0
English muffin	1.0	0
French Slam	60.0	20.0
grits	<1.0	0
ham, 3 oz.	8.0	3.0
Harvest Slam	56.0	16.0
hashed browns	13.0	5.0
International Slam	68.0	21.0
Moons Over My Hammy	66.0	25.0
pancakes, 3, plain	6.0	2.0
sausage, 4 links	22.0	8.0
Scram Slam	91.0	33.0
Senior Grand Slam	24.0	8.0
Senior Starter	45.0	15.0
Southern Slam	71.0	21.0
steak and eggs, w/out bread	51.0	17.0
toast, 2 pieces, w/out butter	2.0	0
breakfast omelettes:		
chili cheese	33.0	4.0
Denver	63.0	21.0
ham 'n' cheddar	34.0	5.0
Mexican	41.0	9.0
senior	57.0	11.0
ultimate	64.0	23.0
vegetable	48.0	16.0
sandwiches:		
BLT	37.0	8.0
bacon Swiss burger, w/out lettuce and tomatoes	45.0	19.0
cheese, grilled	49.0	15.0
cheese, grilled, senior	25.0	10.0
chicken, grilled	34.0	4.0

	total fat (grams)	saturated fat (grams)
chicken melt	41.0	17.0
club	35.0	6.0
Dennyburger	25.0	8.0
French dip	40.0	6.0
Mega Melt	63.0	17.0
patty melt	58.0	14.0
Prime Time	70.0	18.0
roast beef, deluxe	56.0	8.0
Superbird	35.0	5.0
tuna melt supreme	58.0	8.0
tuna salad, senior	17.0	2.0
turkey, senior	27.9	3.9
veggie cheese/veggie cheese melt	40.0	7.0
works burger, w/out lettuce and tomatoes	66.0	14.0
quesadillas:		
chicken	31.0	5.0
Denny's	28.0	4.0
entrees (entree only):		
catfish, 2–4 oz., grilled	43.0	10.0
catfish, senior	32.0	6.0
chicken:		
fried, 4 pieces	27.0	8.0
fried, senior	23.0	6.0
grilled, senior	7.0	2.0
stir-fry, with rice	21.0	6.0
chicken breast, grilled, 4 oz.	3.0	<1.0
chicken breast, grilled, 6 oz.	5.0	1.0
chicken fried steak	38.0	19.0
chicken fried steak, senior	23.0	10.0
liver, w/bacon and onions	41.0	16.0
liver, w/bacon and onions, senior	27.0	10.0
prime rib, 8 oz.	46.0	18.0
roast beef, with bread, gravy, potato	19.0	6.0
roast beef, senior, w/out vegetable	9.0	3.0

	total fat (grams)	saturated fat (grams)

Denny's, entrees *(cont.)*

sirloin tips, senior	5.0	1.0
spaghetti:		
w/meatballs	38.0	14.0
w/sauce	9.0	<1.0
senior, w/out salad, bread	25.0	5.0
trout, grilled rainbow	34.0	12.0
turkey, w/gravy and stuffing	26.0	5.0
turkey, roast, w/stuffing, senior	16.0	2.0
salads:		
Caesar	23.0	3.0
chef	26.0	10.0
garden	4.0	1.0
chicken, crispy	55.0	17.0
chicken, grilled, California	12.0	1.0
chicken, grilled, Caesar	41.0	5.0
taco, w/shell	55.0	14.0
taco, w/out shell	25.0	6.0
salad dressings, 1 oz.:		
bleu cheese	14.0	3.0
French	12.0	3.0
French, light	4.0	0
honey mustard	6.0	n.a.
Italian, creamy	10.0	2.0
Italian, light	1.0	0
ranch or Thousand Island	11.0	2.0
side dishes and appetizers:		
buffalo wings, w/out dressing	22.0	6.0
chicken strips, w/out dressing	25.0	7.0
chili fries	25.0	6.0
coleslaw	9.0	2.0
French fries	12.0	3.0
mozzarella sticks, 4 pieces	20.0	10.0
nachos supreme	45.0	10.0

	total fat (grams)	saturated fat (grams)
soups:		
cheese	23.0	15.0
chicken noodle	2.0	<1.0
chili with beans	6.0	2.0
clam chowder	12.0	9.0
cream of broccoli	12.0	10.0
cream of potato	12.0	9.0
vegetable beef	1.0	<1.0
desserts:		
cake, chocolate	17.0	4.0
ice cream, scoop	7.0	4.0
ice cream, shake	24.0	15.0
ice cream, sundae:		
banana split	37.0	15.0
double dip	26.0	9.0
hot fudge	30.0	10.0
hot fudge cake	39.0	10.0
pie:		
apple	30.0	8.0
blueberry cream cheese	37.0	19.0
cherry	30.0	8.0
cherry cream cheese	37.0	19.0
chocolate cream	30.0	18.0
coconut cream	27.0	17.0
key lime	27.0	13.0
Dessert bars, mix* (see also "Brownie mix"), 1 piece, except as noted:		
(*Betty Crocker Easy Layer Bars*)	8.0	4.0
apple crisp (*Betty Crocker Delicious Desserts*), ⅛ pkg.	11.0	3.0
apple streusel (*Pillsbury* Deluxe)	6.0	1.5
Chips Ahoy! (*Pillsbury* Deluxe)	7.0	2.0
chocolate chunk (*Betty Crocker Easy Layer Bars*)	9.0	2.5
fudge swirl cookie (*Pillsbury* Deluxe)	8.0	1.5
lemon cheesecake (*Pillsbury* Deluxe)	10.0	3.5

	total fat (grams)	saturated fat (grams)

Dessert bars *(cont.)*

    Nutter Butter (*Pillsbury* Deluxe) .... 7.0 .... 1.5

    Oreo (*Pillsbury* Deluxe) .... 6.0 .... 1.5

Dill, weed, fresh, ½ cup loosely packed .... .1 .... tr.

Dill, dried:

    seed, 1 tbsp. 1.0 1

    seed, 1 tsp. .... .3 .... <.1

    weed, 1 tbsp. 1 0

Dill dip mix garden (*Knorr*), ½0 pkg. 0 0

Dip, see specific listings

Dishcloth gourd, see "Gourd"

Dock:

    raw, trimmed, chopped, ½ cup 5 0

    boiled, drained, 4 oz. 7 0

Dogfish, see "Shark"

Dolphin fish, meat only:

    raw, 4 oz. 8 2

    baked, broiled, or microwaved, 4 oz. 1.0 3

Domino's Pizza:

    hand-tossed, 2 slices of 12" pie:

        cheese .... 9.5 .... 4.4

        extra cheese and pepperoni .... 18.8 .... 8.6

        ham .... 10.2 .... 4.6

        Italian sausage and mushrooms .... 13.9 .... 6.1

        pepperoni .... 15.1 .... 6.6

        veggie .... 10.4 .... 4.5

    thin crust, ⅓ of 12" pie:

        cheese .... 15.5 .... 6.3

        extra cheese and pepperoni .... 28.0 .... 12.0

        ham .... 16.6 .... 6.6

        Italian sausage and mushrooms .... 21.4 .... 8.6

        pepperoni .... 23.0 .... 9.2

        veggie .... 16.7 .... 6.5

    deep-dish, 2 slices of 12" pie:

        cheese .... 23.8 .... 9.0

	total fat (grams)	saturated fat (grams)
extra cheese and pepperoni	33.1	13.3
ham	24.5	9.3
Italian sausage and mushrooms	28.2	10.8
pepperoni	29.4	11.2
veggie	24.7	9.2
twisty bread, 1 piece	3.2	.5
Donut (see also "Cake, snack"):		
plain:		
(*Awrey's*), 1 piece	30.0	7.0
(*Hostess*), 1-oz. piece	6.0	3.0
(*Hostess* Jumbo), 1.2-oz. piece	7.0	4.0
(*Hostess* Old Fashioned), 1.5-oz. piece	9.0	4.0
(*Tastykake* Assorted), 1.4-oz. piece	11.0	2.0
chocolate, mini (*Hostess*), 2 oz., 5 pieces	9.0	n.a.
cinnamon:		
(*Hostess*), 1-oz. piece	5.0	2.0
(*Hostess Donette Gems*), 3 oz., 6 pieces	14.0	5.0
(*Tastykake* Assorted), 1.7-oz. piece	12.0	2.0
cinnamon sugar (*Entenmann's* Variety), 2.4-oz. piece	19.0	4.0
crumb (*Hostess*), 1-oz. piece	8.0	4.0
crumb (*Hostess Donette Gems*), 3 oz., 6 pieces	11.0	4.0
crumb topped (*Entenmann's*), 2.1-oz. piece	13.0	3.0
crumb topped (*Entenmann's* Variety), 3.4-oz. piece	22.0	5.0
crunch (*Awrey's*), 1 piece	34.0	8.0
devil's food crumb (*Entenmann's*), 2.1-oz. piece	12.0	3.5
frosted:		
(*Hostess*), 1.4-oz. piece	11.0	7.0
(*Hostess* Jumbo), 2-oz. piece	16.0	10.0
(*Hostess Donette Gems*), 3 oz., 6 pieces	15.0	10.0
mini (*Entenmann's*), 1.8 oz., 2 pieces	20.0	6.0
rich (*Entenmann's*), 2-oz. piece	19.0	6.0
rich (*Entenmann's* Variety), 2.8-oz. piece	27.0	8.0
rich (*Tastykake*), 3-oz. piece	16.0	5.0

Corinne T. Netzer

	total fat (grams)	saturated fat (grams)
Donut, frosted *(cont.)*		
rich, mini (*Tastykake*), 3 oz., 6 pieces	23.0	11.0
rich, mini (*Tastykake*), 2 oz., 4 pieces	15.0	7.0
strawberry filled (*Hostess Donnette Gems*), 2 oz., 3 pieces	9.0	4.0
glazed:		
(*Hostess* Old Fashioned), 2.2-oz. piece	12.0	5.0
(*Hostess* Party), 2.3-oz. piece	10.0	5.0
(*Hostess* Whirl), 1.7-oz. piece	7.0	3.0
buttermilk (*Entenmann's*), 2.3-oz. piece	13.0	3.0
orange (*Tastykake*), 3-oz. piece	9.0	1.5
honey wheat:		
(*Hostess* Old Fashioned), 2.2-oz. piece	12.0	5.0
(*Tastykake*), 3-oz. piece	10.0	2.0
mini (*Tastykake*), 2.5 oz., 6 pieces	13.0	2.5
powdered sugar:		
(*Hostess* Jumbo), 1.3-oz. piece	9.0	5.0
(*Hostess* Family Pack), 1-oz. piece	6.0	2.5
(*Hostess Donette Gems*), 6 pieces, 3 oz.	16.0	6.0
(*Tastykake* Assorted), 1.7-oz. piece	11.0	2.0
mini (*Tastykake*), 2.5 oz., 6 pieces	12.0	2.5
mini (*Tastykake*), 2 oz., 5 pieces	10.0	2.0
raspberry filled (*Hostess O's*), 2.3-oz. piece	10.0	4.0
strawberry filled (*Hostess Donette Gems*), 2 oz., 3 pieces	9.0	4.0
sugared (*Awrey's*), 1 piece	35.0	8.0
Donut, frozen:		
glazed (*Rich's*), 1 piece	7.0	1.5
honey bun (*Rich's*), 1 piece	11.0	2.0
stick (*Downyflake* Dunkin' Stix), 2.75 oz.	23.0	10.0
Dopiaza sauce, see "Cooking sauce"		
Drum, meat only:		
raw, 4 oz.	5.6	1.3
baked, broiled, or microwaved, 4 oz.	7.2	1.6

	total fat (grams)	saturated fat (grams)
Duck, domesticated, roasted:		
meat w/skin, ½ duck, 13.5 oz. (1.3 lbs. w/bone)	108.3	36.9
meat w/skin, 4 oz.	32.1	11.0
meat only, ½ duck, 7.8 oz. (1.3 lbs. w/bone, skin and separable fat)	24.8	9.2
meat only, 4 oz.	12.7	4.7
Duck wild, raw:		
meat w/skin, 4 oz.	17.2	5.7
breast meat only, 4 oz.	4.8	1.6
Duck fat, 1 tbsp.	12.8	4.3
Duck liver, see "Liver"		
Duck sauce, see "Sweet and sour sauce"		
Dumplings, see specific listings		

E

	total fat (grams)	saturated fat (grams)
Eclair, chocolate, 1 piece:		
(*Entenmann's*)	9.0	2.0
(*Sweet Celebrations*)	5.0	1.5
frozen (*Rich's*)	9.0	7.0
Eel, mixed species, meat only:		
raw, 4 oz.	13.2	2.7
baked, broiled, or microwaved, 4 oz.	17.0	3.4
Egg, chicken:		
raw:		
whole, 1 large, about 1.75 oz.	5.0	1.6
white from 1 large egg	0	0
yolk from 1 large egg	5.0	1.6
hard-boiled, chopped, 1 cup	14.4	4.4
Egg, duck, 1 egg, about 2.5 oz.	9.6	2.6
Egg, goose, 1 egg, about 5.1 oz.	19.1	5.2
Egg, quail, 1 egg, about .3 oz.	1.0	.3
"Egg," substitute, frozen or refrigerated:		
(*Egg Beaters*), ¼ cup	0	0
(*Healthy Choice*), 1.9 oz.	<1.0	0
(*Morningstar Farms Better'n Eggs*), ¼ cup	.3	.1
(*Morningstar Farms Scramblers*), 2 oz.	.4	0

	total fat (grams)	saturated fat (grams)
Egg, turkey, 1 egg, about 2.8 oz.	9.4	2.9
Egg breakfast, freeze-dried, ½ cup:		
w/bacon (*Mountain House*)	9.0	3.0
precooked, w/bacon (*Mountain House*)	7.0	2.0
omelette, cheese, (*Mountain House*)	11.0	5.0
Egg breakfast, frozen (see also "Egg breakfast sandwich"), scrambled:		
w/bacon:		
cheese, gravy (*Schwan's Bright Starts*), 5.4 oz.	25.0	9.0
sausage, peppers (*Schwan's Bright Starts* Western), 5.4 oz.	24.0	9.0
home fries (*Great Starts*), 5.25 oz.	19.0	9.0
w/home fries (*Great Starts* Budget), 4.25 oz.	12.0	8.0
Egg breakfast sandwich (see also "Bacon sandwich" and "Sausage sandwich"), frozen:		
English muffin		
(*Weight Watchers*), 4 oz.	7.0	2.0
w/Canadian bacon and cheese (*Great Starts*), 4.1 oz.	15.0	6.0
w/ham steak (*Schwan's*), 1 piece	10.0	4.0
omelet:		
classic (*Weight Watchers*), 3.8 oz.	5.0	1.0
garden (*Weight Watchers*), 3.6 oz.	6.0	2.0
ham and cheese (*Weight Watchers*), 4 oz.	6.0	3.0
Egg roll, frozen:		
(*Empire* Kosher Large), 3-oz. piece	6.0	1.0
(*Empire* Kosher Miniature), 6 pieces, 4.9 oz.	8.0	1.5
chicken:		
(*Chun King*), ½ of 7.5-oz. pkg.	7.0	1.5
(*La Choy* Restaurant Style), 3-oz. piece	5.0	2.5
(*Schwan's*), 2 pieces, 4 oz.	7.0	2.0
mini (*La Choy*), ½ of 7.5-oz. pkg.	6.0	1.5
sweet and sour (*Yu Sing* Snacks), 6-oz. pkg.	12.0	3.0
lobster (*La Choy*), ½ of 7.5-oz. pkg.	6.0	1.0

	total fat (grams)	saturated fat (grams)

Egg roll, frozen *(cont.)*

    meat and shrimp (*LaChoy*), ½ of 7.5-oz. pkg. .... | 9.0 | 2.0

    pork:

        (*La Choy* Restaurant Style), 2-oz. piece ...... | 6.0 | 1.5

        (*Schwan's*), 2 pieces, 4 oz. .... | 11.0 | 3.5

        mu shu (*La Choy* Restaurant Style),

            2-oz. piece .... | 7.0 | 1.5

    pork and shrimp:

        (*Chun King*), ½ of 7.5-oz. pkg. .... | 8.0 | 2.0

        (*Yu Sing* Snacks), 6-oz. pkg. .... | 9.0 | 3.0

        mini (*La Choy*), ½ of 7.5-oz. pkg. .... | 6.0 | 1.5

    shrimp

        (*Chun King*), ½ of 7.5-oz. pkg. .... | 6.0 | 1.0

        (*La Choy* Restaurant Style), 2-oz. piece ...... | 4.0 | 5

        (*Schwan's*), 2 pieces, 4 oz. .... | 4.5 | 5

        (*Yu Sing* Snacks), 6-oz. pkg. .... | 11.0 | 3.0

        mini (*La Choy*), ½ of 7.5-oz. pkg. .... | 4.0 | 1.0

    sweet and sour (*La Choy* Restaurant Style),

        2-oz. piece .... | 4.0 | 1.0

    vegetable, Szechuan (*Yu Sing* Snacks), 6-oz. pkg. ... | 12.0 | 4.0

    vegetarian (*Worthington*), 3-oz. piece .... | 8.0 | 1.5

Egg roll wrapper (*Nasoya*), 1.6 oz., 2 pieces .... | 0 | 0

Eggnog, nonalcoholic, dairy:

    1 cup .... | 19.0 | 11.3

    (*Crowley/Weeks*), ½ cup .... | 9.0 | 5.0

    (*Crowley/Weeks* Light), ½ cup .... | 2.0 | 1.0

Eggnog flavor beverage mix, 1 oz. powder .... | .3 | 1

Eggplant:

    raw, untrimmed, 1 medium, about 4.5 oz. .... | .1 | .... <.1

    boiled, drained, 1" cubes, ½ cup .... | .1 | .... <.1

Eggplant appetizer:

    (*Progresso* Caponata), 2 tbsp. .... | 2.0 | 0

    baby, stuffed (*Krinos*), 2 pieces .... | 2.0 | 3

	total fat (grams)	saturated fat (grams)
Eggplant entree, frozen:		
cutlets (*Celentano*), 5 oz., about ¾ cup	23.0	4.0
parmigiana:		
(*Celentano*), 10-oz. tray	27.0	9.0
(*Celentano*), ½ of 14-oz. tray	21.0	5.0
(*Celentano*), 1 cup, 8 oz.	25.0	5.0
rolettes (*Celentano* Great Choice), 10-oz. tray	15.0	4.0
rolettes (*Celentano* Selects), 10-oz. tray	22.0	4.5
El Pollo Loco, 1 serving:		
chicken:		
breast	6.0	2.0
leg	5.0	1.5
thigh	12.0	4.0
wing	6.0	2.0
burritos:		
bean, rice and cheese	13.0	5.0
chicken	11.0	2.0
chicken, classic or spicy hot	20.0	8.0
chicken, whole wheat	16.0	5.0
chicken, *Loco Grande*	30.0	12.0
steak	22.0	9.0
steak, grilled	29.0	13.0
vegetarian	11.0	2.0
fajitas and tacos:		
fajita meal, chicken	18.0	3.0
fajita meal, steak	38.0	14.0
taco, chicken	7.0	1.0
taco, steak	12.0	4.0
side dishes and salads:		
beans	2.5	.5
coleslaw	8.0	1.0
corn	2.0	1.0
potato salad	10.0	1.5
rice	1.5	0
salad, chicken	4.0	1.0

	total fat (grams)	saturated fat (grams)

El Pollo Loco, side dishes and salads *(cont.)*

salad, side	1.0	0

dressings:

blue cheese	6.0	1.0
Italian, reduced calorie	2.0	0
French, deluxe	4.0	0
honey Dijon mustard	.5	0
ranch	6.0	0
Thousand Island	10.0	0

condiments and tortillas:

cheddar cheese	5.0	3.0
guacamole	6.0	0
salsa	0	0
sour cream	6.0	4.0
tortilla, corn, 1 piece	.5	0
tortilla, flour, 1 piece	2.5	1.5
dessert, cheesecake	18.0	9.0
dessert, churro	8.0	2.0

Elderberries, ½ cup

	.4	0

Enchilada dinner, frozen:

beef (*Banquet* Meals), 11 oz.	12.0	5.0
beef (*Healthy Choice*), 13.4 oz.	5.0	2.0
beef (*Patio*), 12 oz.	8.0	3.0
cheese (*Banquet* Meals), 11 oz.	6.0	2.5
cheese (*Patio*), 12 oz.	8.0	3.0
chicken (*Banquet* Meals), 11 oz.	10.0	3.0
chicken (*Healthy Choice*), 13.4 oz.	6.0	3.0
chicken (*Patio*), 12 oz.	9.0	3.0

Enchilada entree, frozen:

beef:

(*Patio* Family), 15.5 oz.	7.0	2.5
(*Patio* Family), ⅓ of 17-oz. pkg.	4.0	1.5
w/cheese (*Banquet* Family), ⅙ of 28-oz. pkg.	4.0	1.5
and cheese (*Patio* Family), 15.5 oz.	6.0	2.5

	total fat (grams)	saturated fat (grams)
cheese (*Patio* Family), ⅓ of 17-oz. pkg.	4.0	2.0
cheese, and rice (*Stouffer's*), 9¾ oz.	14.0	5.0
chicken:		
(*Healthy Choice*), 9.5 oz.	9.0	3.0
nacho grande (*Weight Watchers*), 9 oz.	8.0	2.5
w/rice (*Stouffer's*), 10 oz.	14.0	3.5
Suiza (*Weight Watchers*), 9 oz.	8.0	3.0
Suiza, w/rice (*Lean Cuisine*), 9 oz.	5.0	2.0
Enchilada sauce:		
(*La Victoria*), ¼ cup	1.0	0
green chili (*Las Palmas*), ¼ cup	1.5	0
green chili (*Old El Paso*), 2 tbsp.	1.5	n.a.
hot (*Old El Paso*), ¼ cup	1.5	n.a.
hot or original (*Las Palmas*), ¼ cup	.5	0
mild (*Old El Paso*), ¼ cup	1.0	n.a.
Enchilada seasoning/sauce mix:		
(*Durkee/French's*), ⅛ pkg.	0	0
(*Lawry's*), 2 tsp.	0	0
(*McCormick*), ⅛ pkg.	0	0
(*Old El Paso*), 2 tsp.	0	0
Endive:		
1 head, about 1.3 lbs., untrimmed	1.0	.2
chopped, ½ cup	.1	<.1
Endive, Belgian, see "Chicory, witloof"		
Eppaw, trimmed, 1 oz.	.5	0
Escarole, see "Endive"		

F

	total fat (grams)	saturated fat (grams)
Fajita entree, canned:		
beef (*Nalley* Superba), 7.5-oz. cup	6.0	2.5
chicken (*Nalley* Superba), 7.5-oz. cup	6.0	2.0
Fajita entree, frozen, chicken		
(*Healthy Choice*), 7 oz.	3.0	1.0
Fajita sauce:		
and marinade, Mexican style (*World Harbors*)		
(Guadalupe Mountain), 1 tbsp.	0	0
skillet (*Lawry's*), 2 tbsp.	0	0
Fajita seasoning mix:		
(*French's*), ⅛ pkg.	0	0
(*Lawry's* Spices & Seasonings), 2 tsp.	0	0
beef (*Durkee* "Easy" Pouch), ⅙ pkg.	0	0
marinade (*McCormick*), ⅙ pkg.	0	0
Falafel mix:		
(*Casbah*), 1.2 oz. dry	3.0	0
(*Fantastic Foods* Falafil), ½ cup	4.0	.5
(*Near East*), 2½ patties fried*	15.0	2.0
Farina (see also "Cereal"), whole grain 1 oz. dry		
or ½ cup cooked	.1	<.1
Fast food restaurants, see specific listings		

	total fat (grams)	saturated fat (grams)
Fat, see specific listings		
Fava beans, see "Broad beans"		
Feioja:		
1 average, 2.3 oz. w/skin	.4	0
puree, ½ cup	1.0	n.a.
Fennel, fresh:		
raw, 1 bulb, 8.3 oz.	.5	0
raw, trimmed, sliced, ½ cup	.2	0
Fennel seeds:		
1 tbsp.	.9	<.1
1 tsp.	.3	0
Fenugreek seeds, 1 tbsp.	.7	0
Fettuccine, plain, see "Pasta"		
Fettuccine dishes, mix:		
(*Golden Grain Noodle Roni*), 1 cup	26.0	6.0
Alfredo (*Country Inn Recipes*) 2.5 oz.	7.0	4.0
mushroom (*Country Inn Recipes*), 2 oz.	3.5	2.0
Fettuccine entree, freeze-dried (*AlpineAire* Leonardo		
da Fettuccine), 1⅓ cups*	3.0	n.a
Fettuccine entree, frozen:		
Alfredo:		
(*Healthy Choice Quick Meal*), 8 oz.	7.0	2.0
(*Lean Cuisine*), 9 oz.	7.0	3.0
(*Stouffer's*), 10 oz.	39.0	21.0
w/broccoli (*Weight Watchers*), 8.5 oz.	6.0	2.5
w/four cheeses (*The Budget Gourmet*),		
11.5 oz.	24.0	13.0
beef, broccoli (*Healthy Choice Generous Servings*),		
12 oz.	3.0	1.0
chicken:		
(*Armour Classics*), 10 oz.	8.0	4.0
(*Healthy Choice*), 8.5 oz.	4.0	2.0
(*Lean Cuisine*), 9 oz.	6.0	2.5
(*Stouffer's* Homestyle), 10.5 oz.	15.0	4.0
(*Weight Watchers*), 8.25 oz.	9.0	3.0

	total fat (grams)	saturated fat (grams)

Fettuccine entree, frozen, chicken *(cont.)*

    w/broccoli (*Lean Cuisine Lunch Express*),

      10¼ oz. .... 8.0 .... 3.5

  primavera:

    (*Green Giant Garden Gourmet Right for Lunch*),

      9.5 oz. .... 8.0 .... 3.0

    (*Lean Cuisine*), 10 oz. .... 8.0 .... 2.5

    (*Stouffer's Lunch Express*), 10¼ oz. .... 25.0 .... 12.0

Field cress, see "Cress, garden,"

Fig:

  fresh, 1 lb. 1.4 3

  fresh, 1 large, 2.3 oz. .... .2 .... <.1

  canned, in water or syrup, ½ cup .... .1 .... <.1

  dried:

    10 figs, 6.6 oz. 1.2 2

    (*Blue Ribbon*), 2 oz. 3 0

    white mission (*Sonoma*), 1.4 oz., 3–4 pieces .. 0 0

Filberts, shelled:

  dried:

    unblanched, 1 oz. .... 17.8 .... 1.3

    unblanched, chopped, ½ cup .... 36.0 .... 2.7

    blanched, 1 oz. .... 19.1 .... 1.4

  dry-roasted, 1 oz. .... 18.8 .... 1.4

  oil-roasted, 1 oz. .... 18.1 .... 1.3

File powder, see "Gumbo file powder"

Finnan haddie, see "Haddock, smoked"

Finocchio, see "Fennel"

Fish, see specific listings

"Fish," vegetarian, frozen, (*Worthington* Fillets), 3

  oz., 2 pieces .... 10.0 .... 2.0

"Fish," vegetarian, mix (*Loma Linda* Ocean Platter),

  ⅓ cup 1.0 0

Fish dinner, frozen, lemon pepper (*Healthy Choice*),

  10.7 oz. .... 5.0 .... 1.0

	total fat (grams)	saturated fat (grams)

Fish entree, frozen (see also specific fish listings):

in butter-flavored sauce (*Mrs. Paul's*), 1 piece	5.0	.... 1.5
divan (*Lean Cuisine*), 10⅜ oz.	6.0	.... 1.0

fillets, battered:

(*Mrs. Paul's*), 1 piece w/¼ tsp. relish mix	10.0	.... 2.5
(*Van de Kamp's*), 1 piece	11.0	.... 1.5
crispy (*Gorton's*), 2 pieces	19.0	.... 5.0

fillets, breaded:

(*Healthy Choice*), 2 pieces	5.0	.... <1.0
(*Mrs. Paul's Healthy Treasures*), 1 piece	3.0	.... 1.5
(*Van de Kamp's*), 2 pieces	19.0	.... 3.0
(*Van de Kamp's* Crisp & Healthy), 2 pieces ...	2.5	5
crispy (*Gorton's*), 2 pieces	19.0	.... 5.0
crispy, crunchy (*Mrs. Paul's*), 2 pieces w/1 tsp. relish mix	10.0	.... 2.5
crunchy (*Gorton's*), 2 pieces	17.0	.... 5.0
crunchy, garlic and herb (*Gorton's*), 2 pieces ...	14.0	.... 1.5
crunchy, hot and spicy (*Gorton's*), 2 pieces ...	14.0	.... 1.5
Italian herb, grilled (*Gorton's*), 1 piece	6.0	.... 1.0
lemon pepper (*Gorton's*), 2 pieces	16.0	.... 2.0
lemon pepper, grilled (*Gorton's*), 1 piece	6.0	.... 1.0
potato (*Gorton's*), 2 pieces	20.0	.... 5.0
Southern fried (*Gorton's*), 2 pieces	16.0	.... 2.0

fillet, fried (*Weight Watchers Smart Ones*),

7.7 oz	8.0	.... 2.5

fillet, w/macaroni and cheese (*Stouffer's*

Homestyle), 9 oz.	21.0	.... 5.0
and chips (*Swanson*), 5.5 oz.	12.0	.... 5.0
and chips (*Swanson*), 10 oz.	20.0	.... 15.0
and fries (*Van de Kamp's*), 1 pkg.	18.0	.... 3.0
nuggets, battered (*Van de Kamp's*), 8 pieces	18.0	.... 2.5

portions:

battered (*Gorton's* Value Pack), 1 piece	10.0	.... 2.0
battered (*Van de Kamp's*), 2 pieces	22.0	.... 3.5
breaded (*Mrs. Paul's*), 2 pieces	15.0	.... 2.0
breaded (*Van de Kamp's*), 3 pieces	21.0	.... 3.0

	total fat (grams)	saturated fat (grams)

Fish entree, frozen, portions *(cont.)*

breaded, crunchy (*Gorton's* Value Pack),

1/10 pkg. .... | 12.0 | .... | 3.0

sandwich, see "Fish sandwich"

sticks (*Kid Cuisine*), 8.5 oz. .... | 9.0 | .... | 2.0

sticks, battered:

(*Van de Kamp's*), 6 pieces .... | 16.0 | .... | 3.0

crispy (*Gorton's*), 5 pieces .... | 20.0 | .... | 5.0

sticks, breaded:

(*Gorton's* Value Pack), 7 pieces .... | 12.0 | .... | 1.0

(*Healthy Choice*), 8 pieces .... | 4.0 | .... | <1.0

(*Van de Kamp's*), 6 pieces .... | 17.0 | .... | 2.5

(*Van de Kamp's* Crisp & Healthy), 6 pieces ... | 3.0 | .... | .5

(*Van de Kamp's* Snack/Value Pack), 6 pieces .. | 14.0 | .... | 2.5

crispy (*Gorton's*), 5 pieces .... | 20.0 | .... | 5.0

crispy, crunchy (*Mrs. Paul's*), 6 sticks w/1 tsp.

relish mix .... | 9.0 | .... | 2.5

crispy, crunchy (*Mrs. Paul's* 18/32-pack),

6 sticks w/1/4 tsp. relish mix .... | 9.0 | .... | 2.5

crunchy (*Gorton's*), 6 sticks .... | 16.0 | .... | 4.0

mini (*Gorton's*), 13 pieces .... | 13.0 | .... | 4.0

mini (*Van de Kamp's*), 13 pieces .... | 14.0 | .... | 2.0

potato (*Gorton's*), 6 pieces .... | 16.0 | .... | 4.0

Fish oil, see specific listings

Fish sandwich, frozen (*Hormel Quick Meal*),

1 piece .... | 16.0 | .... | 4.0

Fish seasoning:

(*Shake'N Bake*), 1/4 pkg. .... | 1.5 | .... | 0

cornmeal, spicy (*Seafood Solutions*), 1 tbsp. ..... | 0 | .... | 0

herb (*Seafood Solutions*), 1 tbsp. .... | 0 | .... | 0

lemon butter (*French's*), 1/4 pkg. .... | .5 | .... | 0

lemon butter dill (*Seafood Solutions*), 1 tbsp. .... | 0 | .... | 0

lemon pepper dill (*Durkee* "Easy"), 1/6 pkg. ...... | .5 | .... | 0

tempura, golden (*Seafood Solutions*), 1 tbsp. .... | 0 | .... | 0

	total fat (grams)	saturated fat (grams)
tomato basil (*Durkee* "Easy"), ½ pkg.	0	0
Fish sticks, see "Fish entree"		
Five spice, see "Oriental seasoning"		
Flatfish, meat only:		
raw, 4 oz.	1.4	.3
baked, broiled, or microwaved, 4 oz.	1.7	.4
Flauta, see "Apple flauta"		
Flavor enhancer, all varieties (*Ac'cent/Sa-son Ac'cent*),		
¼ tsp.	0	0
Flax seed (*Arrowhead Mills*), 3 tbsp.	10.0	1.0
Flax seed oil (*Arrowhead Mills*), 1 tbsp.	14.0	1.0
Flounder, fresh, see "Flatfish"		
Flounder, frozen:		
(*Van de Kamp's* Natural), 4-oz. fillet	2.0	0
fillets (*Schwan's*), 4 oz.	1.5	0
Flounder entree, frozen:		
breaded (*Mrs. Paul's* Premium), 1 piece w/1 tsp.		
relish mix	13.0	3.5
breaded (*Schwan's*), 3.5-oz. fillet	9.0	1.5
breaded, lightly (*Van de Kamp's*), 1 fillet	11.0	1.5
Flour, see "Wheat flour" and specific grain listings		
Flour, mixed grain (*Arrowhead Mills* Multi Blend),		
¼ cup	.5	0
Frankfurter:		
(*Healthy Choice*), 1.6 oz.	1.0	<1.0
(*Healthy Choice* Bunsun Size/Jumbo), 2 oz.	2.0	1.0
(*Hillshire Farm* Bun Size), 2 oz.	16.0	n.a.
(*Hillshire Farm* Light & Mild), 1 link	7.0	n.a.
(*Hillshire Farm* Light & Mild Jumbo), 1 link	8.0	n.a.
(*Hillshire Farms* Lit'l Wieners), 2 oz.	16.0	n.a.
(*Hillshire Farm* Natural Casing), 2 oz.	17.0	n.a.
(*Hormel Light & Lean*)	1.0	.5
(*Hormel Wranglers*), 2 oz.	16.0	6.0
(*Oscar Mayer Big & Juicy* Original Hot Dog),		
2.7-oz. link	23.0	9.0

	total fat (grams)	saturated fat (grams)

Frankfurter *(cont.)*

(*Oscar Mayer Big & Juicy* Hot 'N Spicy),
  2.7-oz. link .... 20.0 .... 8.0
(*Oscar Mayer Big & Juicy* Light Wieners),
  2-oz. link .... 8.0 .... 3.0
(*Oscar Mayer Big & Juicy* Little Wieners),
  2 oz., 6 links .... 17.0 .... 6.0
(*Schwan's* Old Fashioned Weiners), 1 link .... 15.0 .... 5.0
(*Schwan's* Skinless), 1 link .... 13.0 .... 5.0
(*Thorn Apple Valley*), 1 link .... 14.0 .... n.a.
beef (see also "Knockwurst"):
  (*Boar's Head* Giants), 2 oz. .... 14.0 .... 5.0
  (*Boar's Head* Lite), 1.5 oz. .... 6.0 .... 2.5
  (*Boar's Head* Skinless), 1.5 oz. .... 11.0 .... 5.0
  (*Healthy Choice*), ⅛ oz. .... 1.0 .... <1.0
  (*Hebrew National*), 1.7-oz. link .... 14.0 .... 5.0
  (*Hebrew National* Bulk Deli), 2.7-oz. link ... 22.0 .... 8.0
  (*Hebrew National* Convenience/Picnic Pack),
    1.6-oz. link .... 13.0 .... 5.0
  (*Hebrew National* Family Pack), 2-oz. link ..... 16.0 .... 6.0
  (*Hebrew National* Reduced Fat), 2.6-oz. link ... 15.0 .... 6.0
  (*Hebrew National* Reduced Fat), 1.7-oz. link ... 10.0 .... 4.0
  (*Hebrew National* Cocktail), 2 oz., 4 links ..... 16.0 .... 6.0
  (*Hebrew National* Cocktail Club Pack), 1.8 oz.,
    6 links .... 15.0 .... 6.0
  (*Hebrew National* Jumbo/Quarter Pound Dinner),
    4-oz. link .... 34.0 .... 12.0
  (*Hillshire Farm* Bun Size), 2 oz. .... 16.0 .... n.a.
  (*Hillshire Farm* Lit'l Beef), 2 oz. .... 16.0 .... n.a.
  (*Hormel Light & Lean*), 1 link 1.0 5
  (*Hormel Wranglers*), 2 oz. .... 15.0 .... 6.0
  (*Oscar Mayer Big & Juicy* Deli Style Hot Dog),
    2.7-oz. link .... 23.0 .... 10.0
  (*Oscar Mayer Big & Juicy* Franks),
    1.6-oz. link .... 13.0 .... 6.0

	total fat (grams)	saturated fat (grams)
(*Oscar Mayer Big & Juicy* Franks Light), 2-oz. link	8.0	3.0
(*Oscar Mayer Big & Juicy* Original Hot Dogs), 2.7-oz. link	21.0	9.0
(*Oscar Mayer Big & Juicy* Quarter Pound), 4-oz. link	32.0	13.0
(*Oscar Mayer Big & Juicy Bun-Length*), 2-oz. link	17.0	7.0
(*Thorn Apple Valley*), 1 link	14.0	n.a.
(*Thorn Apple Valley* Griddle Hot Dogs), 1 link	25.5	n.a.
cheese (*Oscar Mayer Big & Juicy*), 1.6-oz. link	14.0	5.0
chicken, see "Chicken frankfurter"		
cocktail (*Boar's Head*), 1.9 oz., 5 links	15.0	6.0
corn dog, see "Frankfurter, coated" and " 'Frankfurter,' vegetarian"		
hot and spicy (*Oscar Mayer Big & Juicy*), 2.7-oz. link	20.0	8.0
pork and beef (*Boar's Head/Boar's Head* Giant), 2 oz.	14.0	5.0
pork and turkey weiners:		
(*Oscar Mayer Big & Juicy*), 1.6-oz. link	13.0	5.0
(*Oscar Mayer Big & Juicy Bun-Length*), 2-oz. link	17.0	6.0
and beef (*Oscar Mayer Big & Juicy* Light), 2-oz. link	8.0	3.0
sandwich, see "Frankfurter sandwich"		
smoked (*Oscar Mayer Big & Juicy* Links), 2.7-oz. link	18.0	7.0
turkey, see "Turkey frankfurter"		
Frankfurter, coated, frozen:		
bagel dog:		
(*Boar's Head*), 4 oz.	27.0	11.0
(*Hebrew National*), 5-oz. piece	17.0	6.0

	total fat (grams)		saturated fat (grams)

Frankfurter, coated, bagel dog *(cont.)*

w/cheese (*Schwan's*), 1 piece .... 18.0 .... 9.0

corn dog:

(*Hormel Quick Meal*), 1 piece .... 11.0 .... 3.0

(*Schwan's*), 1 piece .... 11.0 .... 3.5

mini (*Hormel Quick Meal*), 5 pieces .... 15.0 .... 5.0

"Frankfurter," vegetarian, canned (see also
" 'Sausage,' vegetarian, canned"):

(*Loma Linda* Big Franks), 1.8-oz. link .... 7.0 .... 1.0

(*Loma Linda* Linkettes), 1.2-oz. link 4.5 5

(*Loma Linda* Little Links), 1.6 oz., 2 links .... 6.0 .... 1.0

(*Worthington Veja-Links*), 1.1-oz. link 3.0 5

(*Worthington* Super Links), 1.7-oz. link .... 8.0 .... 1.0

"Frankfurter," vegetarian, frozen (see also " 'Sausage,'
vegetarian, frozen"):

(*Morningstar Farms* Deli Franks), 1.6-oz. link ..... 7.0 .... 1.0

(*Natural Touch* Vege-Frank), 1.6-oz. link .... 6.0 .... 1.0

(*Worthington* Leanies), 1.4-oz. link .... 8.0 .... 1.5

corn dog (*Loma Linda*), 2.5-oz. piece .... 9.5 .... 1.5

Frankfurter sandwich (see also "Frankfurter, coated"),
frozen, 1 piece:

cheese (*Hormel Quick Meal* Cheesey Dog) .... 17.0 .... 5.0

chili, w/cheese (*Hormel Quick Meal*) .... 20.0 .... 7.0

corn dog, see "Frankfurter, coated" and
" 'Frankfurter,' vegetarian"

jumbo (*Hormel Quick Meal*) .... 21.0 .... 7.0

French beans:

dry, ½ cup 1.9 2

cooked, ½ cup 7 1

French-cut beans, see "Green bean"

French toast, frozen

(*Aunt Jemima* Original), 2 pieces .... 6.0 .... 1.5

cinnamon (*Aunt Jemima*), 2 pieces .... 6.0 .... 2.0

cinnamon (*Farm Rich*), 3 pieces .... 17.0 .... 3.0

	total fat (grams)	saturated fat (grams)
regular or cinnamon swirl (*Downyflake*), 2 pieces ...	6.0	1.5
sticks:		
(*Farm Rich* 33.5 oz.), 3.75 oz., 4 pieces	12.0	2.0
(*Farm Rich* 7.5 oz), 3.8 oz., 5 pieces	19.0	3.0
apple cinnamon (*Schwan's*), 3.8 oz., 5 pieces	22.0	1.0
French toast breakfast, frozen, w/syrup (*Great Starts*), 4.25 oz.	10.0	5.0
Frosting, ready-to-use, 2 tbsp., except as noted:		
caramel pecan (*Pillsbury Frosting Supreme/Creamy Supreme*)	8.0	2.0
chocolate, all varieties (*Betty Crocker Creamy Deluxe*)	6.0	1.5
chocolate, all varieties (*Pillsbury Frosting Supreme/ Creamy Supreme*)	6.0	1.5
chocolate, lowfat (*Betty Crocker Creamy Deluxe*) ..	1.0	.5
chocolate chip (*Pillsbury Frosting Supreme/Creamy Supreme*)	4.0	1.0
chocolate fudge (*Pillsbury Frosting Supreme/ Funfetti/Creamy Supreme*)	6.0	2.0
chocolate fudge (*Pillsbury Frosting Supreme/ Creamy Supreme Reduced Fat*)	3.5	1.0
chocolate fudge or milk (*Pillsbury Frosting Supreme/Creamy Supreme Lovin' Lites*)	3.0	1.0
coconut almond (*Pillsbury Frosting Supreme/ Creamy Supreme*)	9.0	4.0
coconut pecan (*Pillsbury Frosting Supreme/Creamy Supreme*)	10.0	4.0
cream cheese:		
(*Betty Crocker Creamy Deluxe*)	5.0	1.5
(*Pillsbury Frosting Supreme/Creamy Supreme*)	6.0	1.5
strawberry (*Betty Crocker Creamy Deluxe*)	6.0	1.5
creamy candy (*Pillsbury Frosting Supreme/Creamy Supreme*)	7.0	2.0

	total fat (grams)	saturated fat (grams)

Frosting *(cont.)*

lemon or strawberry (*Pillsbury Frosting Supreme/ Creamy Supreme*) .... 6.0 .... 1.5

rainbow chip (*Betty Crocker Creamy Deluxe*) ..... 6.0 .... 3.0

vanilla (*Betty Crocker Whipped*) .... 5.0 .... 1.5

vanilla (*Pillsbury Frosting Supreme/Creamy Supreme Lovin' Lites*) .... 3.0 .... 1.0

vanilla, all varieties (*Pillsbury Frosting Supreme/ Funfetti/Creamy Supreme*) .... 6.0 .... 1.5

vanilla, lowfat (*Betty Crocker Creamy Deluxe*) 5 5

vanilla/French vanilla (*Betty Crocker Creamy Deluxe*) .... 5.0 .... 1.5

white, sour cream (*Betty Crocker Creamy Deluxe*) ... 6.0 .... 1.5

Fructose, 1 tsp. 0 0

Fruit, see specific listings

Fruit, mixed:

canned:

all varieties (*Del Monte*), ½ cup 0 0

all varieties (*Del Monte* Snack Cups), 1 can ... 0 0

all varieties (*Libby* Lite), ½ cup 0 0

tropical, salad (*Dole*), ½ cup 0 0

dried (*Del Monte*), ⅓ cup 0 0

dried (*Sonoma*), 1.4 oz., 5–8 pieces or ⅓ cup diced 0 0

frozen (*Schwan's*), 1¼ cups 0 0

frozen (*Stilwell*), 1 cup 0 0

Fruit bar, frozen (see also "Ice bar" and "Yogurt bar"), 1 piece:

all varieties:

(*Frozen Joy*) 0 0

(*Pop-Ice*) 0 0

(*Starburst*) 0 0

(*Welch's*) 0 0

except coconut (*Edy's* Tropical Fruit Bars) 0 0

	total fat (grams)	saturated fat (grams)
except coconut and pine-coconut (*Dole*), 1 piece	0	0
banana (*Frozfruit*)	7.0	4.5
cantaloupe, cherry, kiwi-strawberry, lemon, lime, orange, pineapple, raspberry, strawberry juice, or watermelon (*Frozfruit*)	0	0
coconut:		
(*Blue Bell Bullets*)	3.0	3.0
(*Dole*)	7.0	5.0
(*Edy's* Tropical Fruit Bars)	8.0	n.a.
(*Frozfruit*)	12.0	9.0
and cream, all varieties (*Welch's*), 1.75-oz. bar	2.0	n.a.
piña colada (*Frozfruit*)	8.0	6.0
pine-coconut (*Dole*)	4.0	4.0
strawberry cream (*Frozfruit*)	7.0	4.0
strawberry-banana (*Frozfruit*)	7.0	4.5
Fruit dip, caramel or chocolate (*Smucker's* Fat Free), 2 tbsp.	0	0
Fruit juice or drink, all blends and brands, 8 fl. oz.	0	0
Fruit and nut mix, see "Trail mix"		
Fruit pectin (*Sure-Jell*), ¼ tsp.	0	0
Fruit protector (*Ever-Fresh*), ¼ tsp.	0	0
Fruit punch, all blends and brands, 8 fl. oz.	0	0
Fruit snack (see also specific listings):		
all varieties		
(*Fruit By The Foot*), 1 oz.	1.5	0
(*Gushers*), .9-oz pouch	1.0	0
(*Nature's Choice*), 1 bar	0	0
(*Smart Snackers*), .5 oz.	0	0
(*Stretch Island Fruit Leather*), 2 pieces	0	0
(*Sunkist*), 1 roll	0	0
except strawberry and berry-banana (*Fruit Roll Ups*), 1 oz.	0	0
strawberry and berry-banana (*Fruit Roll Ups*), 1 oz.	1.0	0

	total fat (grams)	saturated fat (grams)
Fruit spread (see also "Jams and preserves"), all varieties, all brands, 1 tbsp.	0	0
Fruit spritzer, all varieties (*R.W. Knudsen*), 8 fl. oz.	0	0
Fruit syrup (*Smucker's* Light/Natural), ¼ cup	0	0
Fudge, see "Candy"		
Fudge topping, see "Chocolate topping"		

G

	total fat (grams)		saturated fat (grams)
Garbanzo beans, see "Chickpeas"			
Garbanzo flour (*Arrowhead Mills*), ¼ cup	1.0	...	0
Garlic:			
trimmed, 1 oz.	.1	....	<.1
1 clove, .1 oz.	<.1	....	tr.
marinated (*Frieda's*), 1 oz.	0	...	0
Garlic, liquid (*Durkee*), ¼ tsp.	0	....	0
Garlic bread, see "Bread, frozen"			
Garlic bread seasoning (*Spice Islands*), ½ tsp.	0	...	0
Garlic dip (*Nalley*), 2 tbsp.	13.0	....	2.0
Garlic flakes and chips (*Durkee/Spice Islands*),			
¼ tsp.	0	...	0
Garlic herb sauce mix (*Knorr* Pasta Sauces), ⅙ pkg.	2.0	....	.5
Garlic herb seasoning:			
(*Perc*), 1 tsp.	0	...	0
Italian herb (*Smart Seas*), ½ tsp.	0	...	0
w/parsley (*Smart Seas*), ¼ tsp.	0	....	0
Garlic and oil (*Hain*), 1 tbsp.	14.0	....	2.0
Garlic pepper:			
(*Durkee/Spice Islands*), ¼ tsp.	0	....	0

	total fat (grams)		saturated fat (grams)
Garlic pepper *(cont.)*			
(*Lawry's*), ¼ tsp.	0	....	0
Garlic powder:			
1 tbsp.	.1	....	0
(*Durkee/Spice Islands*), ¼ tsp.	0	....	0
w/parsley (*Lawry's*), ¼ tsp.	0	....	0
Garlic puree (*Progresso*), 1 tsp.	<1.0	....	0
Garlic salt:			
(*Durkee/Spice Islands*), ¼ tsp.	0	....	0
(*Lawry's*), ¼ tsp.	0	....	0
Garlic spread:			
concentrate (*Lawry's*), 2 tsp.	6.0	....	2.5
ready-to-spread (*Lawry's*), 1 tbsp.	10.0	....	5.0
Gelatin, unflavored, ¼ oz.	0		0
Gelatin dessert, all flavors (*Del Monte* Snack Cups), 1 container	0	....	0
Gelatin dessert mix, ½ cup*:			
all flavors (*D-Zerta*)	0	....	0
all flavors (*Jello-O*)	0	....	0
strawberry (*Jell-O 1-2-3*)	1.5	....	1.0
Ginger, root:			
untrimmed, 4 oz.	.8	....	.2
trimmed, ¼ cup sliced or 5 slices, 1" × ⅛"	<.1	....	0
Ginger, ground:			
1 tbsp.	.3	....	.1
(*Durkee/Spice Island*), ¼ tsp.	0	....	0
Ginger, pickled, Japanese, 1 oz.	<.1	....	tr.
Ginkgo nut:			
raw, in shell, 4 oz.	1.5	....	.3
raw, shelled, 1 oz.	.5	....	.1
dried, in shell, 4 oz.	1.7	....	.3
dried, shelled, 1 oz.	.8	....	.1
canned, dried, 1 oz., 14 medium or 9 large	.5	....	.1
Goat, meat only:			
roasted, 12 oz. (1 lb. raw boneless)	10.3	....	3.2

	total fat (grams)	saturated fat (grams)
roasted, 4 oz.	3.4	1.1
Goatfish, meat only, raw, 4 oz.	1.1	n.a.
Godfather's Pizza:		
original crust cheese:		
mini, ¼ pie	4.0	n.a.
small, ⅙ pie	7.0	n.a.
medium, ⅛ pie	7.0	n.a.
large, ⅒ pie	8.0	n.a.
jumbo, ⅒ pie	12.2	7.4
original crust combo:		
mini, ¼ pie	5.0	n.a.
small, ⅙ pie	11.0	n.a.
medium, ⅛ pie	12.0	n.a.
large, ⅒ pie	12.0	n.a.
jumbo, ⅒ pie	18.8	9.7
original crust pepperoni:		
mini, ¼ pie	4.8	2.6
small, ⅙ pie	9.0	4.8
medium, ⅛ pie	9.7	5.1
large, ⅒ pie	11.5	6.2
jumbo, ⅒ pie	17.2	9.2
golden crust cheese:		
small, ⅙ pie	7.9	3.9
medium, ⅛ pie	9.1	4.1
large, ⅒ pie	10.9	4.9
golden crust combo:		
small, ⅙ pie	12.0	n.a.
medium, ⅛ pie	13.0	n.a.
large, ⅒ pie	15.0	n.a.
golden crust pepperoni:		
small, ⅙ pie	10.7	4.9
medium, ⅛ pie	12.3	5.3
large, ⅒ pie	14.3	6.2
Goose, domesticated, roasted:		
meat w/skin, ½ goose, 1.7 lbs. (2.4 lbs. w/bone)	169.7	53.2

	total fat (grams)	saturated fat (grams)
Goose *(cont.)*		
meat w/skin, 4 oz.	24.9	7.8
meat only, ½ goose, 1.3 lbs, (2.4 lbs. w/bone, skin, and visible fat)	74.9	26.9
meat only, 4 oz.	14.4	5.2
Goose fat, 1 tbsp.	12.8	3.5
Goose liver, see "Liver"		
Goose liver pâté, see "Pâté"		
Gooseberry:		
fresh, ½ cup	.4	<.1
canned in light syrup, ½ cup	.3	<.1
canned, in syrup *(Wilderness)*, ½ cup	0	0
Goosefish, see "Monkfish"		
Goulash recipe mix *(Knorr)*, ⅙ pkg.	1.0	.5
Gourd (see also "Wax gourd"), ½ cup:		
dishcloth, boiled, drained, 1" slices	.3	<.1
white-flowered, boiled, drained, 1" cubes	<.1	tr.
Grain, see specific listings		
Grain dishes, mix, 3-grain pilaf, w/herbs *(Fantastic Foods* Quick Pilaf), ⅓ cup	2.0	0
Granadilla, see "Passion fruit"		
Granola, see "Cereal"		
Granola and cereal bars, 1 bar, except as noted:		
all varieties:		
(Health Valley Fat Free)	0	0
(Kellogg's Low Fat)	1.5	0
(Kellogg's Nutri-Grain)	3.0	.5
(Nature's Choice Real Fruit /Granola Fat Free)	0	0
(Sunbelt Fruit Boosters)	2.0	0
(Sunbelt Fruit Gammers)	1.0	.5
apple berry *(Quaker* Lowfat)	2.0	.5
banana nut *(Sunbelt)*, 2 oz.	9.0	4.0
blueberry *(Kudos* Lowfat)	1.5	0
caramel apple *(Quaker)*	3.5	1.0

	total fat (grams)	saturated fat (grams)
carob chip (*Nature's Choice* Granola)	2.0	0
chocolate chip:		
(*Barbara's Grrr-Nola Treats*)	2.0	0
(*Carnation* Breakfast Bar)	6.0	2.5
(*Kudos*)	5.0	2.5
(*Quaker*)	3.5	1.5
(*Rice Krispies*), 1 oz.	4.0	1.5
chewy (*Sunbelt*), 1.25 oz.	7.0	3.0
fudge dipped, chewy (*Sunbelt*), 2 oz.	8.0	4.0
chocolate chunk:		
(*Carnation* Breakfast Bar)	5.0	2.0
(*Kudos* Whole Grain)	3.0	1.0
(*Quaker* Lowfat)	2.0	.5
cinnamon:		
and oats (*Barbara's* Granola)	15.0	4.0
raisin (*Nature's Choice* Granola)	2.0	0
toast (*Barbara's Grrr-Nola Treats*)	2.0	0
coconut almond (*Barbara's* Granola)	20.0	8.0
w/cococut, fudge-dipped (*Sunbelt Macaroo*), 1.4 oz.	13.0	7.0
fruit and nut (*Sunbelt*), 2 oz.	7.0	2.5
honey and oats (*Carnation* Breakfast Bar)	4.0	1.5
low-fat (*Sunbelt*), 2 oz.	3.0	1.0
milk and cookies (*Kudos*)	5.0	2.5
muesli (*Sunbelt*), 2 oz.	2.0	.5
nutty fudge (*Kudos*)	5.0	2.5
nutty trail mix (*Quaker*)	5.0	1.0
oats and honey (*Nature's Choice* Granola)	2.0	0
oats and honey, chewy (*Sunbelt*)	5.0	2.0
peanut butter:		
(*Barbara's* Granola)	15.0	4.0
(*Kudos*)	5.0	2.5
(*Nature's Choice* Granola)	3.0	0
(*Quaker*)	4.0	1.0
(*Sunbelt Naturals*), 1.25 oz.	13.0	2.0

	total fat (grams)	saturated fat (grams)

Granola and cereal bars, peanut butter *(cont.)*

chocolate chip (*Carnation* Breakfast Bar)	5.0	2.0
chocolate chip (*Quaker*)	4.5	1.5
and jelly (*Barbara's Grrr-Nola Treat*)	3.0	0
w/peanuts, fudge dipped, chewy (*Sunbelt*), 1.5 oz.	12.0	3.0
w/raisins, chewy (*Sunbelt*)	6.0	2.0
S'mores (*Quaker*)	3.5	1.5
squares (*Rice Krispies Treats*)	2.0	0
strawberry (*Kudos* Lowfat)	1.5	0
tutti-frutti (*Barbara's Grrr-Nola Treat*)	2.0	0

Grape, fresh:

American type or slipskin (Concord, Delaware, etc.):		
untrimmed, 1 lb.	.9	.3
10 medium, 1.4 oz.	.1	<.1
European type (Thompson seedless, Tokay, etc.):		
seeded, untrimmed, 1 lb.	2.3	.8
seedless, untrimmed, 1 lb.	2.5	.8
seedless, 10 medium, 1.75 oz.	.3	.1

Grape, canned

in water or syrup, ½ cup	.1	<.1

Grape drink or juice, all blends and brands,

8 fl. oz.	0	0

Grape leaf, in jars (*Krinos*), 5 leaves | .5 | 0 |

Grapefruit:

fresh, ½ of 3" diameter fruit	.1	<.1
fresh, sections, w/juice, ½ cup	.1	<.1
canned, in water or syrup, ½ cup	.1	<.1

Grapefruit drink, all blends and brands, 8 fl. oz. | 0 | 0 |

Grapefruit juice:

fresh, 6 fl. oz.	.1	<.1
canned, frozen, or refrigerated, all brands,		
8 fl. oz.	0	0

Grapeseed oil, 1 tbsp. | 13.6 | 1.3 |

Gravy, see specific listings

Gray snapper, see "Snapper"

	total fat (grams)	saturated fat (grams)
Great northern beans:		
dry, 1 oz.	.3	.1
dry, boiled, ½ cup	.4	.1
canned:		
(*Allens*), 1.2 cup	.5	0
(*Eden* Organic), ½ cup	0	0
(*Green Giant/Joan of Arc*), ½ cup	.5	0
(*Hain*), 4 oz.	1.0	0
(*Stokely*), ½ cup	.5	0
w/sausage (*Trappey's*), ½ cup	1.0	.5
Green bean:		
fresh, raw, untrimmed, 1 lb.	.5	.1
fresh, boiled, drained, ½ cup	.2	<.1
canned or packaged, ½ cup:		
all varieties and cuts (*Del Monte*)	0	0
all varieties and cuts (*Seneca*)	0	0
all varieties and cuts, (*Green Giant*)	0	0
whole (*Allens/Sunshine*)	0	0
cut (*Allens/Sunshine*)	.5	0
cut (*Allens* No Salt Added)	0	0
cut or whole (*Del Monte*)	0	0
French style or shell outs (*Allens*)	0	0
Italian (*Allens*)	.5	0
and potatoes (*Allens*)	0	0
freeze-dried (*Mountain House*), ½ cup*	0	0
frozen:		
(*Green Giant*), ¾ cup	0	0
cut (*Green Giant Harvest Fresh*), ⅔ cup	0	0
cut (*McKenzie's*), ⅓ cup	0	0
cut (*Stilwell*), ⅔ cup	0	0
w/almonds (*Green Giant Harvest Fresh*), ⅔ cup	3.0	0
Green bean-mushroom casserole, frozen (*Stouffer's* Side Dish), ½ cup	8.0	2.0
Green pepper, see "Pepper, sweet"		

	total fat (grams)	saturated fat (grams)
Grenadine syrup:		
(*Rose's*), 2 tbsp.	0	0
(*Mr. and Mrs. "T"*), 2 tbsp.	0	0
Grits, see "Corn grits"		
Ground cherry:		
in husk, 1 lb.	3.0	n.a.
trimmed, ½ cup	.5	tr.
Grouper, mixed species, meat only:		
raw, 4 oz.	1.2	.3
baked, broiled, or microwaved, 4 oz.	1.5	.3
Guacamole dip (see also "Avocado dip"), spicy		
(*Nalley*), 2 tbsp.	12.0	1.5
Guacamole dip mix, mild or spicy (*McCormick*),		
2 tsp.	0	0
Guacamole seasoning mix:		
(*Lawry's*), ½ tsp.	0	0
(*Old El Paso*), ½ pkg.	0	0
Guava:		
common, untrimmed, 1 lb.	2.2	.6
common, 1 medium, 4 oz.	.5	.2
strawberry, untrimmed, 1 lb.	2.3	.7
strawberry, 1 medium, .2 oz.	.1	tr.
Guava drink, all varieties (*Mauna La'I Island Guava*),		
8 fl. oz.	0	0
Guava nectar (*Kern's*), 11.5-oz. can	0	0
Guava sauce, cooked, ½ cup	.2	<.1
Guinea hen, fresh:		
raw, meat w/skin, ½ hen, 12.2 oz. (14.6 oz. w/bone)	22.3	n.a.
raw, meat only, 4 oz.	2.8	n.a.
Gumbo file powder, 1 tsp.	.2	<.1
Gyro burger mix (*Casbah*), .6 oz. dry	0	0

H

	total fat (grams)	saturated fat (grams)
Häagen-Dazs Ice Cream Shops, ½ cup:		
ice cream:		
cappuccino	18.0	8.0
cherry brandied	15.0	<1.0
chocolate chocolate, Belgian	18.0	n.a.
chocolate Swiss almond	21.0	1.0
coffee chip	20.0	1.0
macadamia nut	24.0	n.a.
maple walnut	26.0	6.0
pralines and cream	18.0	2.0
vanilla chip	20.0	10.0
sorbet, lemon, orange, or raspberry	0	0
yogurt, soft serve:		
chocolate, strawberry, or vanilla	0	0
coffee or raspberry	4.0	2.0
Haddock, meat only:		
raw, 4 oz.	.8	.2
baked, broiled, or microwaved, 4 oz.	1.1	.2
smoked, 4 oz.	1.1	.2

	total fat (grams)	saturated fat (grams)

Haddock entree, frozen:
  fillets:
    battered (*Schwan's* Fish-N-Batter), 2 pieces,

about 4 oz.	19.0	.... 3.0
battered (*Van de Kamp's*), 2 pieces	16.0	.... 2.5

    battered, crunchy (*Mrs. Paul's*), 2 pieces

w/1 tsp. relish mix	12.0	.... 2.5

    breaded (*Mrs. Paul's* Premium), 1 piece

w/1 tsp. relish mix	11.0	.... 2.5
breaded (*Van de Kamp's*), 2 pieces	17.0	.... 3.0
lightly breaded (*Van de Kamp's*), 1 piece	11.0	.... 2.0

  squares, breaded (*Schwan's*), 1 piece, about

4 oz.	8.0	.... 1.0
sticks, breaded (*Schwan's*), 3 oz., 3 sticks	7.0	.... 1.0

Hake, fresh, see "Whiting"

Hake, frozen, blue, loins (*Schwan's*), 4 oz.	0	 0

Hake entree, frozen, breaded (*Schwan's*),

3-oz. portion	8.0	.... 1.5

Halibut, meat only, 4 oz.:

Atlantic and Pacific, raw	2.6	4
Atlantic and Pacific, broiled, or microwaved	3.3	5
Greenland, raw	15.7	.... 2.8
Greenland, baked, broiled, or microwaved	20.1	.... 3.5

Halibut, frozen, Alaskan:

fillets (*Peter Pan*), 4 oz., about 1 fillet	3.0	5
steaks (*Peter Pan*), 4 oz., about 1 fillet	3.0	5

Halibut entree, frozen, fillets, battered (*Van de*

Kamp's), 3 pieces	21.0	.... 3.0
Halvah, chocolate or marble (*Joyva*), 2 oz.	25.0	.... 4.0

Ham, meat only (see also "Ham luncheon meat"):
  fresh, whole leg, roasted:

lean and fat, 4 oz.	23.5	.... 8.5
lean and fat, diced, 1 cup	29.0	.... 10.5
lean only, 4 oz.	12.5	.... 4.3
lean only, diced, 1 cup	15.4	.... 5.3

	total fat (grams)	saturated fat (grams)
fresh, rump half, roasted:		
lean and fat, 4 oz.	20.2	7.3
lean and fat, diced, 1 cup	24.9	9.1
lean only, 4 oz.	12.1	4.2
lean only, diced, 1 cup	14.9	5.1
fresh, shank half, roasted:		
lean and fat, 4 oz.	25.1	9.1
lean and fat, diced, 1 cup	31.0	11.3
lean only, 4 oz.	11.9	4.1
lean only, diced, 1 cup	14.7	5.1
cured, whole leg:		
unheated, lean and fat, 4 oz.	21.2	7.6
unheated, lean and fat, diced, 1 cup	25.9	9.3
unheated, lean only, 4 oz.	6.4	2.0
unheated, lean only, diced, 1 cup	7.7	2.6
roasted, lean and fat, 4 oz.	19.0	6.8
roasted, lean and fat, diced, 1 cup	23.5	8.4
roasted, lean only, 4 oz.	6.2	2.1
roasted, lean only, diced, 1 cup	7.7	2.6
cured, regular and extra lean:		
unheated, 4 oz.	9.6	3.2
unheated, diced, 1 cup	11.8	3.8
roasted, 4 oz.	8.7	3.0
roasted, diced, 1 cup	10.7	3.7
cured, regular (approx. 11% fat):		
unheated, 4 oz.	12.0	4.0
unheated, diced, 1 cup	14.8	4.8
roasted, 4 oz.	10.2	3.5
roasted, diced, 1 cup	12.6	4.4
cured, extra lean (approx. 5% fat):		
unheated, 4 oz.	5.6	2.0
unheated, diced, 1 cup	6.9	2.3
roasted, 4 oz.	6.3	2.1
roasted, diced, 1 cup	7.7	2.5

	total fat (grams)	saturated fat (grams)

Ham, canned:

regular (approx. 13% fat):

unheated, 4 oz.	14.8	4.8
unheated, diced, 1 cup	18.2	6.0
roasted, 4 oz.	17.2	5.7
roasted, diced, 1 cup	21.3	7.1

extra lean and regular:

unheated, 4 oz.	8.4	2.8
unheated, diced, 1 cup	10.4	3.4
roasted, 4 oz.	9.6	3.2
roasted, diced, 1 cup	11.8	3.9

extra lean (approx. 4% fat):

unheated, 4 oz.	5.2	1.6
unheated, diced, 1 cup	6.4	2.1
roasted, 4 oz.	5.5	1.8
roasted, diced, 1 cup	6.8	2.3
(*Black Label*), 3 oz.	5.0	2.0
(*Cure 81* Half Ham), 3 oz.	5.0	1.5
(*Hormel Curemaster* Ham), 3 oz.	3.0	1.0
(*Hormel Light & Lean* Ham), 3 oz.	2.5	1.0
(*Supreme Cut*), 1 oz.	1.0	<1
chunk (*Hormel*), 2 oz.	6.0	2.0
patties (*Hormel*), 2-oz. patty	17.0	6.0
patties, w/cheese (*Hormel*), 2-oz. patty	17.0	6.0

Ham, frozen or refrigerated, 3 oz., except as noted:

(*Jones Dairy Farm* Dainty/Family)	4.0	1.0
(*Jones Dairy Farm* Fully Cooked)	21.0	7.0
(*Jones Dairy Farm* Homestead)	8.0	3.0
(*Jones Dairy Farm* Old Fashioned)	18.0	6.0
(*Jones Dairy Farm* Skinless/Shankless)	11.0	4.0
(*Jones Dairy Farm* Semi-Boneless)	13.0	5.0
baby, Black Forest (*Boar's Head/Boar's Head Maple Glazed Honey Coat*)	1.5	0
baby, Virginia smoked (*Boar's Head*)	1.0	0

slice:

dinner (*Oscar Mayer*)	3.0	1.0

	total fat (grams)	saturated fat (grams)
dinner (*Louis Rich*), 3.3-oz. slice	1.5	.5
sweet (*Boar's Head Maple Glazed Honey Coat*)	5.0	2.0
sweet, boneless (*Boar's Head*)	5.0	2.0
smoked, bone-in (*Boar's Head*)	7.0	3.0
spiral sliced (*Jones Dairy Farm*)	11.0	4.0
steak:		
(*Jones Dairy Farm* Lean Choice)	4.0	1.0
(*Oscar Mayer*), 2-oz. steak	2.0	.5
(*Rock River*)	4.0	1.0
Virginia (*Boar's Head*)	3.0	1.0
Ham and asparagus entree, frozen:		
au gratin (*The Budget Gourmet*), 8.7 oz.	13.0	5.0
bake (*Stouffer's*), 9.5 oz.	36.0	14.0
Ham bologna (*Boar's Head*), 2 oz.	4.0	1.5
Ham and cheese loaf (*Oscar Mayer*), 1-oz. slice	5.0	2.5
Ham and cheese sandwich, see "Ham sandwich"		
Ham entree, packaged, escalloped potatoes (*Hormel Micro Cup*), 7.5 oz.	16.0	6.0
Ham glaze (*Chelten House*), 2 tbsp.	0	0
Ham luncheon meat (see also "Ham, frozen or refrigerated"):		
all varieties (*Healthy Choice Deli Meats*), 1 oz.	<1.0	<1.0
all varieties, except jalapeño (*Hansel 'n Gretel Healthy Deli*), 2 oz.	1.5	.5
(*Alpine Lace* Reduced Fat /Sodium), 2 oz.	2.0	1.0
(*Boar's Head* Deluxe/Lower Sodium), 2 oz.	1.0	0
(*Healthy Choice* Natural or Water Added), 2 oz.	2.0	1.0
(*Hillshire Farm*), 1 oz.	1.0	n.a.
(*Hillshire Farm* Lower Salt), 1 oz.	1.0	n.a.
(*Hormel Deli*), 1 oz.	1.0	n.a.
(*Jones Dairy Farm* Lean Choice), 1.8 oz., 2 slices	1.5	0
(*Oscar Mayer* Lower Sodium), 2.2 oz., 3 slices	2.5	1.0
(*Patrick Cudahy* Classic), 2 oz.	2.5	1.0
(*Patrick Cudahy* Lower Salt), 2 oz.	2.0	1.0

	total fat (grams)	saturated fat (grams)

Ham luncheon meat *(cont.)*

(*Patrick Cudahy* Royale), 2 oz.	3.0	1.0
(*Thumann's*), 1 oz.	1.1	n.a.
baked:		
(*Healthy Choice* Natural or Water Added), 2 oz.	2.0	1.0
(*Hillshire Farm Deli Select*), 1 slice	<1.0	n.a.
(*Louis Rich Carving Board*), 2 slices, 1.5 oz.	1.0	0
(*Oscar Mayer*), 2.2 oz., 3 slices	1.0	.5
(*Oscar Mayer Healthy Favorites*), 4 slices, 1.8 oz.	1.0	0
brown sugar (*Hillshire Farm* Flavor Pack), .6-oz. slice	<1.0	n.a.
brown sugar (*Hillshire Farm Deli Select*), 1 slice	<1.0	n.a.
Cajun (*Hillshire Farm Deli Select*), 1 slice	<1.0	n.a.
Black Forest, smoked (*Boar's Head*), 2 oz.	.5	0
boiled (*Oscar Mayer*), 2.2 oz., 3 slices	2.5	1.0
boiled (*Oscar Mayer Deli-Thin*), 1.8 oz., 4 slices	2.0	.5
cappy (*Boar's Head*), 2 oz.	1.5	0
chopped:		
(*Black Label*), 1 oz.	6.0	2.0
(*Oscar Mayer*), 1-oz. slice	3.5	1.0
fresh, roasted, seasoned (*Boar's Head*), 2 oz.	3.0	2.0
honey/honey-roasted:		
(*Boar's Head Maple Glazed Honey Coat*), 2 oz.	1.0	0
(*Healthy Choice* Natural Juices), 2 oz.	2.0	1.0
(*Healthy Choice* Water Added), 2 oz.	2.0	<1.0
(*Hillshire Farm*), 1 oz.	1.0	n.a.
(*Hillshire Farm* Flavor Pack), .6-oz. slice	<1.0	n.a.
(*Hillshire Farm Deli Select*), 1 slice	<1.0	n.a.
(*Louis Rich Carving Board*), 1.5 oz., 2 slices	1.5	.5
(*Louis Rich Carving Board* Thin Carve), 2.1 oz., 6 slices	2.0	1.0
(*Oscar Mayer*), 2.2 oz., 3 slices	2.5	1.0

	total fat (grams)	saturated fat (grams)
(*Oscar Mayer Deli-Thin*), 1.8 oz., 4 slices	2.0	.5
(*Oscar Mayer Healthy Favorites*), 1.8 oz., 4 slices	1.5	.5
(*Patrick Cudahy ReaLean*), 3 oz.	2.5	1.0
jalapeño (*Hansel 'n Gretel Healthy Deli*), 2 oz.	1.5	0
pepper (*Boar's Head*), 2 oz.	2.0	1.0
smoked:		
(*Boar's Head* Gourmet), 2 oz.	.5	0
(*Healthy Choice* Natural Juices), 2 oz.	2.0	<1.0
(*Healthy Choice* Water Added), 2 oz.	2.0	1.0
(*Hillshire Farm* Flavor Pack), .6-oz. slice	<1.0	n.a.
(*Hillshire Farm Deli Select*), 1 slice	<1.0	n.a.
(*Louis Rich Carving Board*), 1.5 oz., 2 slices	1.5	.5
(*Oscar Mayer*), 2.2 oz., 3 slices	2.5	1.0
(*Oscar Mayer Deli Thin*), 1.8 oz., 4 slices	2.0	.5
(*Oscar Mayer Healthy Favorites*), 1.8 oz., 4 slices	1.5	.5
(*Patrick Cudahy ReaLean*), 3 oz.	2.5	1.0
hickory (*Louis Rich*), 1-oz. slice	1.0	0
spiced (*Boar's Head*), 2 oz.	10.0	5.0
turkey, see "Turkey ham"		
Virginia (*Boar's Head*), 2 oz.	1.0	0
Ham patties:		
unheated, 1 oz.	8.0	2.9
grilled, 2.1-oz. patty (2.3 oz. unheated)	18.4	6.6
Ham sandwich, frozen, 1 piece:		
and cheese, bagel (*Weight Watchers*), 3 oz.	5.0	2.0
and cheese, pocket (*Weight Watchers*), 5 oz.	7.0	2.5
smoked, w/cheddar (*Weight Watchers*), 4 oz.	8.0	3.0
Ham spread, canned:		
(*Libby Spreadables*), ¼ cup	4.5	1.0
deviled:		
(*Hormel*), 4 tbsp.	12.0	4.0
(*Underwood*), 2 oz., ¼ cup	14.0	4.5

	total fat (grams)	saturated fat (grams)

Ham spread, deviled *(cont.)*

    and crackers (*Underwood Red Devil Snackers*),

      1 pkg. | 22.0 | 6.0

    honey (*Underwood*), 2 oz., ¼ cup | 16.0 | 6.0

    honey, and crackers (*Underwood Red Devil*

      Snackers), 1 pkg. | 24.0 | 7.0

    salad, 1 tbsp. | 2.3 | 8

"Ham," vegetarian, frozen (*Worthington Wham*),

    2 slices, 1.6 oz. | 5.0 | 1.0

Hamburger, see "Beef, ground," "Beef patties," and

    "Beef sandwich"

Hamburger entree mix, dry:

    beef noodle (*Hamburger Helper*), ⅔ cup | 1.5 | 0

    beef taco (*Hamburger Helper*), 1.5 oz. | 2.0 | 5

    cheddar, garden (*Hamburger Helper*), ⅔ cup | 4.0 | 1.0

    cheddar bacon (*Hamburger Helper*), ⅔ cup | 5.0 | 1.5

    cheese, three (*Hamburger Helper*), 1.7 oz. | 6.0 | 2.0

    cheeseburger macaroni (*Hamburger Helper*),

      ⅓ cup | 4.0 | 1.0

    fettuccine Afredo (*Hamburger Helper*), 1.6 oz. | 4.0 | 2.0

    Italian, zesty (*Hamburger Helper*), ½ cup | 1.0 | 0

    lasagna (*Hamburger Helper*), ⅔ cup | .5 | 0

    noodles, cheesy (*Hamburger Helper*), 1.6 oz. | 4.0 | 1.0

    noodles, creamy (*Hamburger Helper*), 1.7 oz. | 6.0 | 2.0

    pizza pasta (*Hamburger Helper*), ½ cup | 2.0 | 0

    rigatoni (*Hamburger Helper*), ½ cup | 1.0 | 0

    Salisbury (*Hamburger Helper*), ¾ cup | 1.0 | 0

Hardee's, 1 serving:

    breakfast:

      Big Country Breakfast, w/bacon | 43.0 | 13.0

      Big Country Breakfast, w/sausage | 61.0 | 19.0

      biscuit, bacon and egg | 27.0 | 9.0

      biscuit, bacon, egg, and cheese | 31.0 | 11.0

      biscuit, chicken fillet | 25.0 | 7.0

      biscuit, *Cinnamon 'N' Raisin* | 18.0 | 5.0

	total fat (grams)	saturated fat (grams)
Biscuit 'N' Gravy	28.0	9.0
biscuit, ham	20.0	6.0
biscuit, ham, country	22.0	6.0
biscuit, ham, egg, and cheese	27.0	10.0
biscuit, Rise 'N' Shine	21.0	6.0
biscuit, Rise 'N' Shine Canadian	32.0	11.0
biscuit, sausage	31.0	10.0
biscuit, sausage and egg	35.0	11.0
biscuit, steak	32.0	10.0
blueberry muffin	17.0	4.0
Frisco breakfast sandwich, ham	22.0	8.0
Hash Rounds, regular	14.0	3.0
pancakes, 3	2.0	1.0
pancakes, 3, w/2 bacon strips	9.0	3.0
pancakes, 3, w/1 sausage patty	16.0	6.0
sandwiches and burgers:		
bacon cheeseburger	36.0	15.0
Big Deluxe burger	30.0	13.0
Big Roast Beef	16.0	7.0
cheeseburger	13.0	7.0
cheeseburger, ¼ lb. (precooked weight)	25.0	12.0
chicken fillet	14.0	4.0
Fisherman's Fillet	22.0	6.0
Frisco burger	50.0	18.0
Frisco grilled chicken	34.0	10.0
hamburger	9.0	4.0
hot dog	20.0	6.0
Hot Ham 'N' Cheese	30.0	9.0
Mushroom 'N' Swiss burger	27.0	13.0
roast beef, regular	11.0	5.0
fried chicken and sides:		
chicken breast	15.0	4.0
chicken leg	7.0	2.0
chicken thigh	15.0	4.0
chicken wing	8.0	2.0

	total fat (grams)	saturated fat (grams)
Hardee's, fried chicken and sides *(cont.)*		
coleslaw, 4 oz.	20.0	3.0
mashed potatoes, 4 oz.	<1.0	<1.0
gravy, 1.5 oz.	<1.0	<1.0
salads and fries:		
chef salad	12.0	7.0
Crispy Curls	16.0	3.0
french fries, small	10.0	3.0
french fries, medium	15.0	4.0
french fries, large	18.0	5.0
garden salad	13.0	9.0
grilled chicken salad	3.0	1.0
peppercorn steak salad	5.0	2.0
side salad	<1.0	<1.0
salad dressings:		
French or honey Dijon, fat-free	0	0
Italian	24.0	4.0
Parmesan peppercorn	34.0	5.0
ranch	29.0	4.0
Thousand Island	23.0	3.0
shakes and desserts:		
Big Cookie	12.0	4.0
Cool Twist cone, chocolate or chocolate/vanilla	2.0	1.0
Cool Twist cone, vanilla	2.0	1.0
Cool Twist sundae, hot fudge	6.0	3.0
Cool Twist sundae, strawberry	2.0	1.0
shake, chocolate	5.0	3.0
shake, peach	4.0	3.0
shake, strawberry	4.0	3.0
shake, vanilla	5.0	3.0
Hawaiian yam, see "Yam, mountain"		
Hazelnut, see "Filberts"		
Hazelnut butter (*Roaster Fresh*), 1 oz.	18.9	1.7
Hazelnut oil:		
1 tbsp.	13.6	1.0

	total fat (grams)	saturated fat (grams)
(*Arrowhead Mills*), 1 tbsp.	14.0	1.0
Head cheese (*Oscar Mayer*), 1-oz. slice	4.0	1.5
Heart, simmered or braised:		
beef, 4 oz.	6.4	1.9
chicken, 4 oz.	9.0	2.6
chicken, .1 oz.	.3	.1
lamb, 4 oz.	9.0	3.6
pork, 4 oz.	5.7	1.5
turkey, 4 oz.	6.9	2.0
veal, 4 oz.	7.7	2.1
Herb brown gravy mix, see "Brown gravy mix"		
Herb and garlic pasta sauce mix (*McCormick Pasta Prima*), ¼ pkg.	0	0
Herb seasoning, all-purpose (*Perc*), ¼ tsp.	<.1	0
Herbs, see specific listings		
Herbs, mixed (*Lawry's* Pinch of Herbs), ¼ tsp.	0	0
Herring, meat only, 4 oz.:		
Atlantic, raw	10.3	2.3
Atlantic, baked, broiled, or microwaved	13.1	3.0
Pacific, raw	15.8	3.7
Pacific, baked, broiled, or microwaved	20.2	4.7
Herring, canned, see "Sardine"		
Herring, kippered, Atlantic:		
4 oz.	14.0	3.2
1 piece, 4⅜" × 1¾" × ¼"	5.0	1.1
Herring, lake, see "Cisco"		
Herring, pickled, Atlantic:		
4 oz.	20.4	2.7
1 piece, 1¾" × ⅞" × ½"	2.7	.4
Herring, pickled, in jars:		
(*Vita* Homestyle), 2 oz., about ¼ cup	8.0	1.5
(*Vita* Party Snacks), 2 oz., about ¼ cup	5.0	1.5
roll mops (*Vita*), 2.5 oz., about 1 roll mop	7.0	4.0
sliced (*Vita* Lunch Herring), 2 oz., about ¼ cup	8.0	1.5
in sour cream (*Elf*), 3 oz.	10.0	n.a.

	total fat (grams)	saturated fat (grams)

Herring, pickled, in jars *(cont.)*

    in sour cream (*Vita*), 2.25 oz., ¼ cup .... 7.0 .... 4.0

    Swedish style, in dill sauce (*Elf*), 3 oz. .... 8.0 .... n.a.

    in wine sauce (*Elf*), 3 oz. .... 8.0 .... n.a.

Herring oil, 1 tbsp. .... 13.6 .... 2.9

Herring salad (*Vita*), ¼ cup .... 4.0 .... 1.0

Hickory nut, dried:

    in shell, 4 oz. .... 23.4 .... 2.6

    shelled, 1 oz. .... 18.3 .... 2.0

Hog plum, seeded, 1 oz. 6 0

Hoisin sauce (*House of Tsang*), 1 tsp. 0 0

Hollandaise sauce mix (*Durkee/French's*), ¹⁄₁₀ pkg. .. 0 0

Homestyle gravy mix:

    (*Durkee/French's*), ¼ pkg. 5 0

    (*Pillsbury*), 2 tsp. 0 0

Hominy, canned, ½ cup:

    golden (*Allens*) 5 0

    Mexican (*Allens*) 1 0

    white (*Allens*) 5 0

    white or yellow (*Van Camp's*) 1.0 0

    white or yellow 7 1

Hominy grits, see "Corn grits"

Honey, 1 tbsp. 0 0

Honey bun, see "Bun, honey"

Honey butter (*Downey's*), 1 tbsp. 1.0 5

Honey loaf, 1-oz. slice:

    (*Oscar Mayer*) 1.0 0

    pork and beef 1.3 4

Honey roll sausage, 1-oz. slice .... 3.0 .... 1.2

Honeydew melon:

    untrimmed, 1 lb. 2 0

    cubed, 1 cup 1 0

Horse bean seeds, dried, whole, 1 oz. .... .4 .... n.a.

Horseradish, prepared:

    (*Axelrod/Crowley*), 1 oz. .... <1.0 0

	total fat (grams)	saturated fat (grams)
(*Heluva* Good), 1 tsp.	0	0
(*Kraft*), 1 tsp.	0	0
(*Kraft Sauceworks*), 1 tsp.	1.5	0
w/beets (*Gold's*), 1 tsp.	0	0
cream style (*Kraft*), 1 tsp.	0	0
grated in vinegar (*Boar's Head*), 1 tsp.	0	0
Japanese, see "Wasabi"		
red or white (*Hebrew National/Rosoff*), 1 tbsp.	0	0
Horseradish mustard (*Heluva* Good), 1 tsp.	2.0	0
Horseradish sauce (*Heinz*), 1 tsp.	2.5	0
Horseradish tree:		
leafy tips, raw, trimmed, chopped, ½ cup	.1	0
leafy tips, boiled, drained, chopped, ½ cup	.2	n.a.
pods, raw, 1 pod, .7 oz.	<.1	0
pods, boiled, drained, sliced, ½ cup	.1	0
Hot dog, see "Frankfurter"		
Hot sauce, see "Pepper sauce" and specific listings		
Hubbard squash:		
raw, untrimmed, 1 lb.	1.5	.3
raw, cubed, ½ cup	.3	.1
baked, cubed, ½ cup	.6	.1
boiled, drained, mashed, ½ cup	.4	.1
Hummus:		
1 oz., about 2 tbsp.	2.4	.4
½ cup	10.4	1.6
(*Casbah Timeless Cuisine*), 1 oz.	4.5	n.a.
Hummus mix:		
(*Casbah*), 1 oz. dry, ½ cup*	5.0	0
dip (*Fantastic Foods*), about 2 tbsp.	2.0	0
Hunter gravy mix (*Knorr Gravy Classics*), ⅕ pkg.	1.0	0
Hush puppies, frozen:		
(*Delta Pride*), 2 oz.	5.0	1.0
(*Schwan's*), 3 pieces, 2.3 oz.	6.0	1.0
jalapeño (*Delta Pride*), 2 oz.	4.5	1.0

	total fat (grams)	saturated fat (grams)
Hyacinth bean:		
raw, untrimmed, 1 lb.	.8	.4
boiled, drained, ½ cup	.1	.1
dried, raw, 1 oz.	.5	n.a.
dried, boiled, ½ cup	.6	n.a.

I

	total fat (grams)		saturated fat (grams)
Ice:			
all varieties (*Ben & Jerry's*), ½ cup	0	....	0
cherry or orange freeze (*Blue Bell* Snack Cups),			
3 fl. oz.	0	....	0
Italian, all flavors (*Luigi's*), 1 cup	0	....	0
Ice bar (see also "Fruit bar"), 1 piece:			
all varieties:			
(*Blue Bell Bullet /Freeze/Frostbite*/Rainbow/Twin			
Pop)	0	....	0
(*Great American Chilly Pops*)	0	....	0
(*LifeSavers*)	0	....	0
(*Nestlé Cool Creations*)	0	....	0
(*Schwan's*), all flavors	0	....	0
tea w/lemon (*Frozfruit*)	0	....	0
Ice cream (see also "*Baskin-Robbins*" and "*Häagen-Dazs*" Ice Cream Shops"), ½ cup, except as noted:			
all flavors:			
(*Edy's Grand* Fat Free)	0	....	0
(*Edy's Grand* No Sugar Added)	4.0	....	2.5
except chocolate chip cookie dough (*Borden/ Meadow Gold* Low Fat)	2.0	....	1.0

	total fat (grams)	saturated fat (grams)

Ice cream, all flavors *(cont.)*

except country vanilla, rocky road, and tropical

fruit (*Blue Bell Diet*)	0	0
Almond Affair (*Edy's Grand*)	8.0	5.0
Almond Joy (*Weeks*)	10.0	6.0
almond praline (*Edy's Grand*)	8.0	4.0
almond praline (*Edy's Grand* Light)	4.0	2.0
banana:		
nut (*Blue Bell*)	9.0	5.0
pudding (*Blue Bell*)	9.0	6.0
split (*Blue Bell*)	8.0	5.0
split (*Blue Bell* Light)	2.0	1.0
split (*Edy's Grand*)	10.0	5.0
Black Forest cake (*Blue Bell*)	8.0	6.0
black raspberry (*Schwan's*)	7.0	4.5
black raspberry (*Weeks*)	8.0	5.0
black walnut (*Blue Bell*)	9.0	6.0
blueberry cheesecake (*Blue Bell*)	8.0	5.0
bubble gum (*Weeks*)	8.0	5.0
butter crunch (*Schwan's*)	8.0	5.0
butter crunch (*Schwan's* Lite)	3.5	2.0
butter crunch (*Weeks*)	9.0	5.0
butter pecan:		
(*Ben & Jerry's*)	26.0	11.0
(*Blue Bell*)	13.0	6.0
(*Crowley*)	10.0	5.0
(*Edy's Grand*)	10.0	5.0
(*Edy's Grand* Light)	5.0	2.0
(*Häagen-Dazs*)	17.0	9.0
(*Schwan's*)	9.0	5.0
(*Weeks*)	11.0	6.0
butterscotch parfait (*Weeks*)	8.0	5.0
butterscotch ripple (*Schwan's*)	7.0	4.5
café au lait (*Edy's Grand* Light)	4.0	2.5
candy bar classic (*Weeks*)	10.0	5.0

	total fat (grams)	saturated fat (grams)
Cappuccino Commotion (*Häagen-Dazs Exträas*) ...	22.0	10.0
Caramel Cone Explosion (*Häagen-Dazs Exträas*) ...	21.0	10.0
caramel nut sundae (*Häagen-Dazs*)	21.0	n.a.
caramel pecan fudge (*Blue Bell*)	11.0	8.0
caramel sundae crunch (*Blue Bell*)	10.0	7.0
Carrot Cake Passion (*Häagen-Dazs Exträas*)	21.0	n.a.
cashew caramel turtle (*Weeks*)	9.0	5.0
cheesecake chunk (*Edy's Grand* Light)	5.0	3.0
cherry:		
(*Crowley* Premium *White House*)	7.0	4.5
Amaretto cordial (*Blue Bell*)	9.0	6.0
chocolate chip (*Edy's Grand*)	8.0	5.0
cobbler (*Blue Bell*)	7.0	4.0
dark, sweet (*Schwan's*)	6.0	4.5
nut (*Schwan's*)	7.0	4.5
vanilla (*Ben & Jerry's*)	17.0	10.0
vanilla (*Schwan's*)	7.0	4.5
vanilla (*Weeks*)	8.0	5.0
vanilla fudge (*Blue Bell* Light)	2.0	1.0
Cherry Garcia (*Ben & Jerry's*)	16.0	10.0
chocolate:		
(*Crowley* Premium)	8.0	5.0
(*Edy's Grand*)	9.0	5.0
(*Häagen-Dazs*)	17.0	8.0
(*Häagen-Dazs*), 3.5-fl.-oz. container	15.0	7.0
(*Schwan's*)	7.0	4.5
(*Weeks*)	9.0	6.0
chunky supreme (*Schwan's*)	8.0	5.0
decadence (*Blue Bell*)	11.0	9.0
deep (*Häagen-Dazs*)	20.0	7.0
deep dark (*Ben & Jerry's* Smooth)	15.0	9.0
Dutch (*Blue Bell*)	9.0	6.0
Dutch (*Blue Bell* Light)	2.0	1.0
milk (*Blue Bell*)	10.0	7.0
triple (*Blue Bell*)	9.0	6.0

	total fat (grams)	saturated fat (grams)

Ice cream, chocolate *(cont.)*

    Triple Chocolate Tornado (*Weight Watchers*

Light)	3.5	1.5
wickedly (*Weeks*)	10.0	6.0

chocolate almond:

(*Schwan's*)	8.0	4.5
fudge (*Edy's Grand* Light)	5.0	2.5
marshmallow (*Blue Bell*)	11.0	6.0
Swiss (*Weeks*)	10.0	5.0
white (*Blue Bell*)	11.0	7.0

chocolate chip:

(*Blue Bell*)	10.0	6.0
(*Crowley* Premium)	9.0	6.0
(*Edy's Grand* Chips!)	9.0	5.0
(*Edy's Grand* Light)	5.0	2.5
(*Schwan's*)	8.0	5.0
(*Weeks*)	9.0	6.0
chocolate (*Edy's Grand*)	10.0	6.0
chocolate (*Häagen-Dazs*)	20.0	10.0
cookie dough (*Ben & Jerry's*)	17.0	9.0
cookie dough (*Blue Bell*)	10.0	5.0
cookie dough (*Borden/Meadow Gold* Low Fat)	2.5	1.5
cookie dough (*Schwan's*)	8.0	4.5
cookie dough (*Weeks*)	9.0	5.0
mint (*Blue Bell*)	10.0	6.0
mint (*Edy's Grand* Chips!)	9.0	5.0
mint (*Schwan's*)	8.0	5.0
mint (*Weeks*)	9.0	6.0
mint, chocolate (*Häagen-Dazs*)	20.0	n.a.
w/chocolate chunks (*DoveBar*)	19.0	9.0

chocolate fudge:

brownie (*Ben & Jerry's*)	14.0	9.0
deep (*Häagen-Dazs*)	15.0	9.0
double (*Ben & Jerry's*)	16.0	9.0
mousse (*Edy's Grand*)	8.0	5.0

	total fat (grams)	saturated fat (grams)
mousse (*Edy's Grand* Light)	4.0	2.5
ripple (*Schwan's*)	7.0	4.5
sundae (*Edy's Grand*)	8.0	4.0
chocolate marshmallow:		
(*Crowley* Premium)	7.0	4.5
ripple (*Schwan's*)	5.0	3.5
chocolate peanut butter, deep (*Häagen-Dazs*)	19.0	n.a.
chocolate and praline (*Crowley* Premium)	9.0	4.5
chocolate sundae (*Blue Bell*)	9.0	6.0
Chunky Monkey (*Ben & Jerry's*)	19.0	10.0
cinnamon (*Ben & Jerry's*)	13.0	8.0
coconut almond (*Ben & Jerry's*)	16.0	7.0
coconut almond fudge chip (*Ben & Jerry's*)	25.0	14.0
coffee:		
(*Ben & Jerry's Aztec Harvest* Smooth)	16.0	10.0
(*Blue Bell*)	8.0	6.0
(*Edy's Grand*)	8.0	5.0
(*Häagen-Dazs*)	17.0	8.0
(*Häagen-Dazs*), 3.5-fl.-oz. container	15.0	7.0
(*Weeks*)	9.0	5.0
coffee almond fudge (*Ben & Jerry's*)	20.0	9.0
coffee toffee crunch (*Ben & Jerry's*)	19.0	10.0
coffee toffee crunch (*Häagen-Dazs*)	19.0	9.0
cookie dough (*Edy's Grand*)	9.0	5.0
cookie dough (*Edy's Grand* Light)	4.0	2.5
Cookie Dough Craze (*Weight Watchers* Light)	3.5	2.0
Cookie Dough Dynamo (*Häagen-Dazs Exträas*)	18.0	7.0
cookies and chocolate mint (*Blue Bell*)	10.0	7.0
cookies and cream:		
(*Blue Bell*)	10.0	7.0
(*Blue Bell* Light)	3.0	3.0
(*Edy's Grand*)	8.0	5.0
(*Edy's Grand* Light)	4.0	2.5
(*Häagen-Dazs*)	18.0	n.a.
(*Schwan's*)	8.0	4.5

	total fat (grams)	saturated fat (grams)
Ice cream, cookies and cream *(cont.)*		
(*Weeks*)	9.0	5.0
crunchy cone (*Edy's Grand*)	9.0	6.0
Dreamy Caramel Cream (*Edy's Grand* Light)	4.0	2.5
egg nog (*Weeks*)	8.0	5.0
English toffee crunch (*Ben & Jerry's*)	21.0	12.0
espresso chip (*Edy's Grand*)	9.0	6.0
French Silk (*Edy's Grand* Light)	5.0	3.0
fruit, tropical (*Blue Bell Diet*)	4.0	3.0
fruit special (*Blue Bell*)	8.0	5.0
fudge:		
brownie, double (*Edy's Grand*)	9.0	5.0
brownie nut (*Blue Bell*)	9.0	6.0
parfait (*Weeks*)	8.0	5.0
ripple (*Crowley* Premium)	7.0	4.0
walnut (*Weeks*)	10.0	5.0
fudgescotch swirl (*Edy's Grand* Light)	4.0	2.5
Heath bar crunch (*Crowley* Premium)	9.0	5.0
Heath bar crunch (*Weeks*)	11.0	6.0
heavenly hash (*Crowley* Premium/*Weeks*)	8.0	5.0
honey vanilla (*Häagen-Dazs*)	16.0	8.0
honey vanilla (*Häagen-Dazs*), 3.5-fl.-oz. container	14.0	7.0
ice cream sandwich (*Edy's Grand*)	8.0	5.0
M&M candy (*Weeks*)	9.0	6.0
macadamia nut brittle (*Häagen-Dazs*)	18.0	n.a.
malt ball 'n fudge (*Edy's Grand*)	8.0	5.0
malt ball 'n fudge (*Edy's Grand* Light)	4.0	2.5
maple nut (*Schwan's*)	9.0	5.0
maple walnut (*Weeks*)	10.0	5.0
marble fudge (*Edy's Grand*)	7.0	5.0
marble fudge (*Edy's Grand* Light)	4.0	2.5
(*Milky Way* Lowfat)	3.0	2.0
Milky Way (*Weeks*)	9.0	5.0
mint chocolate cookie (*Ben & Jerry's*)	17.0	10.0
mint fudge (*Edy's Grand* Light)	4.0	2.5

	total fat (grams)	saturated fat (grams)
Mississippi mud (*Weeks*)	10.0	6.0
mocha, Dutch (*Weeks*)	8.0	4.5
mocha almond fudge (*Edy's Grand*)	9.0	4.0
mocha almond fudge (*Edy's Grand* Light)	5.0	2.0
mocha fudge (*Ben & Jerry's* Smooth)	18.0	10.0
Neapolitan:		
(*Blue Bell*)	9.0	6.0
(*Blue Bell* Light)	2.0	1.0
(*Crowley* Premium)	8.0	5.0
(*Schwan's*)	7.0	5.0
New York Super Fudge Chunk (*Ben & Jerry's*)	20.0	11.0
Oreo cookie (*Crowley* Premium)	8.0	5.0
orange tango (*Crowley* Premium)	4.5	3.0
peach (*Crowley* Premium)	7.0	4.5
peach (*Schwan's*)	6.0	4.0
peach (*Schwan's Premium Extra Lite* Nonfat)	0	0
peaches and homemade vanilla (*Blue Bell*)	8.0	5.0
Peanut Butter Burst (*Häagen-Dazs Exträas*)	22.0	9.0
peanut butter cup (*Ben & Jerry's*)	26.0	12.0
peanut butter cup (*Edy's Grand*)	10.0	5.0
peanut butter fudge ripple (*Schwan's*)	7.0	4.5
pecan praline sundae (*Schwan's*)	7.0	4.5
pecan praline and cream (*Blue Bell*)	11.0	8.0
pecan praline and cream (*Blue Bell* Light)	3.0	2.0
peppermint (*Blue Bell*)	9.0	6.0
peppermint stick (*Schwan's*)	7.0	4.5
peppermint stick (*Weeks*)	9.0	5.0
pink divinity (*Schwan's*)	7.0	4.0
pistachio:		
California (*Weeks*)	10.0	6.0
almond (*Blue Bell*)	11.0	6.0
almond (*Blue Bell* Light)	2.0	1.0
Positively Praline Crunch (*Weight Watchers* Light)	3.0	1.5
praline almondine sundae (*Schwan's* Lite)	3.5	2.0

	total fat (grams)	saturated fat (grams)
Ice cream *(cont.)*		
Rainforest Crunch *(Ben & Jerry's)*	23.0	11.0
raspberry delight *(Schwan's)*	5.0	3.5
raspberry ripple *(Schwan's)*	7.0	4.5
rocky road:		
(*Blue Bell*)	10.0	6.0
(*Blue Bell* Diet /Reduced Calorie)	4.0	2.0
(*Blue Bell* Light)	3.0	1.0
(*Edy's Grand*)	10.0	5.0
(*Edy's Grand* Light)	5.0	2.5
Reckless Rocky Road (*Weight Watchers* Light)	3.0	1.5
(*Schwan's*)	6.0	4.0
rum raisin (*Häagen-Dazs*)	17.0	8.0
rum raisin (*Weeks*)	8.0	5.0
(*Schwan's* Summer Dream)	5.0	3.5
(*Snickers*)	11.0	5.0
strawberry:		
(*Blue Bell*)	7.0	4.0
(*Crowley* Premium)	7.0	4.0
(*Häagen-Dazs*)	15.0	8.0
(*Schwan's*)	7.0	4.5
(*Schwan's* Premium Extra Lite Nonfat)	0	0
(*Weeks*)	8.0	5.0
and cream (*Blue Bell*)	7.0	5.0
real (*Edy's Grand*)	6.0	4.0
sundae (*Blue Bell* Light)	2.0	1.0
strawberry cheesecake:		
(*Blue Bell*)	8.0	5.0
(*Edy's Grand*)	8.0	5.0
(*Weeks*)	7.0	4.5
Tangerine Dream (*Edy's Grand* Light)	4.0	2.0
tin roof (*Blue Bell*)	10.0	6.0
tin roof sundae (*Weeks*)	9.0	5.0

	total fat (grams)	saturated fat (grams)
Triple Brownie Overload (*Häagen-Dazs Exträas*) ...	22.0	n.a.
vanilla:		
(*Ben & Jerry's* Smooth)	17.0	10.0
(*Blue Bell* Light)	2.0	1.0
(*Crowley* Premium)	8.0	5.0
(*Edy's Grand*)	10.0	6.0
(*Edy's Grand* Light)	4.0	2.5
(*Häagen-Dazs*)	17.0	8.0
(*Häagen-Dazs*), 3.5-fl.-oz. container	15.0	7.0
Oh! So Very Vanilla! (*Weight Watchers* Light) ...	2.5	1.5
(*Schwan's*)	7.0	5.0
(*Schwan's* Premium Lite)	3.0	2.0
(*Schwan's Premium Extra Lite* Nonfat)	0	0
bean (*Ben & Jerry's* Smooth)	17.0	10.0
bean (*Edy's Grand*)	9.0	6.0
bean, natural (*Blue Bell*)	11.0	7.0
bean or regular (*Weeks*)	9.0	5.0
country (*Blue Bell*)	9.0	6.0
country (*Blue Bell Diet*)	4.0	2.0
w/chocolate chunks (*DoveBar*)	20.0	10.0
w/toffee chunks (*Nestlé Crunch*)	19.0	14.0
w/toffee chunks (*Nestlé Crunch* Lite), 2.5 oz. ..	7.0	5.0
vanilla, French:		
(*Blue Bell*)	9.0	6.0
(*Crowley* Premium)	7.0	4.5
(*Edy's Grand*)	10.0	6.0
(*Schwan's*)	9.0	6.0
(*Weeks*)	9.0	5.0
vanilla caramel fudge (*Ben & Jerry's* Smooth)	17.0	10.0
vanilla fudge (*Blue Bell* Light)	2.0	2.0
vanilla fudge (*Häagen-Dazs*)	17.0	n.a.
vanilla peanut butter swirl (*Häagen-Dazs*)	20.0	8.0
vanilla Swiss almond (*Häagen-Dazs*)	19.0	10.0
vanilla-chocolate-strawberry (*Edy's Grand*)	7.0	5.0
Wavy Gravy (*Ben & Jerry's*)	24.0	10.0

	total fat (grams)	saturated fat (grams)

Ice cream *(cont.)*

White Russian (*Ben & Jerry's* Smooth)	16.0	10.0

"Ice cream," substitute and nondairy:

all varieties, except chocolate chip mint and praline and caramel (*Healthy Choice*), 4 oz.	2.0	1.0

bars:

chocolate (*Rice Dream*), 1 bar	16.0	n.a.
chocolate, w/nuts (Nutty *Rice Dream*), 1 bar	23.0	n.a.
strawberry (*Rice Dream*), 1 bar	14.8	n.a.
vanilla (*Rice Dream*), 1 bar	15.8	n.a.
vanilla, w/nuts (Nutty *Rice Dream*), 1 bar	23.0	n.a.
carob (*Rice Dream*), ½ cup	5.0	n.a.
carob almond, carob chip, or mint carob chip (*Rice Dream*), ½ cup	6.0	n.a.
cappuccino (*Rice Dream*), ½ cup	5.0	n.a.
chocolate chip mint (*Healthy Choice*), ½ cup	2.0	2.0
cocoa marble fudge (*Rice Dream*), ½ cup	6.0	n.a.
lemon (*Rice Dream*), ½ cup	5.0	n.a.
peanut butter fudge (*Rice Dream*), ½ cup	7.0	n.a.
pie, oatmeal cookie, all varieties (*Rice Dream*), 1 pie	19.0	n.a.
praline and caramel (*Healthy Choice*), 4 oz.	2.0	0
strawberry or wildberry (*Rice Dream*), ½ cup	5.0	n.a.
vanilla (*Rice Dream*), ½ cup	5.0	n.a.
vanilla fudge (*Rice Dream*), ½ cup	6.0	n.a.
vanilla Swiss almond (*Rice Dream*), ½ cup	6.0	n.a.

Ice cream bar, 1 bar, except as noted:

almond (*Blue Bell*)	15.0	10.0
almond praline (*Edy's Grand*)	17.0	n.a.
Arctic D'Lites (*Weight Watchers*)	7.0	3.5
(*Blue Bell* Krunch), 2.2-oz. bar	13.0	10.0
(*Blue Bell* Krunch), 1.8-oz. bar	11.0	8.0
(*Blue Bell* Eskimo Pie)	12.0	9.0
(*Blue Bell* Eskimo Pie Take Home Snacks)	5.0	3.0
(*Blue Bell* Mooo)	13.0	11.0

	total fat (grams)	saturated fat (grams)
(*Blue Bell Mooo* Diet)	8.0	6.0
(*Blue Bell Mooo* Mini)	6.0	5.0
banana fudge (*Blue Bell*)	4.0	4.0
berries and cream mousse (*Weight Watchers*), 2 bars	1.5	0
caramel almond crunch (*Häagen-Dazs*)	18.0	7.0
caramel nut (*Weight Watchers*)	8.0	3.5
cappuccino (*Frozfruit*)	10.0	6.0
cherry cream (*Blue Bell*)	2.0	1.0
cherry royale (*DoveBar* Bite Size), 5 pieces	23.0	15.0
chocolate:		
(*Blue Bell* Stick Slices)	7.0	4.0
Chocolate Treat (*Weight Watchers*)	1.0	0
(*Nestlé Crunch*), 3-oz. bar	14.0	9.0
(*3Musketeers*), 1.6-oz. bar	8.0	4.0
(*3Musketeers*), 2.2-oz. bar	11.0	6.0
w/dark chocolate (*DoveBar*), 2.8-oz. bar	17.0	10.0
w/dark chocolate (*DoveBar*), 3.5-oz. bar	21.0	13.0
w/dark chocolate (*Häagen-Dazs*)	27.0	15.0
dip (*Weight Watchers*)	6.0	3.0
double (*Blue Bell*)	12.0	8.0
double (*DoveBar* Bit Size), 5 pieces	23.0	15.0
eclair (*Good Humor*)	9.0	3.0
fudge (*Blue Bell*)	5.0	5.0
malt (*Schwan's Push-Ems*)	2.5	1.5
mousse (*Weight Watchers*), 2 bars	1.0	.5
peanut butter crunch (*Häagen-Dazs*)	21.0	7.0
sundae crunch (*Schwan's*)	9.0	5.0
chocolate chip cookie dough, (*Ben & Jerry's*)	28.0	15.0
coffee almond crunch (*Häagen-Dazs*)	26.0	15.0
cookies and cream (*Edy's Grand*)	17.0	n.a.
cookies and cream, mini (*Blue Bell*)	4.0	3.0
eggnog w/dark chocolate (*DoveBar Bite Size*), 5 pieces	22.0	14.0

	total fat (grams)	saturated fat (grams)

Ice cream bar *(cont.)*

fudge:

    (*Blue Bell*) .... 4.0 .... 4.0

    (*Blue Bell* Diet) .... 1.0 .... 1.0

    (*Blue Bell Blast*) .... 6.0 .... 6.0

    (*Häagen-Dazs* Pops) .... 14.0 .... 7.0

    (*Schwan's*) .... 10.0 .... 2.0

    (*Schwan's Trim Creations*) 0 0

    double (*Blue Bell*) .... 12.0 .... 8.0

    mini (*Blue Bell*) .... 3.0 .... 2.0

(*Milky Way* Reduced Fat) .... 7.0 .... 3.0

(*Milky Way* Lowfat Shake), 8-oz. cup .... 3.0 .... 2.0

mint, w/fudge truffle (*DoveBar*) .... 17.0 .... 11.0

(*Nestlé Butterfinger*) .... 12.0 .... 7.0

(*Nestlé Cool Creations* Mickey Mouse), 2.5 oz. ... 7.0 .... 3.0

(*Nestlé Cool Creations* Mickey Mouse), 4 oz. ..... 11.0 .... 4.0

(*Nestlé Flintstones* Push-up Pebbles), 2.75 oz. ... 6.0 .... 4.0

(*Nestlé Heath*) .... 12.0 .... 8.0

New York Super Fudge Chunk (*Ben & Jerry's*) ... 31.0 .... 13.0

orange and cream (*Häagen-Dazs* Pops) .... 6.0 .... 3.0

orange and cream (*Schwan's Rainbow Stick*) ..... 1.0 .... 1.0

Orange Vanilla Treat (*Weight Watchers*), 2 bars ... 1.0 5

peanut (*Schwan's*) .... 14.0 .... 10.0

peanut butter and chocolate crisp (*Häagen-Dazs*) ... 28.0 .... 7.0

peppermint (*DoveBar* Bite Size), 5 pieces .... 22.0 .... 14.0

pralines 'n cream, crispy (*Weight Watchers*) ..... 7.0 .... 3.5

pudding, chocolate (*Schwan's*) .... 9.0 .... 5.0

root beer float (*Schwan's*) .... 2.0 .... 1.5

rocky road (*Edy's Grand*) .... 19.0 .... n.a.

(*Schwan's*) .... 14.0 .... 11.0

(*Schwan's Gold 'N' Nugit*) .... 16.0 .... 10.0

(*Schwan's Krispie Krunch*) .... 8.0 .... 6.0

(*Schwan's Silver Mint*) .... 10.0 .... 7.0

(*Snickers*) .... 12.0 .... 4.0

(*Snickers* Snack Size), 4 bars, 3.8 oz. .... 25.0 .... 9.0

strawberry shortcake (*Good Humor*) .... 8.0 .... 4.0

	total fat (grams)	saturated fat (grams)
toffee, English (*Schwan's*)	14.0	10.0
toffee, English (*Weight Watchers*)	7.0	3.5
toffee crunch, English (*Ben & Jerry's*)	23.0	15.0
vanilla:		
(*Ben & Jerry's*)	28.0	15.0
(*Blue Bell* Homemade)	17.0	13.0
(*Blue Bell* Stick Slices)	7.0	5.0
(*DoveBar* Bite Size), 5 pieces	24.0	16.0
(*Nestlé Crunch*), 3-oz. bar	14.0	9.0
(*Nestlé Crunch* Nuggets), 8 pieces	20.0	10.0
(*3Musketeers*), 1.6-oz. bar	7.0	4.0
(*3Musketeers*), 2.2-oz. bar	10.0	6.0
caramel and brittle (*DoveBar*)	16.0	11.0
caramel and brittle (*Häagen-Dazs*)	25.0	14.0
dark chocolate-coated (*Nestlé Bon Bons*),		
5 pieces	13.0	8.0
French (*DoveBar* Bite Size), 5 pieces	23.0	15.0
milk chocolate-coated (*Nestlé Bon Bons*),		
5 pieces	14.0	8.0
mocha cashew crunch (*DoveBar*)	17.0	10.0
w/almonds (*DoveBar*), 2.8-oz. bar	19.0	11.0
w/almonds (*DoveBar*), 3.5-oz. bar	24.0	14.0
w/dark chocolate (*DoveBar*), 2.7-oz. bar	17.0	11.0
w/dark chocolate (*DoveBar*), 3.4-oz. bar	21.0	14.0
w/dark chocolate (*Häagen-Dazs*)	27.0	15.0
w/milk chocolate (*DoveBar*), 2.7-oz. bar	17.0	11.0
w/milk chocolate (*DoveBar*), 3.4-oz. bar	21.0	15.0
w/mild chocolate (*Häagen-Dazs*)	24.0	14.0
w/white chocolate (*DoveBar*)	17.0	11.0
sandwich bar (*Weight Watchers*)	3.5	2.0
vanilla and almonds (*Edy's Grand*)	20.0	n.a.
vanilla and almonds (*Häagen-Dazs*)	27.0	14.0
vanilla crisp crunch (*Häagen-Dazs*)	16.0	6.0
Ice cream cone and cup, unfilled, 1 piece:		
(*Comet* Cup/Sugar Cone)	0	0

	total fat (grams)	saturated fat (grams)

Ice cream cone and cup *(cont.)*

(*Comet* Waffle Cone)	.5	0
chocolate (*Oreo*)	1.0	0
cinnamon graham (*Teddy Grahams*)	.5	0

Ice cream cone, filled, 1 piece:

(*Blue Bell* Mini Country Cones)	6.0	4.0
(*Nestlé Cool Creations*)	14.0	9.0
(*Schwan's Sundae Cone*)	10.0	7.0
caramel almond crunch (*Edy's Grand*)	20.0	n.a.
chocolate (*Nestlé Drumstick*)	19.0	10.0
chocolate, dipped (*Nestlé Drumstick*)	17.0	10.0
chocolate fudge, double (*Edy's Grand*)	27.0	n.a.
cookies and cream (*Edy's Grand*)	20.0	n.a.
pecan praline (*Schwan's Sundae Cone*)	12.0	7.0
vanilla (*Blue Bell* Country Cone)	18.0	12.0
vanilla (*Nestlé Crunch*)	16.0	10.0
vanilla (*Nestlé Drumstick*)	20.0	11.0
vanilla, w/caramel (*Nestlé Drumstick*)	20.0	12.0
vanilla fudge (*Nestlé Drumstick*)	21.0	11.0
vanilla fudge sundae (*Edy's Grand*)	19.0	n.a.

Ice cream cup, filled, 3 fl. oz., except as noted:

(*Blue Bell* Twist O Line Snack Cups)	5.0	3.0
(*Milky Way* Lowfat) 2.2-oz. cup	2.0	1.5
(*Schwan's*), 1.9-oz. cup	6.0	4.0
caramel fudge a la mode (*Weight Watchers*), 6.1 oz.	3.0	1.0
cherry freeze (*Blue Bell* Snack Cups)	0	0
chocolate or strawberry (*Blue Bell* Snack Cups)	5.0	3.0
chocolate or strawberry (*Schwan's*), 1.9 oz.	5.0	3.5
chocolate chip cookie dough (*Weight Watchers*), 5.4 oz.	4.0	1.5
cookies and cream (*Blue Bell*), 3-fl.-oz. cup	7.0	4.0
strawberry (*Carnation*), 5 oz.	8.0	5.0
strawberry or vanilla (*Schwan's* Nonfat), 2.6 oz.	0	0

	total fat (grams)	saturated fat (grams)
sundae, cherry, chocolate, fiesta, or strawberry (*Blue Bell* Snack Cups)	5.0	3.0
vanilla, homemade (*Blue Bell* Snack Cups)	8.0	5.0
vanilla or sprinkle twist (*Blue Bell* Snack Cups)	5.0	4.0
Ice cream sandwich, 1 piece:		
(*Blue Bell*)	6.0	4.0
(*Good Humor Sidewalk Sundae*), 3.5 fl. oz.	8.0	4.0
(*Schwan's*)	7.0	4.0
cookies and cream (*Blue Bell*)	7.0	5.0
cookies and cream (*Nestlé Cool Creations*), 3.5 oz.	11.0	4.0
mini (*Nestlé Cool Creations*), 2.3 oz.	5.0	2.0
Neapolitan (*Blue Bell*)	8.0	6.0
Ice cream and sorbet, see "Sorbet"		
Icing, cake, see "Frosting"		
Italian beans, canned (*Green Giant/Joan of Arc*), ½ cup	1.5	0
Italian sausage:		
(*Jones Dairy Farm*), 2-oz. link cooked	10.0	4.0
hot (*Hillshire Farm*), 2 oz.	17.0	n.a.
mild (*Hillshire Farm*), 2 oz.	11.0	n.a.
mild or hot (*Hillshire Farm* Light), 2 oz.	11.0	n.a.
pork:		
raw, 3.2-oz. link, 5 links per lb.	28.5	10.3
raw, 4-oz. link, 4 links per lb.	35.4	12.7
cooked, 2.4-oz. link (3.2-oz. link raw)	17.2	6.1
cooked, 3-oz. link (4-oz. link raw)	21.3	7.5
smoked (*Hillshire Farm* Flavorseal), 2 oz.	18.0	n.a.
turkey, see "Turkey sausage"		
Italian seasoning:		
1 tsp.	.1	<.1
(*Perc*), 1 tsp.	.1	0

J

	total fat (grams)	saturated fat (grams)
Jack-in-the-Box, 1 serving:		
breakfast:		
Breakfast Jack	12.0	5.0
croissant, sausage	48.0	19.0
croissant, supreme	36.0	15.0
Country Crock Spread	3.0	.5
grape jelly	0	0
hash browns	11.0	2.5
pancake platter	12.0	3.0
pancake syrup, 1.5 oz.	0	0
scrambled egg pocket	21.0	8.0
sourdough breakfast sandwich	20.0	7.0
ultimate breakfast sandwich	35.0	11.0
sandwiches:		
bacon bacon cheeseburger	45.0	15.0
burger, ¼ lb.	27.0	10.0
burger, colossus	84.0	28.0
burger, grilled sourdough	43.0	16.0
cheeseburger, regular	15.0	6.0
cheeseburger, double	24.0	12.0
cheeseburger, ultimate	79.0	26.0

	total fat (grams)	saturated fat (grams)
chicken	18.0	4.0
chicken Caesar	26.0	6.0
chicken, spicy crispy	27.0	5.0
chicken fajita pita	8.0	3.0
chicken fillet, grilled	19.0	5.0
chicken supreme	36.0	11.0
fish supreme	34.0	6.0
hamburger	11.0	4.0
Jumbo Jack burger	32.0	10.0
Jumbo Jack burger, w/cheese	40.0	14.0
The Outlaw Burger	40.0	17.0
The Really Big Chicken Sandwich	56.0	14.0
roast beef, Monterey	30.0	9.0
finger foods:		
egg rolls, 3 pieces	24.0	7.0
egg rolls, 5 pieces	41.0	12.0
chicken strips, breaded, 4 pieces	13.0	3.0
chicken strips, breaded, 6 pieces	20.0	5.0
jalapeños, stuffed, 7 pieces	27.0	12.0
jalapeños, stuffed, 10 pieces	39.0	16.0
potato wedges, bacon and cheddar	58.0	16.0
dipping sauces:		
barbecue dipping sauce, 1 oz.	0	0
buttermilk house dipping sauce, .9 oz.	13.0	5.0
sour cream, 1 oz.	6.0	4.0
sweet and sour dipping sauce, 1 oz.	0	0
Mexican food:		
guacamole, .9 oz.	4.0	.5
salsa, 1 oz.	0	0
taco	11.0	4.0
taco, super	17.0	6.0
teriyaki bowl, chicken	1.5	<1.0
salads and dressings:		
garden chicken salad	9.0	4.0
side salad	4.0	2.5

	total fat (grams)	saturated fat (grams)

Jack-in-the-Box, salads and dressings *(cont.)*

bleu cheese dressing, 2 oz.	18.0	3.5
buttermilk house dressing, 2 oz.	30.0	11.0
Italian, low calorie, dressing, 2 oz.	1.5	.0
Thousand Island dressing, 2 oz.	24.0	4.0
croutons	2.0	.5

side dishes:

french fries, small	11.0	2.5
french fries, regular	17.0	4.0
french fries, jumbo	19.0	5.0
french fries, curly, seasoned	20.0	5.0
french fries, super scoop	29.0	7.0
onion rings	23.0	6.0

condiments:

cheese, American, 1 slice	3.5	2.5
cheese, Swiss, 1 slice	3.0	2.0
hot sauce, ketchup, or soy sauce packet	0	0
mayonnaise packet	17.0	2.5
mustard packet, regular or Chinese hot	0	0
salsa	0	0
tartar dipping sauce	15.0	1.0

desserts and shakes:

apple turnover, hot	19.0	4.0
cheesecake	18.0	9.0
chocolate chip cookie dough cheesecake	18.0	8.0
shake, chocolate, regular	6.0	3.5
shake, strawberry or vanilla, regular	7.0	4.0

Jackfruit:

untrimmed, 1 lb.	.4	n.a.
trimmed, 1 oz.	.1	0

Jalapeño, see "Pepper, jalapeño"

Jalapeño dip:

(*Kraft*), 2 tbsp.	4.0	3.0
bean (*Doritos*)	1.0	.5

	total fat (grams)	saturated fat (grams)
bean (*Old El Paso*)	1.0	0
cheddar, see "Cheese dip"		
Jalapeño relish (*Old El Paso*), 1 tbsp.	0	0
Jalfrezi sauce, see "Cooking sauce"		
Jam and preserves, fruit, all varieties, all brands,		
1 tbsp.	0	0
Jamaican jerk:		
marinade base and dry seasoning (*Helen's Tropical*		
Exotics), 1 tbsp.	0	0
dipping sauce (*Helen's Tropical Exotics*), 2 tbsp. ...	0	0
Jambalaya mix (*Casbah*), 10 fl. oz.*	0	0
Jamaican jerk (see also "Marinade seasoning"):		
dipping sauce (*Helen's Jerk*), 2 tbsp.	0	0
marinade base or dry seasoning (*Helen's Jerk*),		
1 tbsp.	0	0
Java plum:		
w/seeds, 1 lb.	.9	n.a.
3 medium, about .4 oz.	<.1	0
seeded, ½ cup	.2	0
Jelly, fruit, all varieties, all brands, 1 tbsp.	0	0
Jelly, pepper (*Tabasco/Mchenny*), 1 tbsp.	0	0
Jerusalem artichoke:		
untrimmed, 1 lb.	<.1	0
sliced, ½ cup	<.1	0
Jicama, see "Yam bean tuber"		
Jowl, pork, raw, 1 oz.	19.7	7.2
Jujube:		
raw, w/seeds, 1 lb.	.8	n.a.
dried, 1 oz.	.3	n.a.
Jute:		
raw, untrimmed, 1 lb.	.7	.1
raw, trimmed, ½ cup	.1	<.1
boiled, drained, ½ cup	.1	<.1

K

	total fat (grams)	saturated fat (grams)
Kale:		
raw, untrimmed, 1 lb.	1.9	.3
raw, chopped, ½ cup	.2	<.1
boiled, drained, chopped, ½ cup	.3	<.1
canned (*Allens/Sunshine*), ½ cup	.5	0
frozen, 10-oz. pkg.	1.3	.2
frozen, boiled, drained, chopped, ½ cup	.3	<.1
Kale, Scotch:		
raw, untrimmed, 1 lb.	1.7	.2
raw, chopped, ½ cup	.2	<.1
boiled, drained, ½ cup	.3	<.1
Kamut, grain (*Arrowhead Mills*), ¼ cup	1.0	0
Kamut flour (*Arrowhead Mills*), ¼ cup	.5	0
Kamut pasta, see "Pasta"		
Kanpyo:		
1 lb.	2.5	.2
½ cup	.2	<.1
Kasha, see "Buckwheat groats"		
KFC, 1 serving:		
Original Recipe chicken:		
breast	20.0	5.0

	total fat (grams)	saturated fat (grams)
drumstick	7.0	2.0
thigh	17.0	5.0
whole wing	8.0	3.0
Colonel's Rotisserie Gold chicken, quarter:		
breast and wing, as served	18.7	5.4
breast and wing, skin and wing removed	5.9	1.7
thigh and leg, as served	23.7	6.6
thigh and leg, skin removed	12.2	3.5
Extra Tasty Crispy chicken:		
breast	28.0	7.0
drumstick	11.0	3.0
thigh	25.0	6.0
whole wing	13.0	4.0
Hot & Spicy chicken:		
breast	35.0	8.0
drumstick	11.0	3.0
thigh	27.0	7.0
whole wing	15.0	4.0
chicken snackables:		
BBQ flavored chicken sandwich, value	8.0	1.0
Colonel's chicken sandwich	27.0	6.0
Hot Wings, 6 pieces	33.0	8.0
Kentucky Nuggets, 6 pieces	18.0	4.0
side dishes:		
BBQ baked beans	2.0	1.0
biscuit, 1 piece	12.0	3.0
coleslaw	6.0	1.0
corn on the cob	12.0	2.0
cornbread, 1 piece, 2 oz.	6.4	1.4
garden rice	1.0	0
green beans	1.0	0
macaroni and cheese	8.0	3.0
mashed potatoes w/gravy	5.0	<1.0
Mean Greens	2.0	1.0
potato salad	11.0	2.0

	total fat (grams)	saturated fat (grams)

KFC, side dishes *(cont.)*

potato wedges	9.0	3.0
red beans and rice	3.0	1.0

Kidney bean, dried:

all varieties, raw, 1 oz.	.2	.1
all varieties, boiled, ½ cup	.4	.1
red (*Arrowhead Mills*), ¼ cup	.5	0
red (*Van Camp's*), ½ cup	0	0
canned, red, ½ cup		
(*Eden* Organic)	0	0
dark (*Allens/East Texas Fair*)	.5	0
dark or light (*Brooks*)	.5	0
dark or light (*Green Giant/Joan of Arc*)	0	0
dark or light (*Stokely*)	.5	0
dark or light (*Van Camp's*), ½ cup	0	0
drained (*Progresso*)	.5	0
light (*Allens*)	.5	0
w/bacon, New Orleans style (*Trappey's*)	1.0	.5
w/chili gravy (*Trappey's*)	1.0	0
w/jalapeños (*Trappey's*)	1.0	0
canned, white (*Progresso* Cannellini), ½ cup	.5	0

Kidney bean, sprouted, mature seeds:

raw, lb.	2.3	.3
raw, ½ cup	.5	.1
boiled, drained, 4 oz.	.7	.1

Kidney, simmered or braised:

beef, 4 oz.	3.9	1.2
lamb, 4 oz.	4.1	1.4
pork, 4 oz.	5.3	1.7
veal, 4 oz.	6.4	2.0

Kielbasa (see also "Polish sausage"), 2 oz.,
   except as noted:

(*Boar's Head*)	10.0	4.0
(*Healthy Choice* Low Fat Polska)	2.0	1.0
(*Hillshire Farm*)	17.0	n.a.

	total fat (grams)	saturated fat (grams)
(*Hillshire Farm* Bun Size)	16.0	n.a.
(*Hillshire Farm* Links 80% Fat Free)	10.0	n.a.
(*Hillshire Farm* Lit'l Polska)	16.0	n.a.
(*Hillshire Farm* Lower Fat)	11.0	n.a.
(*Hillshire Farm* Polska Links)	17.0	n.a.
(*Hillshire Farm* Polska Links Light), 2.7 oz.	15.0	n.a.
(*Hillshire Farm Flavorseal* Polska Regular or Mild)	17.0	n.a.
(*Hillshire Farm Flavorseal* Light)	11.0	n.a.
(*Thorn Apple Valley*), 2 oz.	16.0	n.a.
(*Thorn Apple Valley* Skinless), 3 oz. link	24.0	n.a.
beef (*Hillshire Farm Flavorseal* Polska)	17.0	n.a.
pork and beef, 1 oz.	7.7	2.8
Kishka (*Hebrew National*), 2 oz.	11.0	5.0
Kiwi:		
untrimmed, 1 lb.	1.7	n.a.
1 large, about 3.7 oz.	.4	0
dried (*Sonoma*), 1 oz., 7–8 pieces	1.0	0
Knockwurst:		
(*Hillshire Farm* Links), 2 oz.	16.0	n.a.
beef (*Boar's Head*), 4 oz.	27.0	11.0
beef (*Hebrew National*), 3-oz. link	25.0	9.0
pork and beef, 2.4-oz. link	18.9	6.9
Kohlrabi:		
raw, untrimmed, 1 lb.	.4	<.1
raw, sliced, ½ cup	.1	<.1
boiled, drained, sliced, ½ cup	.1	<.1
Kumbu, see "Seaweed"		
Kumquat:		
untrimmed, 1 lb.	.4	<.1
1 medium, about .7 oz.	<.1	0

L

	total fat (grams)	saturated fat (grams)
Lamb, choice grade, meat only, 4 oz., except as noted:		
cubed for stew or kabob (leg and shoulder):		
braised or stewed	10.0	3.6
broiled	8.3	3.0
foreshank, braised or stewed:		
lean and fat	15.3	6.4
lean only	6.8	2.4
ground:		
raw, 1 oz.	6.7	2.9
broiled	22.3	9.2
broiled, 1 cup, approx. 4.1 oz.	23.1	9.4
leg, roasted:		
whole, lean and fat	18.7	7.8
whole, lean only	8.8	3.1
shank half, lean and fat	14.1	5.8
shank half, lean only	7.6	2.7
sirloin half, lean and fat	23.4	9.9
sirloin half, lean only	10.4	3.7
loin chop, broiled:		
lean and fat, 1 chop, 2.25 oz. (4.2 oz. w/bone)	14.7	6.3

	total fat (grams)	saturated fat (grams)
lean and fat	26.2	11.1
lean only, 1 chop, 1.6 oz. (4.2 oz. w/bone and fat)	4.5	1.6
lean only	11.0	3.9
loin, roasted, lean and fat	26.8	11.6
loin, lean only	11.1	4.2
rib:		
broiled, lean and fat	33.6	14.4
broiled, lean only	14.7	5.3
roasted, lean and fat	33.8	14.5
roasted, lean only	15.1	5.4
shoulder, whole:		
braised, lean and fat	27.8	11.7
braised, lean only	10.0	7.0
broiled, lean and fat	21.8	9.1
broiled, lean only	11.9	4.4
roasted, lean and fat	22.6	9.6
roasted, lean only	12.2	4.6
shoulder, arm, braised or stewed:		
lean and fat, 1 chop, 2.5 oz. (5.6 oz. w/bone)	16.9	7.0
lean only, 1 chop, 1.9 oz. (5.6 oz. w/bone and fat)	7.7	2.8
lean and fat	27.2	11.2
lean only	16.0	5.7
shoulder, arm, broiled:		
lean and fat, 1 chop, 3.3 oz. (5.6 oz. w/bone)	18.2	7.8
lean only, 1 chop, 2.6 oz. (5.6 oz. w/bone and fat)	6.7	2.5
lean and fat	22.2	9.5
lean only	10.2	3.9
shoulder, arm, roasted:		
lean and fat	23.0	9.9

	total fat (grams)	saturated fat (grams)
Lamb, shoulder, arm, roasted *(cont.)*		
lean only	10.5	4.1
shoulder, blade:		
braised or stewed, lean and fat	28.0	11.7
braised or stewed, lean only	18.9	7.2
broiled, lean and fat	22.6	9.3
broiled, lean only	12.8	4.6
roasted, lean and fat	23.4	9.8
roasted, lean only	13.1	4.9
Lamb, New Zealand, frozen, 4 oz., except as noted:		
foreshank, braised or stewed:		
lean and fat	18.0	8.9
lean only	6.8	3.0
leg, whole, roasted:		
lean and fat	17.6	8.6
lean only	7.9	3.5
loin, broiled:		
lean and fat, 1 chop, 1.5 oz. (3 oz. w/bone)	10.2	5.2
lean only, 1 chop, 1.1 oz. (3 oz. w/bone and fat)	2.5	1.1
lean and fat	27.1	13.6
lean only	9.3	4.1
rib, roasted:		
lean and fat	32.6	16.4
lean only	11.5	5.0
shoulder, whole, braised or stewed:		
lean and fat	29.8	14.4
lean only	17.6	7.7
Lamb's-quarter:		
raw, trimmed, 1 oz.	.2	<.1
boiled, drained, chopped, ½ cup	.6	<.1
Lard, pork:		
1 tbsp.	12.8	5.0
(*Patrick Cudahy*), 1 tbsp.	13.0	5.0
Lasagna, noodles, see "Pasta"		

	total fat (grams)	saturated fat (grams)

Lasagna entree, canned or packaged:

(*Hormel*), 7.5-oz. can	14.0	.... 7.0
(*Hormel* Micro Cup), 1 cup	7.0	.... 2.0
(*Libby's Diner*), 7.75 oz.	7.0	.... 3.5
(*Nalley*), 7.5 oz.	6.0	.... 3.0
and beef, w/tomato sauce (*Hormel* Micro Cup), 1 cup	19.0	.... 7.0
w/beef (*Nalley*), 7.5 oz.	6.0	.... 2.5
w/beef and three cheeses (*Nalley*), 7.5 oz.	6.0	.... 3.0
Italian (*Hormel Top Shelf*), 1 bowl	15.0	.... 8.0
w/meat and sauce (*Dinty Moore American Classics*), 1 bowl	4.0	.... 2.0

Lasagna entree, freeze-dried

(*Mountain House*), 1 cup*	9.0	.... 4.0

Lasagna entree, frozen:

(*Celentano*), 10 oz.	14.0	.... 6.0
(*Celentano*), ½ of 14-oz. tray	10.0	.... 5.0
(*Celentano*, 25 oz.), 8 oz., 1 cup	17.0	.... 9.0
(*Celentano* Value Pack), 8 oz., 1 cup	11.0	.... 5.0
(*Healthy Choice*), 10 oz.	5.0	.... 2.0
w/beef in sauce (*Schwan's*), 1 cup	11.0	.... 6.0
cheese:		
(*Lean Cuisine* Classic), 11.5 oz.	6.0	.... 3.0
four (*Stouffer's*), 10¾ oz.	19.0	.... 10.0
three (*The Budget Gourmet*), 10.5 oz.	16.0	.... 10.0
casserole (*Lean Cuisine* Lunch Express), 9.5 oz.	7.0	.... 2.5
w/chicken scalloppini (*Lean Cuisine* Cafe Classics), 10 oz.	8.0	.... 2.5
chicken Alfredo (*Schwan's*), 1 cup	12.0	.... 6.0
Florentine (*Weight Watchers Smart Ones*), 10 oz.	2.0	5
garden (*Weight Watchers*), 11 oz.	5.0	.... 1.0
w/Italian cheese (*Weight Watchers*), 11 oz.	8.0	.... 3.0

	total fat (grams)	saturated fat (grams)
Lasagna entree, frozen *(cont.)*		
w/Italian vegetables (*Weight Watchers Smart Ones*),		
9.5 oz.	2.0	.5
w/meat sauce:		
(*Banquet*), 7 oz.	8.0	4.0
(*The Budget Gourmet* Light & Healthy), 9.4 oz.	7.0	3.0
(*Lean Cuisine*), 10¼ oz.	6.0	2.5
(*Stouffer's*), 10½ oz.	13.0	5.0
(*Stouffer's*), ⅓ of 21-oz. pkg.	10.0	4.0
(*Stouffer's*), ⅕ of 40-oz. pkg.	10.0	4.0
(*Stouffer's*), 1/13 of 96-oz. pkg.	12.0	6.0
(*Stouffer's Lunch Express*), 10¼ oz.	10.0	5.0
(*Weight Watchers*), 10.25 oz.	7.0	2.5
sausage, Italian (*The Budget Gourmet*), 10.5 oz.	21.0	9.0
vegetable, 10 oz., except as noted:		
(*The Budget Gourmet* Light & Healthy),		
10.5 oz.	10.0	5.0
(*Celentano* Great Choice)	2.5	1.0
(*Celentano* Great Choice Primavera)	7.0	4.0
(*Celentano* Selects Primavera)	4.0	1.5
(*Schwan's*), 1 cup	10.0	6.0
(*Stouffer's*), 10.5 oz.	19.0	5.0
(*Stouffer's*), 1/12 of 96-oz. pkg.	12.0	5.0
California style (*Schwan's*), 1 cup	10.0	5.0
zucchini:		
(*Healthy Choice Quick Meal*), 11.5 oz.	3.0	2.0
(*Lean Cuisine*), 11 oz.	4.0	1.5
Leaf fat, raw, 1 oz.	26.7	12.8
Leek:		
raw, untrimmed, 1 lb.	.6	.1
raw, 1 medium, about 9.9 oz.	.4	.1
boiled, drained, 1 medium, about 4.4 oz.	.3	<.1
boiled, drained, chopped, ½ cup	.1	<.1
Leek, freeze-dried, 1 tbsp.	.2	tr.
Lekvar, see "Prune-plum pastry filling"		

	total fat (grams)	saturated fat (grams)
Lemon:		
whole, 1 medium, 3.9 oz.	.3	<.1
peeled, 1 medium	.2	<.1
Lemon drink, all varieties, all brands, 8 fl. oz.	0	0
Lemon juice, fresh, 1 fl. oz.	0	0
Lemon peel, 1 tbsp.	<.1	0
Lemon pepper marinade, 1 tbsp.:		
(*Lawry's*)	.5	0
and garlic (*World Harbors* Acadia)	0	0
Lemon pepper seasoning:		
(*Lawry's*), ¼ tsp.	0	0
(*Perc*), 1 tsp.	.1	0
Lemon spice seasoning (*Perc*), 1 tsp.	0	0
Lemonade, all blends and brands, 8 fl. oz.	0	0
Lentil:		
raw:		
1 oz.	.3	<.1
½ cup	.9	.1
green or red (*Arrowhead Mills*), ¼ cup	0	0
boiled, ½ cup	.4	.1
Lentil, sprouted:		
raw, ½ cup	.2	<.1
stir-fried, w/out fat, 4 oz.	.5	.1
Lentil entree, canned, 1 cup:		
w/garden vegetables (*Health Valley*)	1.0	0
tofu (*Health Valley* Vegetarian Cuisine)	1.0	0
Lentil mix:		
chili, see "Chili, mix"		
hearty, and wild rice (*Spice Islands*), 1 pkg.	2.5	0
pilaf (*Casbah*), 1 oz. dry, ½ cup*	0	0
pilaf (*Near East*), 1 cup*	4.0	1.0
Lentil rice loaf, frozen (*Natural Touch*), 3.2 oz., 1" slice	9.0	2.5
Lettuce:		
bibb, Boston or butterhead, untrimmed, 1 lb.	.7	.1

	total fat (grams)	saturated fat (grams)

Lettuce *(cont.)*

bibb, Boston or butterhead, 1 medium head ..... | .4 | <.1

iceberg:

    untrimmed, 1 lb. .... | .8 | .1

    6" head, 1¼ lbs. .... | 1.0 | .1

    w/carrots and red cabbage (*Dole*), 3.5 oz. .... | 0 | 0

looseleaf, untrimmed, 1 lb. .... | .9 | .1

looseleaf, shredded, ½ cup .... | .1 | <.1

romaine or cos:

    untrimmed, 1 lb. .... | .9 | .1

    shredded, ½ cup .... | .1 | 0

    and radicchio (*Dole*), 3.5 oz. .... | 1.0 | 0

Lima bean:

raw, untrimmed, 1 lb. .... | 1.7 | .4

raw, trimmed, ½ cup .... | .4 | .1

boiled, drained, ½ cup .... | .3 | .1

dried, ½ cup:

    baby, raw .... | .9 | .2

    baby, boiled .... | .3 | .1

    large, raw .... | .6 | .1

    large, boiled .... | .4 | .1

canned, ½ cup:

    (*Green Giant/Joan of Arc* Butter Beans) ...... | 0 | 0

    (*Seneca*) .... | 0 | 0

    (*Stokely*) .... | 1.0 | 0

    (*Van Camp's*) .... | .5 | 0

    green (*Allens/Butterfield/Sunshine*) .... | .5 | 0

    green (*Del Monte*) .... | 0 | 0

    green, baby, w/bacon (*Allens/Trappey's*) ...... | 1.0 | .5

    green and white (*Allens*) .... | 1.0 | .5

    large (*Sunshine* Butterbeans) .... | .5 | 0

    white, baby, w/bacon (*Allens/Trappey's*) ...... | 1.5 | .5

    white, large, w/sausage (*Allens/Trappey's*) .... | 1.0 | 0

frozen, ½ cup, except as noted:

    (*McKenzie's*) .... | 0 | 0

	total fat (grams)	saturated fat (grams)
(*McKenzie's* Petite)	.5	0
baby (*Green Giant Harvest Fresh*)	0	0
in butter sauce (*Green Giant*), ⅔ cup	2.5	2.0
(*Stilwell/Stilwell* Butter Beans)	0	0
Lima beans and ham, canned, in sauce (*Nalley*), 1 cup	5.0	2.0
Lime, 1 medium, 2.8 oz.	.1	<.1
Lime juice:		
fresh, 1 fl. oz.	<.1	0
sweetened (*Rose's*), 1 tbsp.	0	0
Limeade, all varieties, all brands, 8 fl. oz.	0	0
Ling, meat only:		
raw, 4 oz.	.7	n.a.
baked, broiled, or microwaved, 4 oz.	.9	n.a.
Lingcod, meat only:		
raw, 4 oz.	1.2	.2
baked, broiled, or microwaved, 4 oz.	1.5	.3
Linguine, see "Pasta"		
Linguine dishes, mix:		
w/chicken and broccoli (*Golden Grain Noodle Roni*), 1 cup*	16.0	3.0
herbed (*Country Inn Recipes*), 2 oz.	3.0	1.5
Linguine entree, frozen:		
w/clam sauce (*Lean Cuisine Entree*), 9⅝ oz.	8.0	2.0
w/shrimp, clams (*The Budget Gourmet* Light & Healthy), 9.5 oz.	8.0	5.0
w/shrimp, clams, marinara (*The Budget Gourmet*), 10 oz.	11.0	6.0
w/tomato sauce, Italian sausage (*The Budget Gourmet*), 10.25 oz.	14.0	4.0
Liquor, distilled (bourbon, brandy, rum, rye, scotch, tequila, vodka, etc.), all proofs, 4 fl. oz.	0	0
Litchi nut:		
raw, untrimmed, 1 lb.	1.2	n.a.
raw, shelled and seeded, ½ cup	.4	tr.

	total fat (grams)	saturated fat (grams)

Litchi nut *(cont.)*
dried, 1 oz. .... .3 .... <.1
Liver:
beef:
    raw, 1 oz. 1.1 4
    braised, 4 oz. .... 5.5 .... 2.2
    pan-fried in vegetable oil, 4 oz. .... 9.1 .... 3.0
calves', see "veal," below
chicken, broiler-fryer:
    raw, 1 liver, 1.1 oz. 1.2 4
    simmered, 1 liver, about .7 oz. 1.1 4
    simmered, chopped or diced, 1 cup .... 7.6 .... 2.6
duck, domesticated, raw, 1 oz. 1.3 4
goose, domesticated, raw, 1 medium, 3.3 oz. .... 4.0 .... 1.5
lamb:
    raw, 1 oz. 1.4 6
    braised, 4 oz. .... 10.0 .... 3.9
    pan-fried in vegetable oil, 4 oz. .... 14.3 .... 5.6
pork, raw, 1 oz. 1.0 3
pork, braised, 4 oz. .... 5.0 .... 1.6
turkey:
    raw, 1 oz. 1.1 4
    simmered, 4 oz. .... 6.7 .... 2.1
    simmered, chopped or diced, 1 cup .... 8.3 .... 2.6
veal:
    raw, 1 oz. 1.2 5
    braised, 4 oz. .... 7.8 .... 2.9
    pan-fried in vegetable oil, 4 oz. .... 12.9 .... 4.8
Liver cheese:
(*Oscar Mayer*), 1.3-oz. slice .... 10.0 .... 4.0
pork, 1 oz. .... 7.2 .... 2.5
Liver pâté, see "Liverwurst" and "Pâté"
Liver sausage, see "Liverwurst"
Liverwurst (see also "Braunschweiger"):
(*Boar's Head* Strassburger), 2 oz. .... 15.0 .... 6.0

	total fat (grams)	saturated fat (grams)
(*Hormel*), 4 tbsp.	10.0	3.5
(*Jones Dairy Farm* Sausage Chub), 1-oz. slice	6.0	n.a.
(*Jones Dairy Farm* Sausage Chub Light), 1-oz. slice	3.0	n.a.
(*Jones Dairy Farm* Sausage Sliced), .8-oz. slice	7.0	n.a.
pâté (*Boar's Head*), 2 oz.	12.0	4.0
pork, 1 oz.	8.1	3.0
smoked (*Boar's Head*), 2 oz.	15.0	6.0
Liverwurst, canned (see also "Pâté") (*Underwood*), 2 oz., ¼ cup	14.0	5.0
Lobster, northern, meat only:		
raw, 5.3 oz. (1½ lbs. in shell)	1.4	n.a.
boiled, poached, or steamed, 4 oz.	.7	.1
boiled, poached, or steamed, 1 cup	.9	.2
Lobster, spiny, see "Spiny lobster"		
Lobster sauce, canned, rock (*Progresso*), ½ cup	7.0	1.0
Loganberry:		
trimmed, 1 cup	.9	n.a.
frozen, ½ cup	.2	n.a.
Longan:		
raw, 5 medium, about 1 oz.	<.1	0
dried, 1 oz.	.1	0
Loquat:		
untrimmed, 1 lb.	.6	.1
peeled and seeded, 1 oz.	.1	<.1
Lotte, see "Monkfish"		
Lotus seeds:		
raw, in shell, 1 lb.	1.3	.2
raw, shelled, 1 oz.	.2	<.1
dried, 1 oz., 47 small or 36 large	.6	.1
Lox, see "Salmon, chinook, smoked" and "Salmon, smoked"		
Lunch combinations, 1 pkg.:		
bologna and American:		
(*Hillshire Farm Lunch 'n Munch*)	37.0	n.a.

	total fat (grams)	saturated fat (grams)

Lunch combinations, bologna and American *(cont.)*

(*Hillshire Farm Lunch 'n Munch, Snickers*)	34.0	.... n.a.
(*Oscar Mayer Lunchables*)	37.0	.... 17.0
(*Oscar Mayer Lunchables* Fun Pack)	29.0	.... 14.0

chicken:

Monterey jack (*Oscar Mayer Lunchables* Dessert)	20.0	.... 10.0
and turkey (*Oscar Mayer Lunchables* Deluxe) .	23.0	.... 12.0

chicken, smoked, and Monterey jack:

(*Hillshire Farm Lunch 'n Munch*)	20.0	.... n.a.
(*Hillshire Farm Lunch 'n Munch, Snickers*)	23.0	.... n.a.

ham and American:

(*Oscar Mayer Lunchables* Dessert)	20.0	.... 10.0
(*Oscar Mayer Lunchables* Fun Pack)	20.0	.... 10.0

ham and cheddar:

(*Hillshire Farm Lunch 'n Munch, Snickers*)	23.0	.... n.a.
(*Oscar Mayer Lunchables*)	23.0	.... 12.0

ham w/spreadable cheese, garden vegetable, or
herb and chive (*Oscar Mayer Lunchables Deli-Thin*)

Thin)	21.0	.... 9.0

ham and Swiss:

(*Hillshire Farm Lunch 'n Munch*)	22.0	.... n.a.
(*Hillshire Farm Lunch 'n Munch Oreo*)	21.0	.... n.a.
(*Hillshire Farm Lunch 'n Munch Snickers*)	21.0	.... n.a.
(*Oscar Mayer Lunchables*)	20.0	.... 10.0
(*Oscar Mayer Lunchables* Dessert)	21.0	.... 10.0

pepperoni and American:

(*Hillshire Farm Lunch 'n Munch*)	46.0	.... n.a.
(*Oscar Mayer Lunchables*)	38.0	.... 18.0
salami and American (*Oscar Mayer Lunchables*) ..	34.0	.... 17.0

turkey:

(*Oscar Mayer Lunchables* Fun Pack/Pacific Cooler)	21.0	.... 10.0
(*Oscar Mayer Lunchables* Fun Pack/Surfer Cooler)	16.0	.... 8.0

	total fat (grams)	saturated fat (grams)
turkey and cheddar:		
(*Hillshire Farm Lunch 'n Munch*)	21.0	n.a.
(*Hillshire Farm Lunch 'n Munch*, Brownie)	22.0	n.a.
(*Oscar Mayer Lunchables*)	22.0	12.0
(*Oscar Mayer Lunchables*) Dessert /Jell-O	16.0	9.0
(*Oscar Mayer Lunchables* Dessert /Trail Mix)	23.0	11.0
turkey and spreadable cheese, green onion or ranch and herb (*Oscar Mayer Lunchables Deli-Thin*)	20.0	9.0
turkey and ham (*Oscar Mayer Lunchables* Deluxe)	21.0	11.0
turkey and Monetery jack (*Oscar Mayer Lunchables*)	21.0	11.0
Luncheon meat (see also specific listings):		
spiced (*Oscar Mayer* Loaf), 1-oz. slice	5.0	1.5
canned (*Spam/Spam* Less Salt), 2 oz.	16.0	6.0
canned (*Spam* Lite), 2 oz.	8.0	3.0
Luncheon "meat," vegetarian:		
canned (*Worthington Protose*), 1.9 oz., 3/8" slice	7.0	1.0
frozen (*Worthington Wham*), 1.6 oz., 2 slices	5.0	1.0
Lungs, 4 oz.:		
beef, braised	4.2	1.4
lamb, braised	3.5	n.a.
pork, braised	3.5	1.2
veal, braised	.7	n.a.
Lupin:		
raw, 1 oz.	2.8	.3
raw, ½ cup	8.8	1.0
boiled, ½ cup	2.4	.3
Luxury loaf, pork, 1-oz. slice	1.4	.5
Lychee, see "Litchi nut"		

M

	total fat (grams)		saturated fat (grams)
Macadamia nut, shelled, except as noted:			
dried, in shell, 4 oz.	25.9	....	3.9
dried, 1 oz.	20.9	....	3.1
oil-roasted, 1 oz., 10–12 whole kernels	21.7	....	3.3
oil-roasted, chopped, ½ cup	42.1	....	6.3
Macaroni (see also "Pasta"), dry:			
uncooked, 2 oz.:			
regular, raw	.9	....	.1
vegetable or tri-color	.6	....	.1
whole wheat	.8	....	.1
cooked, 1 cup:			
elbow or spirals	.9	....	.1
small shells	.8	....	.1
vegetable or tri-color, spirals	.1	....	<.1
whole wheat, spirals	.8	....	.1
Macaroni entree, canned or packaged:			
(*Chef Boyardee*), ½ of 15-oz. can	7.0	....	3.0
and beef:			
(*Hormel Kid's Kitchen* Cheezy Mac & Beef),			
7.5-oz. cup	7.0	....	2.5
(*Libby's Diner*), 7.75 oz.	9.0	....	4.0

	total fat (grams)	saturated fat (grams)
(*Nalley*), 7.5 oz.	4.0	1.0
w/vegetables (*Hormel* Micro Cup), 1 cup	8.0	3.0
beefy (*Hormel Kid's Kitchen*), 7.5-oz. cup	6.0	2.5
and cheese:		
(*Franco American*), 1 cup	7.0	3.0
(*Hormel Kid's Kitchen*), 7.5-oz. cup	11.0	6.0
(*Hormel Micro Cup*), 7.5 oz.	11.0	6.0
(*Libby's Diner*), 7.75 oz.	20.0	7.0
(*Nalley*), 7.5 oz.	14.0	10.0
Macaroni entree, frozen:		
and beef:		
(*Banquet* Family), 8 oz.	7.0	3.0
(*Healthy Choice Quick Meal*), 8.5 oz.	3.0	1.0
(*Lean Cuisine*), 10 oz.	8.0	2.0
(*Stouffer's*), 11.5 oz.	12.0	5.0
(*Weight Watchers*), 9.5 oz.	4.5	1.5
and cheese:		
(*Banquet* Family), 8 oz.	10.0	5.0
(*The Budget Gourmet* Homestyle), 10 oz.	20.0	12.0
(*The Budget Gourmet* Side Dish), 6 oz.	13.0	8.0
(*Healthy Choice Quick Meal*), 9 oz.	6.0	3.0
(*Kid Cuisine*), 8.5 oz.	7.0	2.5
(*Lean Cuisine*), 9 oz.	7.0	3.5
(*Morton* Casseroles), 8 oz.	4.0	2.0
(*Schwan's*), 1 cup	20.0	5.0
(*Stouffer's*), ½ of 12-oz. pkg.	16.0	6.0
(*Stouffer's*), 1 cup or ⅕ of 40-oz. pkg.	16.0	6.0
(*Stouffer's*), ⅑ of 76-oz. pkg.	14.0	6.0
(*Swanson*), 9 oz.	14.0	9.0
(*Swanson* Budget), 10.3 oz.	11.0	7.0
(*Swanson* Mac & More), 6 oz.	9.0	4.0
(*Swanson Fun Feast*), 11 oz.	11.0	5.0
(*Tabatchnick*), 7.5 oz.	12.0	6.0
(*Weight Watchers*), 9 oz.	6.0	2.0

	total fat (grams)	saturated fat (grams)

Macaroni entree, frozen, and cheese *(cont.)*

    and broccoli (*Lean Cuisine Lunch Express*),

        9¾ oz. .... 6.0 .... 3.0

    w/broccoli (*Stouffer's Lunch Express*),

        10⅜ oz. .... 19.0 .... 5.0

    w/broccoli (*Swanson* Mac & More), 6 oz. .... 8.0 .... 3.5

    w/cheddar and Parmesan (*The Budget Gourmet*

        Light & Healthy), 10 oz. .... 8.0 .... 5.0

    nacho (*Healthy Choice Quick Meal*), 9 oz. .... 5.0 .... 3.0

    nacho (*Hormel Kid's Kitchen*), 7.5 oz. .... 6.0 .... 2.0

    salsa (*Swanson* Mac & More), 6 oz. .... 8.0 .... 3.0

  pie (*Banquet*), 7 oz. .... 3.0 .... 1.5

  pie (*Morton*), 6.5 oz. .... 3.0 .... 1.5

Macaroni entree, mix (see also "Pasta dishes, mix"):

  (*Kraft* Dinner Original), 2.5 oz. .... 2.5 .... 1.0

  (*Kraft* Dinner Original), about 1 cup* .... 17.0 .... 4.0

  (*Kraft* Deluxe Original Dinner), 3.5 oz., about

    1 cup* .... 10.0 .... 6.0

  (*Kraft* Thick 'N Creamy Dinner), 2.5 oz. .... 2.5 .... 1.0

  (*Kraft* Thick 'N Creamy Dinner), about 1 cup* .... 10.0 .... 6.0

  (*Kraft* Dinosaurs/Santa Mac/Spirals/*Super Mario*

    Bros./Teddy Bears/*The Flintstones* Dinner),

    2.5 oz. .... 3.0 .... 1.5

  (*Kraft* Dinosaurs/Santa Mac/Spirals/*Super Mario*

    Bros./Teddy Bears/*The Flintstones* Dinner),

    about 1 cup* .... 17.0 .... 4.5

  cheddar:

    (*Fantastic*), ⅜ cup 1.5 0

    mild white (*Kraft* Thick 'N Creamy), 2.5 oz. ... 3.0 .... 1.0

    mild white (*Kraft* Thick 'N Creamy), about

      1 cup* .... 17.0 .... 4.0

  Parmesan (*Fantastic*), ⅜ cup 1.5 0

Macaroni and beef or cheese,

  see "Macaroni entree"

	total fat (grams)	saturated fat (grams)
Mace, ground:		
1 tbsp.	1.7	.5
1 tsp.	.6	.2
Mackerel, meat only, 4 oz.:		
Atlantic, raw	15.8	3.7
Atlantic, baked, broiled or microwaved	20.2	4.7
king, raw	2.3	.4
king, baked, broiled, or microwaved	2.9	.5
Pacific and jack, raw	9.0	2.6
Spanish, raw	7.2	2.1
Spanish, baked, broiled, or microwaved	7.2	2.0
Mackerel, canned, jack:		
4 oz.	7.1	2.1
1 cup	12.0	3.5
Mahi-mahi, fresh, see "Dolphin fish"		
Mahi-mahi, frozen, fillets (*Peter Pan*), 4 oz.,		
about 1 fillet	.5	0
Malacca apple, seeded, 1 oz.	<.1	tr.
Malt liquor, all varieties, all brands, 12 fl. oz.	0	0
Mai-tai mixer (*Mr. and Mrs. "T"*), 4.5 fl. oz.	0	0
Malted milk powder, dry:		
(*Kraft*), 3 tbsp.	2.0	1.0
chocolate (*Kraft*), 3 tbsp.	1.0	0
chocolate flavor, ¾ oz. or 3 heaping tsp.	.8	.5
natural flavor, ¾ oz. or 3 heaping tsp.	1.7	.9
Mammy apple:		
untrimmed, 1 lb.	1.4	n.a.
1 medium, about 3 lbs.	4.2	n.a.
Mandarin orange, see "Tangerine"		
Mango:		
untrimmed, 1 lb.	.9	.2
1 medium, about 10.5 oz.	.6	.1
sliced, ½ cup	.2	.1
dried (*Sonoma*), 2 oz., 10–12 pieces	1.0	0
Mango drink or nectar, all varieties, all brands,		
8 fl. oz.	0	0

	total fat (grams)	saturated fat (grams)
Mango-peach juice (*R. W. Knudsen* Tropical Blend), 8 fl. oz.	0	0
Manhattan cocktail mixer (*Holland House*), 2 fl. oz.	0	0
Manicotti entree, frozen:		
(*Celentano*), 7 oz., 2 pieces	15.0	7.0
(*Celentano*), 10 oz., 2 pieces	21.0	8.0
(*Celentano* Great Choice), 10 oz., 2 pieces	2.5	1.0
(*Healthy Choice*), 9.25 oz.	3.0	2.0
cheese:		
(*Stouffer's*), 9 oz.	16.0	7.0
(*Stouffer's*), 1/12 of 61-oz. pkg.	7.0	3.0
(*Weight Watchers*), 9.25 oz.	9.0	3.5
w/meat sauce (*The Budget Gourmet*), 10 oz.	22.0	11.0
Florentine (*Celentano* Great Choice), 10 oz., 2 pieces	6.0	2.0
Florentine (*Celentano* Selects), 10-oz. tray	6.0	1.0
mini, w/out sauce (*Celentano*), 4.8 oz., 2 pieces	12.0	6.0
w/sauce (*Celentano*), 8 oz., 2 pieces	15.0	7.0
w/out sauce (*Celentano*), 7 oz., 2 pieces	19.0	11.0
Maple syrup, pure (see also "Pancake syrup") (*Spring Tree*), 1/4 cup	0	0
Margarine, 1 tbsp.:		
(*Promise* 1/4's)	10.0	2.0
(*Promise* Ultra Fat Free)	0	0
light:		
(*Smart Beat*)	2.0	0
(*Weight Watchers*)	4.0	1.0
unsalted (*Smart Beat*)	3.0	0
reduced fat, sticks (*Weight Watchers*)	7.0	1.5
safflower, all varieties (*Hain*)	11.0	2.0
safflower (*Hollywood*)	11.0	2.0
sodium free, light (*Weight Watchers*)	4.0	1.0

	total fat (grams)	saturated fat (grams)
soft:		
(*Chiffon*)	11.0	7.0
(*Parkay*)	11.0	2.0
(*Parkay* Diet)	6.0	1.0
(*Promise* Ultra)	4.0	0
(*Smart Beat Nucanola*)	7.0	<1.0
vegetable oil:		
(*Imperial*)	10.0	2.0
(*Willow Run* ¼'s)	11.0	2.5
(*Willow Run* Tub)	10.0	2.0
whipped (*Chiffon*)	7.0	1.5
whipped (*Parkay*)	7.0	1.5
blends/spreads:		
(*Country Morning* Blend Stick)	11.0	2.5
(*Country Morning* Blend Tub)	11.0	2.0
(*I Can't Believe It's Not Butter* ¼'s/Squeeze/ Tub)	10.0	2.0
(*Kraft Touch of Butter* 70%)	10.0	2.0
(*Kraft Touch of Butter* 64% Squeeze)	9.0	1.5
(*Kraft Touch of Butter* 47%)	7.0	1.5
(*Land O'Lakes* Spread Stick)	10.0	2.0
(*Land O'Lakes* Spread Tub)	8.0	1.5
(*Mrs. Filberts* Family Soft Spread Tub)	7.0	1.5
(*Parkay* 70%)	10.0	2.0
(*Parkay* 64% Squeeze)	9.0	1.5
(*Parkay* 50%)	7.0	1.5
(*Shedd's Spread* Tub)	7.0	1.5
light (*Country Morning* Blend Tub)	6.0	2.5
light (*I Can't Believe It's Not Butter* Tub)	6.0	1.0
light (*Parkay Light*)	6.0	1.0
light, salted (*Country Morning* Blend Stick)	6.0	3.0
w/sweet cream (*Land O'Lakes* Stick)	10.0	2.0
w/sweet cream (*Land O'Lakes* Tub)	8.0	2.0

	total fat (grams)		saturated fat (grams)

Margarita cocktail mixer:

(*Holland House*), 4 fl. oz.	0	....	0
(*Mr. and Mrs. "T"*), 4 fl. oz.	0	....	0
strawberry (*Holland House*), 3.5 fl. oz.	0	....	0
strawberry (*Mr. and Mrs. "T"*), 3.5 fl. oz.	0	....	0
frozen* (*Bacardi*), 8 fl. oz.	0	....	0

Marinade seasoning (see also "Barbecue sauce" and specific listings), 1 tbsp.:

(*House of Tsang Mandarin*)	0	....	0
Hawaiian (*Lawry's*)	0	....	0
Jamaican style (*World Harbors* Blue Mountain Jerk sauce)	0	....	0
red wine (*Lawry's*), 1 tbsp.	0	....	0
Thai, East Asian style (*World Harbors* Nong Khai Mountain)	0	....	0

Marinara sauce, see "Pasta sauce"

Marjoram, dried:

1 tbsp.	.1	....	0
1 tsp.	<.1	....	0

Marmalade, all varieties, 2 tbsp. | 0 | .... | 0

Marmalade plum, see "Sapote"

Marshmallow, see "Candy"

Marshmallow topping, 2 tbsp.:

(*Smucker's*)	0	....	0
creme (*Kraft*)	0	....	0
regular or raspberry (*Marshmallow Fluff*)	0	....	0

Masa, see "Corn flour"

Matzo, see "Cracker"

Mayonnaise, 1 tbsp.:

(*Hain*)	12.0	....	2.0
(*Hellmann's*)	11.0	....	1.5
(*Kraft*)	11.0	....	2.0
(*Mrs. Filberts*)	12.0	....	2.0
(*Nalley*)	11.0	....	1.0

	total fat (grams)	saturated fat (grams)
(*Nalley* Cholesterol Free)	4.0	.5
(*Nalley* Light)	5.0	.5
canola:		
(*Hain*)	11.0	1.0
(*Hollywood*)	11.0	1.0
super light (*Smart Beat*)	3.0	0
reduced calorie (*Hain*)	5.0	0
eggless (*Hain* No Salt Added)	12.0	1.5
fat free, all brands	0	0
light:		
(*Hain* Low Sodium)	6.0	1.0
(*Kraft Light*)	5.0	1.0
(*Weight Watchers*)	2.0	0
low-sodium (*Weight Watchers*)	2.0	1.0
safflower (*Hain*)	12.0	1.0
safflower (*Hollywood*)	12.0	1.0
spicy (*Tabasco/McIhenny*)	12.0	3.0
Mayonnaise-type dressing, see "Salad dressing"		
McDonald's, 1 serving:		
breakfast biscuit:		
plain	13.0	3.0
bacon, egg, and cheese	26.0	8.0
sausage	28.0	8.0
sausage and egg	34.0	11.0
breakfast dishes:		
burrito	17.0	5.0
eggs, scrambled, 2	10.0	3.0
hash browns	7.0	1.0
hotcakes, plain	4.0	1.0
hotcakes, w/syrup and 2 pats margarine	9.0	1.5
sausage	15.0	5.0
breakfast muffins:		
English	4.0	1.0
Egg McMuffin	11.0	4.0

	total fat (grams)	saturated fat (grams)

McDonald's, breakfast muffins *(cont.)*

Sausage McMuffin	20.0	7.0
Sausage McMuffin, w/egg	25.0	8.0

danish and muffin:

apple bran muffin	0	0
apple danish	16.0	5.0
cheese danish	22.0	8.0
cinnamon raisin danish	22.0	7.0
raspberry danish	16.0	5.0

sandwiches:

Big Mac	27.0	9.0
cheeseburger	13.0	5.0
chicken fajita	8.0	2.0
Filet-O-Fish	18.0	4.0
hamburger	9.0	3.5
McChicken	30.0	6.0
McGrilled Chicken	12.0	4.0
McLean Deluxe	10.0	4.0
McLean Deluxe, w/cheese	14.0	5.0
Quarter Pounder	20.0	8.0
Quarter Pounder, w/cheese	27.0	10.0

Chicken McNuggets:

4 piece	10.0	2.0
6 piece	15.0	3.5
9 piece	23.0	5.0

McNuggets sauces, 1 pkt.:

barbeque, sweet and sour, or honey	0	0
hot mustard	3.5	.5

french fries:

small	12.0	2.5
medium	17.0	3.5
large	22.0	5.0

salads:

chef	9.0	4.0
chicken, fajita	8.0	2.0

	total fat (grams)	saturated fat (grams)
garden	2.0	.5
side	1.0	.5
salad bacon bits, 1 pkg.	1.0	.5
salad croutons, 1 pkg.	2.0	.5
salad dressing, 1 pkg.:		
blue cheese	21.0	5.0
ranch	21.0	3.0
red French, reduced calorie	8.0	1.0
Thousand Island	16.0	3.0
vinaigrette, lite	2.0	0
desserts and shakes:		
baked apple pie	15.0	2.0
Chocolaty Chip cookies, 1 pkg.	15.0	4.0
McDonaldland Cookies, 1 pkg.	9.0	1.0
shake, chocolate, small, 16 fl. oz.	6.0	4.0
shake, strawberry or vanilla, small, 16 fl. oz.	5.0	3.0
sundae nuts, ¼ oz.	3.0	.5
yogurt, lowfat, frozen, vanilla cone	1.0	.5
yogurt, lowfat, frozen, hot caramel sundae	3.0	1.5
yogurt, lowfat, frozen, hot fudge sundae	3.0	2.0
yogurt, lowfat, frozen, strawberry sundae	1.0	.5
Meat, see specific listings		
Meat, canned (see specific listings):		
deviled (*Libby's*), 3-oz. can	13.0	5.0
potted (*Hormel*), 4 tbsp.	7.0	3.0
potted (*Libby's*), 3-oz. can	13.0	5.0
Meat marinade:		
(*French's*), ⅒ pkg.	0	0
(*Kikkoman*), 1 oz.	.3	0
Meatball dinner, frozen, Swedish (*Armour Classics*), 10 oz.	17.0	7.0
Meatball entree, canned:		
stew (*Dinty Moore*), 1 cup	16.0	7.0
stew (*Dinty Moore* Microwave Cup), 1 cup	15.0	7.0
Meatball entree, frozen:		
spaghetti and, see "Spaghetti entrees"		

	total fat (grams)	saturated fat (grams)

Meatball entree, frozen *(cont.)*
  Swedish:
    (*The Budget Gourmet*), 10 oz. .... 34.0 .... 16.0
    (*Stouffer's*), 9¼ oz. .... 23.0 .... 8.0
    (*Weight Watchers Smart Ones*), 9 oz. .... 8.0 .... 3.0
    w/pasta (*Lean Cuisine*), 9⅛ oz. .... 8.0 .... 3.0
    w/pasta (*Stouffer's Lunch Express*), 10¼ oz. .. 32.0 .... 11.0
"Meatball," vegetarian, canned (*Loma Linda Tender*
    Rounds), 2.8 oz., 8 pieces .... 5.0 .... 1.0
Meatball seasoning mix, Italian (*Durkee*),
  ⅕ pkg. 0 0
Meatloaf dinner, frozen:
  (*Armour Classics*), 11.25 oz. .... 10.0 .... 5.0
  (*Banquet Meals*), 9.5 oz. .... 17.0 .... 10.0
  (*Banquet Extra Helping*), 19 oz. .... 38.0 .... 16.0
  (*Morton*), 9 oz. .... 13.0 .... 4.0
Meatloaf entree, packaged, w/mashed potato
    and gravy (*Dinty Moore American Classics*),
    1 bowl .... 13.0 .... 5.0
Meatloaf entree, frozen:
  (*Healthy Choice*), 12 oz. .... 8.0 .... 3.0
  and whipped potatoes:
    (*Lean Cuisine*), 9⅜ oz. .... 7.0 .... 2.0
    (*Stouffer's* Homestyle), 9⅞ oz. .... 24.0 .... 8.0
"Meatloaf," vegetarian, mix (*Natural Touch*),
  4 tbsp. 5 0
Meatloaf seasoning mix:
  (*Durkee/French's*), ⅛ pkg. 0 0
  (*Durkee/French's* Roasting Bag), ⅛ pkg. 0 0
  (*Lawry's* Spices & Seasoning), 1 tbsp. 0 0
  (*McCormick*), ¹⁄₁₀ pkg. 0 0
  (*McCormick Bag'n Season*), ⅛ pkg. 0 0
Melon, see specific listings
Melon balls, frozen:
  cantaloupe and honeydew, ½ cup 2 0

	total fat (grams)	saturated fat (grams)
(*Stilwell*), 1 cup	0	0
Menhaden oil:		
1 tbsp.	13.6	4.1
fully hydrogenated, 1 tbsp.	12.5	12.0
Mexican beans, canned, ½ cup:		
(*Allens/Brown Beauty*)	1.0	0
(*Old El Paso Mexe-Beans*)	.5	0
w/jalapeños (*Allens/Brown Beauty*)	1.0	0
w/jalapeños (*Trappey's*)	1.5	.5
Ranchero (*Chi-Chi's*)	.5	0
Mexican dinner, frozen (see also specific listings):		
(*Banquet* Combo), 11 oz.	11.0	5.0
(*Banquet Extra Helping*), 22 oz.	34.0	14.0
(*Morton*), 10 oz.	7.0	3.0
(*Patio*), 13.25 oz.	15.0	6.0
(*Patio* Fiesta), 12 oz.	9.0	4.0
(*Patio* Ranchera), 13 oz.	15.0	6.0
style (*Banquet* Meals), 11 oz.	13.0	5.0
Mexican entree, frozen, see specific listings:		
Mexican rice seasoning (*Lawry's* Spices & Seasonings), 1½ tbsp.	0	0
Mexican seasoning (*Perc*), 1 tsp.	.5	0
Milk, fluid (see also "Milk, canned"), 8 fl. oz.:		
buttermilk:		
cultured	2.2	1.3
(*Crowley/Axelrod* Lowfat)	4.0	2.5
(*Friendship* Lowfat)	4.0	2.5
whole:		
3.7% fat	8.9	5.6
3.3% fat	8.2	5.1
(*Crowley/Axelrod*)	8.0	5.0
lowfat:		
2% fat	4.7	2.9
2% fat (*Crowley/Axelrod*)	5.0	3.0
1% fat	2.6	1.6

	total fat (grams)	saturated fat (grams)
Milk, lowfat *(cont.)*		
1% fat, regular or acidophilus (*Crowley/ Axelrod*)	2.5	1.5
skim	.4	.3
skim, nonfat (*Weight Watchers*)	0	0
skim, regular or protein added (*Crowley/ Axelrod*)	0	0
Milk, canned:		
condensed, sweet:		
1 cup	26.6	16.8
2 tbsp.	3.4	2.0
(*Carnation*), 2 tbsp.	3.0	2.0
evaporated, whole:		
1 cup	19.1	11.6
2 tbsp.	2.4	1.4
(*Carnation*), 2 tbsp.	2.5	1.5
(*Pet*), 2 tbsp.	2.0	1.0
evaporated, low fat (*Carnation*), 2 tbsp.	.5	0
evaporated, skim:		
1 cup	.5	.3
(*Carnation*), 2 tbsp.	0	0
(*Pet*), 2 tbsp.	0	0
Milk, dry (instant):		
buttermilk, sweet cream, 1 tbsp.	.4	.2
whole, ⅓ cup	11.4	7.1
nonfat, ⅓ cup	.3	.2
nonfat (*Carnation*), ⅓ cup	0	0
Milk, flavored, see specific listings		
Milk, goat, fluid, 1 cup	10.1	6.5
Milk, sheep, fluid, 1 cup	17.2	11.3
Milk, substitute, see "Rice beverage" and "Soy beverage"		
Milkfish, meat only:		
raw, 4 oz.	7.6	n.a.

	total fat (grams)	saturated fat (grams)
baked, broiled, or microwaved, 4 oz.	9.8	n.a.
Millet:		
dry, 1 oz.	1.2	.2
dry, hulled (*Arrowhead Mills*), ¼ cup	1.5	0
cooked, 1 cup	2.4	.4
Millet flour (*Arrowhead Mills*), ¼ cup	1.0	0
Mirin cooking seasoning (*Kikkoman Kotterin*), 1 tbsp.	0	0
Miso:		
1 oz.	1.7	.2
½ cup	8.4	1.2
all varieties, except hacho (*Eden*), 1 tbsp.	1.0	0
w/barely malt, 1 oz.	1.2	n.a.
hacho (*Eden*), 1 tbsp.	1.5	0
w/rice malt, dark yellow, 1 oz.	1.6	n.a.
w/soybean malt, 1 oz.	3.9	n.a.
Mocha flavor drink:		
(*Carnation* Instant Breakfast Café Mocha), 10 fl. oz.	2.5	.5
(*Nescafé* Mocha Cooler), 8 fl. oz.	4.0	3.0
Mocha flavor drink mix (*Carnation* Instant Breakfast Café Mocha), 1 pkt.	.5	0
Molasses, all varieties, all brands, 1 tbsp.	0	0
Monkfish, meat only, 4 oz.:		
raw	1.7	n.a.
baked, broiled, or microwaved	2.2	n.a.
Monosodium glutamate, 1 tbsp.	0	0
Mortadella:		
beef and pork, 1 oz.	7.2	2.7
plain or w/pistachios (*Cinghiale*), 2 oz.	14.0	5.0
Moth bean:		
raw, ½ cup	1.6	.4
boiled, ½ cup	.5	.1
Mousse mix, see "Pudding mix"		

	total fat (grams)	saturated fat (grams)
Muffin (see also "Muffin, sweet"), 1 piece:		
(*Arnold Bran'nola*)	1.5	0
(*Arnold* Extra Crisp)	1.0	0
English:		
(*Arnold/Franklin*)	1.0	0
(*Pepperidge Farm*)	1.0	0
(*Roman Meal* Original)	1.0	0
(*Tastykake* Traditional)	.5	0
(*Thomas'*, 4-Pack)	1.0	<1.0
(*Thomas'* Sandwich Size, 4-Pack)	2.0	0
(*Thomas'* Sandwich Size, Twin-Pack)	1.5	0
cinnamon raisin (*Pepperidge Farm*)	1.0	0
cinnamon raisin (*Tastykake*)	1.0	0
honey wheat (*Thomas'*)	1.0	0
oat bran (*Thomas'*)	1.0	.5
onion (*Thomas'* Sandwich Size Em's)	1.5	0
raisin (*Thomas'*)	1.0	0
7-grain or sourdough (*Pepperidge Farm*)	1.0	0
sourdough (*Tastykake*)	1.0	0
sourdough (*Thomas'*)	1.0	0
sourdough (*Thomas'* Sandwich Size Em's)	2.0	0
wheat (*Thomas'* Sandwich Size Em's)	1.5	0
raisin (*Arnold*)	1.0	0
sourdough (*Arnold*)	1.0	0
Muffin, frozen or refrigerated (see also "Toaster pastries"), 1 piece, except as noted:		
apple oatmeal (*Pepperidge Farm*)	3.5	.5
banana nut (*Weight Watchers*)	5.0	1.5
blueberry (*Pepperidge Farm*)	2.5	0
blueberry (*Weight Watchers*)	5.0	1.0
bran w/raisins (*Pepperidge Farm*)	2.0	.5
bran, harvest honey (*Weight Watchers*)	4.0	1.0
chocolate chip (*Weight Watchers*)	4.0	1.5
corn (*Pepperidge Farm*)	3.0	0
English, plain or honey wheat (*Thomas'*)	1.0	0

	total fat (grams)	saturated fat (grams)
Muffin, mix:		
blueberry (*Pillsbury Lovin' Lites*), 1½ pkg.	1.0	0
blueberry (*Schwan's*), 1½ tube	8.0	2.0
bran (*Arrowhead Mills*), ⅓ cup	2.0	0
corn (*Flako*), ⅓ cup	4.0	1.0
oat, wheat free (*Arrowhead Mills*), ⅓ cup,		
2 muffins	4.0	1.5
Muffin, sweet:		
all varieties (*Health Valley* Fat Free), 2-oz. piece ...	0	0
almond, date, oat bran (*Adventure Foods*),		
3.7 oz.	14.0	1.5
almond poppy seed (*Aunt Fanny's*), 2.75 oz.,		
2 pieces	13.0	2.0
apple:		
(*Adventure Foods*), 4 oz.	4.2	.9
(*Awrey's*), 1.5-oz. piece	6.0	1.0
(*Awrey's*), 2.5-oz. piece	10.0	2.0
bran (*Aunt Fanny's*), 2.75 oz., 2 pieces	11.0	2.0
streusel (*Awrey's* Grande), 4.2-oz. piece	13.0	2.0
banana nut (*Aunt Fanny's*), 2.75 oz., 2 pieces	14.0	2.0
banana nut (*Awrey's* Grande), 4.2-oz. piece	15.0	3.0
banana walnut mini (*Hostess*), 5 pieces	16.0	2.0
blueberry:		
(*Aunt Fanny's*), 2.75 oz., 2 pieces	11.0	2.0
(*Awrey's*), 1.5-oz. piece	5.0	1.0
(*Awrey's*), 2.5-oz. piece	8.0	1.0
(*Awrey's* Grande), 4.2-oz. piece	14.0	2.0
(*Entenmann's*), 2-oz. piece	7.0	1.5
(*Entenmann's* Fat Free), 2-oz. piece	0	0
loaf (*Hostess*), 1 loaf	19.0	3.0
mini (*Hostess*), 5 pieces	13.0	2.0
chocolate chip, mini (*Hostess*), 5 pieces	15.0	5.0
cinnamon apple, mini (*Hostess*), 5 pieces	16.0	2.5
corn (*Awrey's*), 1.5-oz. piece	5.0	1.0

	total fat (grams)	saturated fat (grams)

Muffin, sweet *(cont.)*

    corn (*Awrey's*), 2.5-oz. piece . . . . 8.0 . . . . 1.0

    cranberry (*Awrey's*), 1.5-oz. piece 4.0 0

    oat bran (*Hostess*), 1 piece . . . . 8.0 . . . . 1.0

    oat bran banana nut (*Hostess*), 1 piece . . . . 6.0 . . . . 1.0

    raisin bran:

        (*Awrey's*), 1.5-oz. piece . . . . 4.0 . . . . 1.0

        (*Awrey's*), 2.5-oz. piece . . . . 7.0 . . . . 1.0

        (*Awrey's* Grande), 4.2-oz. piece . . . . 12.0 . . . . 2.0

Muffin sandwich, see specific listings

Mulberries, ½ cup 3 0

Mullet, striped, meat only:

    raw, 4 oz. . . . . 4.3 . . . . 1.3

    baked, broiled, or microwaved, 4 oz. . . . . 5.5 . . . . 1.6

Mung bean, dried:

    raw, ½ cup 1.2 4

    raw (*Arrowhead Mills*), ¼ cup 5 0

    boiled, ½ cup 4 1

Mung bean, sprouted (see also "Bean sprouts"):

    raw, 1 oz. . . . . .1 . . . . <.1

    raw (*Jonathan's Sprouts*), 3 oz., 1 cup 5 0

    boiled and drained, ½ cup .1 . . . . <.1

    canned, drained, ½ cup . . . . <.1 . . . . <.1

Mung bean long rice, dehydrated, 1 oz. . . . . tr. . . . . tr.

Mungo bean, dried:

    raw, ½ cup 1.9 1

    boiled, ½ cup . . . . .5 . . . . <.1

Mushroom:

    fresh:

        raw, untrimmed, 1 lb. 1.9 2

        raw, pieces, ½ cup . . . . .2 . . . . <.1

        boiled, drained, pieces, ½ cup . . . . .4 . . . . <.1

    canned:

        drained, pieces, ½ cup . . . . .2 . . . . <.1

        (*Seneca*), ½ cup 0 0

	total fat (grams)		saturated fat (grams)
all cuts, except garlic (*BinB*), 1 can	0	....	0
all cuts (*Green Giant*), ½ cup	0	....	0
w/garlic, sliced (*BinB*), 1 can	.5	....	0
straw (*Green Giant*), ¼ cup	0	....	0
frozen, breaded:			
(*Empire* Kosher), 7 pieces, 2.8 oz.	1.0	....	0
(*Schwan's*), 1 cup	12.0	....	1.5
Mushroom, shiitake:			
cooked, 4 medium or ½ cup pieces	.2	....	<.1
dried, 1 oz.	.3	....	.1
Mushroom entree, freeze-dried, pilaf, w/vegetables			
(*AlpineAire*), 1½ cups*	2.0	....	n.a.
Mushroom gravy (see also "Mushroom sauce"),			
canned:			
¼ cup	1.6	....	.2
(*Swanson*), ¼ cup	1.0	....	0
Mushroom gravy mix:			
¼ cup*	.2	....	.1
(*Durkee*), ¼ pkg.	0	....	0
(*French's*), ¼ pkg.	.5	....	0
(*Loma Linda Gravy Quik*), 1 tbsp.	.3	....	.1
Mushroom sauce (see also "Cooking sauce") (*House*			
of Tsang), 1 tbsp.	.5	....	0
Mushroom sauce mix (*Knorr* Classic Sauces),			
⅕ pkg.	1.0	....	0
Muskmelon, see "Cantaloupe"			
Mussel, blue, meat only:			
raw, in shell, 1 lb., about 24	10.2	....	1.9
raw, 1 cup	3.4	....	.6
boiled or steamed, 4 oz.	5.1	....	1.0
Mustard, prepared, 1 tsp.:			
(*Boar's Head* Delicatessen Style)	0	....	0
(*Gulden's* Spicy Brown)	0	....	0
(*French's*)	0	....	0
(*Grey Poupon*)	0	....	0

	total fat (grams)	saturated fat (grams)
Mustard, prepared *(cont.)*		
all varieties (*Kraft*)	0	0
blend (*Hellmann's Dijonnaise*)	1.0	0
deli, all varieties (*Hebrew National*)	0	0
honey, zesty (*Nance's*)	0	0
horseradish, see "Horseradish mustard"		
hot (*Eden*)	0	0
hot or sharp and creamy (*Nance's*)	1.0	0
Mustard greens:		
fresh:		
raw, untrimmed, 1 lb.	.8	<.1
raw, trimmed, chopped, ½ cup	.1	tr.
boiled, drained, chopped, ½ cup	.2	tr.
canned (*Allens/Sunshine*), ½ cup	.5	0
frozen:		
10-oz. pkg.	.8	<.1
boiled, drained, ½ cup	.2	<.1
(*Stilwell*), 1 cup	0	0
Mustard oil, 1 tbsp.	14.0	1.6
Mustard powder, 1 tsp.	.6	n.a.
Mustard sauce mix, herb (*Knorr* Classic Sauces), ¼ pkg.	1.5	0
Mustard seeds, yellow, 1 tbsp.	3.2	.2
Mustard spinach:		
raw, untrimmed, 1 lb.	1.3	n.a.
boiled, drained, chopped, ½ cup	.2	n.a.
Mustard tallow, 1 tbsp.	12.8	6.1

N

	total fat (grams)		saturated fat (grams)
Namasu sauce (*House of Tsang*), 1 tsp.	0	....	0
Nan, see "Bread"			
Natto:			
1 oz.	3.1	....	.5
½ cup	9.7	....	1.4
Navy bean:			
dried, raw, ½ cup	1.3	....	.3
dried, boiled, ½ cup	.5	....	.1
canned, ½ cup:			
(*Allens*)	1.0	....	0
(*Eden*)	.5	....	0
(*Stokely*)	.5	....	0
w/bacon (*Allens*)	1.5	....	.5
w/bacon and jalapeño (*Allens/Trappey's*)	1.5	....	5
Navy bean, sprouted:			
raw, ½ cup	.4	....	<.1
boiled, drained, 4 oz.	.9	....	.1
Nectarine:			
untrimmed, 1 lb.	1.9	....	0
1 medium, 2½" diameter, about 5.3 oz.	.6	....	0

	total fat (grams)	saturated fat (grams)

Nectarine *(cont.)*

sliced, ½ cup 3 0

New England Brand sausage:

(*Oscar Mayer*), 1.6 oz., 2 slices .... 2.5 .... 1.0

pork and beef, 1 oz. 2.2 7

New Zealand spinach:

raw, untrimmed, 1 lb. 7 1

raw, trimmed, chopped, ½ cup .... .1 .... tr.

boiled, drained, chopped, ½ cup .... .2 .... <.1

Newburg sauce mix (*Knorr* Classic Sauces),

⅕ pkg. 5 0

Noodle, egg (see also "Pasta"): dry:

2 oz. 2.4 5

all varieties (*Herb's*), 2 oz. 2.0 0

spinach, 2 oz. 2.6 6

cooked, 1 cup 2.4 5

cooked, spinach, 1 cup 2.5 6

Noodle, Chinese:

cellophane or long rice, dehydrated, 2 oz. .... <.1 0

chow mein, 1 oz. .... 8.7 .... 1.2

chow mein, 1 cup .... 13.8 .... 2.0

crispy (*Frieda's*), 1 oz. .... 5.0 .... n.a.

Noodle, Japanese, dry:

soba:

buckwheat, dry, 2 oz. 4 1

buckwheat, dry (*Eden* 100%), 2 oz. 1.5 0

buckwheat, dry (*Eden* 40%), 2 oz. 1.0 0

buckwheat, cooked, 1 cup .... .1 .... <.1

lotus root, dry (*Eden*), 2 oz. 1.0 0

mugwort, dry (*Eden*), 2 oz. 5 0

wild yam, dry (*Eden*), 2 oz. 5 0

somen, wheat, dry, 2 oz. 5 1

somen, wheat, cooked, 1 cup .... .3 .... <.1

udon:

dry (*Eden*), 2 oz. 1.5 0

	total fat (grams)	saturated fat (grams)
brown rice, dry (*Eden*), 2 oz.	1.0	0
wheat, dry, 2 oz.	.7	0
wheat, cooked, 1 cup	.6	0
Noodle dishes, mix:		
Alfredo (*Lipton* Noodles & Sauce), ⅔ cup	7.0	4.0
Alfredo broccoli (*Lipton* Noodles & Sauce), ⅔ cup	7.0	4.0
beef (*Lipton* Noodles & Sauce), ⅔ cup	4.0	1.5
broccoli au gratin (*Golden Grain Noodle Roni*), 1 cup*	10.0	3.0
broccoli and mushroom (*Golden Grain Noodle Roni*), 1 cup*	24.0	6.0
butter (*Lipton* Noodles & Sauce), ⅔ cup	8.0	4.0
butter and herb (*Country Inn Recipes*), 2 oz.	6.0	2.5
butter and herb (*Lipton* Noodles & Sauce), ⅔ cup	6.0	3.0
carbonara Alfredo (*Lipton* Noodles & Sauce), ⅔ cup	7.0	3.0
cheddar (*Kraft*), 1 cup*	21.0	6.0
cheddar, mild (*Golden Grain Noodle Roni*), 1 cup*	11.0	3.5
cheddar bacon (*Lipton* Noodles & Sauce), ⅔ cup	4.0	2.0
cheese (*Lipton* Noodles & Sauce), ⅔ cup	5.0	2.0
cheeses, four (*Golden Grain Noodle Roni*), 1 cup*	19.0	5.0
chicken:		
(*Golden Grain Noodle Roni*), 1 cup*	13.0	3.0
(*Kraft*), 1 cup*	12.0	3.5
(*Lipton* Noodles & Sauce), ⅔ cup	4.0	1.5
creamy (*Lipton* Noodles & Sauce), ⅔ cup	7.0	2.5
chicken broccoli (*Lipton* Noodles & Sauce), ⅔ cup	3.0	1.0
garlic, creamy (*Golden Grain Noodle Roni*), 1 cup*	29.0	7.0

	total fat (grams)	saturated fat (grams)

Noodle dishes, mix, chicken *(cont.)*

herb and butter (*Golden Grain Noodle Roni*), 1
cup* .... 28.0 .... 7.0

Oriental (*Golden Grain Noodle Roni*), 1 cup* .. 12.0 .... 1.5

Oriental (*Knorr*), 1 pkg. 3.0 5

Parmesan (*Lipton* Noodles & Sauce),
⅔ cup .... 7.0 .... 4.0

Parmesano (*Golden Grain Noodle Roni*),
1 cup* .... 17.0 .... 4.5

Romanoff (*Golden Grain Noodle Roni*),
1 cup* .... 19.0 .... 5.0

Romanoff (*Lipton* Noodles & Sauce), ⅔ cup .. 7.0 .... 2.5

sour cream and chive (*Lipton* Noodles & Sauce),
⅔ cup .... 7.0 .... 3.0

Stroganoff (*Golden Grain Noodle Roni*), 1 cup* .. 14.0 .... 4.0

Stroganoff (*Lipton* Noodles & Sauce), ⅔ cup .... 4.0 .... 1.5

Noodle and chicken entree, canned or packaged:

(*Dinty Moore*), 7.5-oz. can .... 8.0 .... 2.0

(*Dinty Moore American Classics*), 1 bowl .... 8.0 .... 4.0

(*Hormel* Micro Cup), 7.5-oz. cup .... 8.0 .... 2.0

(*Hormel* Micro Cup), 10.5-oz. cup .... 11.0 .... 3.0

(*Nalley*), 7.5-oz. cup .... 7.0 .... 2.0

w/vegetables:

(*Chef Boyardee* Classic), 10.5-oz. bowl 1.0 0

(*Nalley*), 7.5-oz. cup .... 6.0 .... 2.0

Noodle entree, canned (*Van Camp's* Noodle Weenee),
1 can .... 8.0 .... 2.0

Noodle entree, frozen:

and chicken (*Banquet* Family), 8 oz. .... 9.0 .... 3.0

Romanoff (*Stouffer's* Entree), 12 oz. .... 25.0 .... 6.0

and turkey, escalloped (*The Budget Gourmet*),
10.75 oz. .... 20.0 .... 10.0

Nori, see "Seaweed"

Nut pastry filling (see also specific listings), fancy
(*Solo*), 2 tbsp. 5.0 5

	total fat (grams)	saturated fat (grams)
Nut topping (*Planters*), 2 tbsp.	9.0	1.0
Nutmeg, ground:		
1 tbsp.	2.5	1.8
1 tsp.	.8	.6
Nutmeg butter oil, 1 tbsp.	13.6	12.2
Nuts, see specific listings		
Nuts, mixed (see also specific listings):		
(*Eagle* With/Without Peanuts), 1 oz., ¼ cup	17.0	3.0
dry-roasted:		
(*Planters*), 1 oz.	14.0	2.0
w/peanuts, 1 oz.	14.6	2.0
w/peanuts, ¼ cup	17.6	2.4
honey-roasted:		
(*Planters*), 1 oz.	13.0	2.0
cashews and peanuts (*Eagle*), 1 oz., ¼ cup	14.0	3.0
cashews and peanuts (*Planters*), 1 oz.	12.0	2.0
oil-roasted:		
(*Planters*), 1 oz.	15.0	2.5
(*Planters* Deluxe), 1 oz.	18.0	2.5
(*Planters* Lightly Salted), 1.25 oz.	19.5	2.5
(*Planters* Unsalted), 1 oz.	15.0	2.0
cashews, almonds, macadamias (*Planters* Select Mix), 1 oz.	16.0	2.5
cashews, almonds, pecans (*Planters* Select Mix), 1 oz.	15.0	2.0
cashews, almonds, peanuts (*Planters* Select Mix), 1 oz.	14.0	2.0
cashews, pecans, peanuts (*Planters* Select Mix), 1 oz.	17.0	2.5
w/peanuts, 1 oz.	16.0	2.5
w/peanuts, ¼ cup	20.2	3.1
sesame nut mix (*Planters*), 1 oz.	12.0	2.0
tamari-roasted (*Eden*), 1 oz.	11.0	1.5

O

	total fat (grams)		saturated fat (grams)
Oat bran (*Arrowhead Mills*), ⅓ cup	2.5	....	0
Oat flour (*Arrowhead Mills*), ¼ cup	2.0	....	0
Oat groats (*Arrowhead Mills*), ¼ cup	3.0	....	.5
Oats (see also "Cereal"):			
whole-grain, 1 oz.	2.0	....	.3
whole-grain, 1 cup	10.8	....	1.9
rolled or oatmeal:			
dry, 1 oz.	1.8	....	.3
dry, 1 cup	5.1	....	.9
dry (*Arrowhead Mills*), ⅓ cup	2.5	....	0
cooked, 1 cup	2.4	....	.4
Oatmeal, see "Cereal" and "Oats"			
Ocean perch, Atlantic, meat only:			
raw, 4 oz.	1.9	....	.3
baked, broiled, or microwaved, 4 oz.	2.4	....	.4
Ocean perch, frozen, fillets (*Schwan's*), 4 oz.	2.0	....	.5
Octopus, meat only, raw, 4 oz.	1.2	....	.3
Oheloberries, ½ cup	.2	....	0
Oil (see also specific oil listings):			
(*Crisco*), 1 tbsp.	14.0	....	1.5
(*Crisco Puritan*), 1 tbsp.	14.0	....	1.0

	total fat (grams)	saturated fat (grams)
(*Hain* All Blend), 1 tbsp.	14.0	1.5
Okra:		
fresh:		
raw, untrimmed, 1 lb.	.4	.1
raw, 8 pods, about 3.9 oz.	.1	<.1
boiled, drained, 8 pods or ½ cup sliced	.1	<.1
canned, ½ cup:		
cut or w/tomatoes (*Allens/Trappey's*)	0	0
w/tomatoes and corn (*Allens/Trappey's*)	0	0
Creole gumbo (*Trappey's*)	0	0
frozen:		
10-oz. pkg.	.7	.2
boiled, drained, sliced, ½ cup	.3	.1
cut (*McKenzie's*), ¾ cup	0	0
cut (*Stilwell*), ¾ cup	0	0
whole (*Stilwell*), 9 pieces	.5	0
frozen, breaded (*Schwan's*), 1 cup	13.0	2.0
Okra, cocktail, hot or mild (*Trappey's*), 1-oz. piece	0	0
Old-fashioned loaf (*Oscar Mayer*), 1-oz. slice	5.0	1.5
Old-fashioned mixer (*Holland House*), 2 fl. oz.	0	0
Olive:		
Alfonso (*Krinos*), 3 olives	3.0	.5
Calamata:		
(*Krinos*), 3 olives	4.0	.5
(*Zorba*), 1 olive	9.0	1.0
green:		
whole, 10 small, select or standard, about 1.2 oz.	3.6	n.a.
whole, 10 large, about 1.6 oz.	4.9	n.a.
whole, pitted, 1 oz.	3.6	n.a.
cracked (*Krinos*), 2 olives	1.0	.5
Spanish (*Zorba*), 2 olives	2.0	.5
Nafplion (*Krinos*), .5 oz., about 7 olives	1.0	.2
ripe:		
Greek (*Zorba*), 1 olive	4.0	1.0
Greek (*Krinos*), 2 olives	3.0	.5

	total fat (grams)	saturated fat (grams)
Olive, ripe *(cont.)*		
Manzanilla or Mission, pitted, 1 oz.	3.0	.4
oil-cured (*Krinos*), 5 olives	6.0	1.0
oil-cured (*Progresso*), 6 pieces	6.0	.5
royal (*Krinos*), 2 olives	2.5	.5
Sevillano or Ascolano, pitted, 1 oz.	1.9	.3
ripe, whole:		
(*Lindsay*), .5 oz., 6 small, 5 medium, or 4 large	2.5	0
(*Lindsay*), .4 oz., 2 jumbo	1.5	0
(*Lindsay*), .5 oz., 2 colossal	2.0	0
(*Lindsay*), .4 oz., 1 super colossal	1.5	0
ripe, pitted:		
(*Lindsay*), .5 oz., 6 small, 5 medium, 4 large, or 3 extra large	2.5	0
(*Lindsay*), .6 oz., 3 jumbo or 2 colossal	2.0	0
(*Lindsay*), .3 oz., 1 super colossal	1.0	0
broken (*Lindsay*), .5 oz., ¼ cup	2.5	0
chopped (*Lindsay*), .5 oz., 1⅓ tbsp.	2.5	0
sliced (*Lindsay*), ¼ cup	2.5	0
wedged (*Lindsay*), ¼ cup	2.0	0
wedged (*Lindsay*), 2 tbsp.	3.0	0
Olive loaf:		
(*Boar's Head*), 2 oz.	12.0	4.5
(*Oscar Mayer*), 1-oz. slice	5.0	1.5
pork, 1 oz.	4.7	1.7
Olive oil:		
1 tbsp.	13.5	1.8
(*Arrowhead Mills*), 1 tbsp.	14.0	2.0
(*Hain*), 1 tbsp.	14.0	2.0
all varieties (*Progresso*), 1 tbsp.	14.0	2.0
Olive salad, drained (*Progresso*), 2 tbsp.	2.5	0
Onion, mature (see also "Onion, green"):		
fresh:		
raw, untrimmed, 1 lb.	.7	.1

	total fat (grams)	saturated fat (grams)
raw, chopped, ½ cup	.2	<.1
raw, chopped, 1 tbsp.	<.1	0
boiled, drained, chopped, ½ cup or 4 oz.	.1	<.1
canned, w/liquid, 4 oz.	.1	<.1
canned, whole (*Green Giant*), ½ cup	0	0
frozen, chopped (*Ore-Ida*), ¾ cup	0	0
Onion, condiment:		
marinated (*Krinos*), 5 onions	.5	0
Vidalia, in sauce (*Boar's Head*), 1 tbsp.	0	0
Onion, dried:		
flakes, 1 tbsp.	<.1	0
minced, flaked, or toasted (*Durkee/Spice Islands*),		
¼ tsp.	0	0
minced (*Lawry's*), ¼ tsp.	0	0
Onion, green (scallion):		
untrimmed, 1 lb.	.8	.1
trimmed, w/top, chopped, ½ cup	.1	<.1
Onion, minced, see "Onion, dried"		
Onion, Welsh:		
untrimmed, 1 lb.	1.2	.2
trimmed, 1 oz.	.1	<.1
Onion dip, 2 tbsp.:		
creamy (*Kraft* Premium)	4.0	2.5
French:		
(*Breakstone's*)	4.0	3.0
(*Doritos*)	5.0	3.0
(*Heluva* Good)	5.0	3.0
(*Heluva* Good Light)	2.0	1.0
(*Knudsen* Premium)	4.0	3.0
(*Kraft*)	4.0	3.0
(*Kraft* Premium)	4.0	2.5
(*Nalley*)	10.0	1.5
(*Sealtest*)	4.0	3.0
yogurt (*Crowley's*)	2.0	1.5
green (*Kraft*)	4.0	3.0

	total fat (grams)	saturated fat (grams)
Onion dip *(cont.)*		
homestyle (*Heluva* Good)	5.0	3.0
toasted (*Breakstone's*)	4.0	3.0
Onion dip mix:		
chive (*Knorr*), ⅟₂₀ pkg.	0	0
toasted (*McCormick Collection*), ⅟₁₆ pkg.	0	0
Onion flakes, see "Onion, dried"		
Onion flavor snack (*Funyuns*), 1 oz., 13 pieces	7.0	1.5
Onion gravy mix:		
¼ cup*	.7	.5
(*Durkee*), ¼ pkg.	0	0
(*French's*), ¼ pkg.	1.0	0
(*Loma Linda Gravy Quik*), 1 tbsp.*	.3	.1
Onion pepper (*Spice Islands*), ¼ tsp.	0	0
Onion powder:		
1 tsp.	<.1	0
(*Durkee/Spice Island*), ¼ tsp.	0	0
Onion rings, frozen:		
(*Ore-Ida Onion Ringers*), 6 pieces	14.0	2.5
(*Schwan's*), 3 oz.	8.0	1.5
breaded, 9-oz. pkg.	36.0	11.6
breaded, oven-heated, 2 rings, .7 oz.	5.3	1.7
breaded, oven-heated (*Mrs. Paul's* Old Fashioned), 3 oz.	12.0	2.5
Onion salt:		
1 tsp.	0	0
(*Durkee/Spice Islands*), ¼ tsp.	0	0
Onion sprouts (*Jonathan's Sprouts*), 3 oz., 1 cup	0	0
Opossum, meat only, roasted, 4 oz.	11.6	n.a.
Orange, all varieties:		
untrimmed, 1 lb.	.4	.1
1 medium, about 6.3 oz.	.2	<.1
sections, ½ cup	.1	0
Orange, mandarin or canned, see "Tangerine"		
Orange drink, all varieties and brands, 8 fl. oz.	0	0

	total fat (grams)	saturated fat (grams)

Orange juice:

fresh, juice from 1 medium orange .... .2 .... <.1

fresh, 6 fl. oz. .... .4 .... <.1

canned, chilled, or bottled:

    (*R.W. Knudsen* Organic), 8 fl. oz. 0 0

    (*Tree Top*), 11.5 fl. oz. 0 0

    from concentrate (*Crowley*), 8 fl. oz. 0 0

    from concentrate (*Mott's*), 10 fl. oz. 5 0

frozen:

    undiluted, 6 fl. oz. 4 1

    diluted, 8 fl. oz. .... .1 .... <.1

    diluted (*Schwan's*), 8 fl. oz. 0 0

Orange juice float (*R.W. Knudsen*), 8 fl. oz. 0 0

Orange peel, 1 tbsp. .... <.1 .... tr.

Orange roughy, see "Roughy"

Orange-mango juice (*R.W. Knudsen* Tropical Blend),

   8 fl. oz. 0 0

Oregano, dried, ground:

1 tsp. 1 0

(*Durkee/Spice Islands*), ¼ tsp. 0 0

(*Krinos* Imported), 1 tsp. 0 0

Oriental seasoning:

(*Perc*), 1 tsp. 0 0

5 spice (*Tone*), 1 tsp. 3 0

Oyster, fresh, meat only:

Eastern:

    raw, 1 cup .... 6.1 .... .1.6

    raw, 6 medium, about 3 oz., 70 per quart 2.1 5

    boiled, poached, or steamed, 6 medium, 1.5 oz.

        (3 oz. raw) 2.1 5

Pacific, 1 medium, about 1¾ oz., 20 per quart ... 1.2 3

Oyster, canned, Eastern w/liquid, 1 cup, about

   8.7 oz. .... 6.1 .... 1.6

Oyster plant, see "Salsify"

Oyster stew, see "Soup, canned, condensed"

P

	total fat (grams)	saturated fat (grams)
Palm kernel oil, 1 tbsp.	13.6	11.1
Palm oil, 1 tbsp.	13.6	6.7
Pancake, frozen, 3 pieces:		
(*Aunt Jemima* Original)	3.0	.5
(*Aunt Jemima* Low Fat)	1.5	0
(*Downyflake*)	7.0	2.0
all varieties, except blueberry (*Hungry Jack* Microwave)	4.0	1.0
blueberry (*Aunt Jemima*)	3.5	.5
blueberry (*Hungry Jack* Microwave)	3.5	.5
buttermilk (*Aunt Jemima*)	3.0	.5
buttermilk (*Schwan's*)	5.0	1.5
Pancake batter, frozen, buttermilk or original (*Aunt Jemima*), ½ cup	3.0	1.0
Pancake breakfast, frozen, w/sausage:		
(*Great Starts*), 6 oz.	25.0	11.0
on stick (*Jimmy Dean Flapsticks*), 1 piece	12.0	n.a.
blueberry, on stick (*Jimmy Dean Flapsticks*), 1 piece	10.0	n.a.
silver dollar, six (*Great Starts* Budget), 3.75 oz.	18.0	9.0

	total fat (grams)	saturated fat (grams)
Pancake and waffle mix, ⅓ cup, except as noted:		
(*Aunt Jemima* Complete)	2.0	.5
(*Aunt Jemima* Original)	.5	0
(*Hungry Jack* Original)	1.5	0
(*Hungry Jack Extra Lights*)	1.5	0
(*Hungry Jack Extra Lights* Complete)	2.0	.5
buckwheat (*Arrowhead Mills*)	1.5	0
buckwheat (*Aunt Jemima*)	1.0	0
buttermilk:		
(*Aunt Jemima* Complete)	2.0	.5
(*Aunt Jemima* Reduced Calorie)	1.5	.5
(*Hungry Jack*)	1.5	0
(*Hungry Jack* Complete)	1.5	0
multi or whole grain (*Arrowhead Mills*), ¼ cup	.5	0
wheat free (*Arrowhead Mills Griddle Lite*), ¼ cup	2.0	0
whole wheat (*Aunt Jemima*), ¼ cup	.5	0
wild rice (*Arrowhead Mills*), ¼ cup	1.0	0
Pancake syrup:		
regular varieties, all brands, 2 tbsp.	0	0
w/butter, 2 tbsp.	.6	.4
Pancreas, braised:		
beef, 4 oz.	19.5	n.a.
lamb, 4 oz.	17.1	7.8
pork, 4 oz.	12.2	n.a.
veal, 4 oz.	16.6	n.a.
Papaya:		
fresh, 1 medium, about 1 lb.	.4	.1
fresh, cubed, ½ cup	.1	<.1
dried (*Sonoma*), 2 oz., 2 pieces	4.0	0
Papaya juice, creamed, concentrate (*R.W. Knudsen*), 8 fl. oz.	0	0
Papaya nectar, canned or bottled:		
6 fl. oz.	.3	.1
(*R.W. Knudsen*), 8 fl. oz.	0	0

	total fat (grams)	saturated fat (grams)
Papaya-lime juice (*R.W. Knudsen* Tropical Blend),		
8 fl. oz.	0	0
Pappadum, see "Cracker"		
Paprika:		
1 tbsp.	.9	.1
1 tsp.	.3	<.1
(*Durkee/Spice Islands*), ¼ tsp.	0	0
Parma rosa sauce mix (*Knorr* Pasta Sauces),		
⅛ pkg.	1.0	0
Parrot fish, meat only, raw, 4 oz.	.5	n.a.
Parsley:		
fresh:		
untrimmed, 1 lb.	3.4	.6
10 sprigs, about .4 oz.	.1	<.1
chopped, ½ cup	.2	<.1
dried, 1 tbsp.	.6	<.1
dried, 1 tsp.	.1	0
freeze-dried, 1 tbsp.	<.1	0
Parsley root, 1 oz.	.2	0
Parsnip:		
raw, untrimmed, 1 lb.	1.2	.2
raw, sliced, ½ cup	.2	<.1
boiled, drained, 1 medium, 9" × 2¼" diameter	.5	.1
boiled, drained, sliced, ½ cup	.2	<.1
Passion fruit, purple:		
untrimmed, 1 lb.	1.7	n.a.
1 medium, about 1.2 oz.	.1	0
Passion fruit juice, fresh:		
purple, 6 fl. oz.	.1	0
yellow, 6 fl. oz.	.3	0
Passion fruit-raspberry juice (*R.W. Knudsen*),		
8 fl. oz.	0	0
Pasta (see also "Macaroni" and "Noodles") dry:		
uncooked, 2 oz.:		
plain	.9	.1
all varieties (*Buckeye*)	1.0	0

	total fat (grams)	saturated fat (grams)
all varieties (*Pritikin*)	1.0	0
artichoke, all varieties (*De Boles*)	1.0	0
basil fettuccine (*Al Dente*)	2.0	n.a.
bean, mung (*Eden*)	0	0
chili, red fettuccine (*Al Dente*)	2.0	n.a.
corn, spaghetti or elbows (*De Boles*)	1.0	0
egg fettuccine or linguine (*Al Dente*)	2.0	n.a.
fennel bell pepper fettuccine (*Al Dente*)	1.5	.5
fettuccine (*Al Dente* Fiesta)	1.5	.5
garlic and parsley, all varieties (*De Boles*)	1.0	0
garlic parsley fettuccine (*Al Dente*)	2.0	.5
kamut, spirals (*Eden*)	1.5	0
lemon chive fettuccine (*Al Dente*)	1.5	.5
mushroom, wild, fettuccine (*Al Dente*)	2.0	.5
orange poppyseed fettuccine (*Al Dente*)	2.0	.5
parsley garlic (*Eden*)	1.0	0
parsley garlic fettuccine (*Herb's*)	2.0	0
pepper, bell, and basil (*Herb's*)	2.0	0
pepper, three, fettuccine (*Al Dente*)	1.5	.5
potato, sweet, and kudzu (*Eden*)	0	0
primavera rotini (*De Boles*)	1.0	0
rice (*Eden*)	.5	0
rice, sesame (*Eden*)	2.0	0
sesame, spicy (*Al Dente*)	2.0	n.a.
spinach fettuccine (*Herb's*)	2.0	0
spinach fettuccine or linguine (*Al Dente*)	2.0	n.a.
spinach fettuccine or spaghetti (*De Boles*)	1.0	0
squid ink fettuccine (*Al Dente*)	1.5	.5
tarragon fettuccine (*Al Dente*)	2.0	n.a.
tomato fettuccine (*Al Dente*)	1.5	.5
tomato and basil, angel hair or rotini (*De Boles*)	1.0	0
tomato and lemon pepper or pesto, angel hair or fettuccine (*De Boles*)	1.0	0

	total fat (grams)	saturated fat (grams)

Pasta, uncooked, 2 oz. *(cont.)*

vegetable (*Eden*)	1.0	0
vegetable (*Herb's* Organic)	1.0	0
vegetables, mixed (*Herb's*)	2.0	0
walnut (*Al Dente*)	3.0	n.a.
wheat, regular, spinach, curry, pesto, all shapes (*Eden*)	1.0	0
whole wheat, all varieties (*De Boles*)	2.0	0
whole wheat, all varieties (*Eden*)	1.5	0
whole wheat fettuccine (*Al Dente*)	1.0	0
cooked, plain, 1 cup	.9	.1

Pasta, fresh, refrigerated:

w/egg, dry, 2 oz.	1.3	.2
w/egg, cooked, 4 oz.	1.2	.2
spinach, w/egg, dry, 2 oz.	1.2	.3
spinach, w/egg, cooked, 4 oz.	1.1	.2

Pasta dishes, frozen (see also "Pasta entree, frozen" and specific pasta listings):

Alfredo (*Green Giant Pasta Accents*), 2 cups	8.0	2.5
Alfredo, w/broccoli (*The Budget Gourmet* Side Dish), 5.8 oz.	11.0	7.0
cheddar (*Green Giant Pasta Accents*), 2⅓ cup	8.0	3.0
cheddar, white (*Green Giant Pasta Accents*), 1¾ cups	12.0	3.5
cheddar bake w/ (*Lean Cuisine* Entree), 9 oz.	6.0	2.0
and chicken marinara (*Lean Cuisine Lunch Express*), 9⅛ oz.	6.0	1.5
garden herb (*Green Giant Pasta Accents*), 2 cups	7.0	4.0
garlic (*Green Giant Pasta Accents*), 2 cups	10.0	5.0
Florentine (*Green Giant Pasta Accents*), 2 cups	9.0	3.0
marinara twist (*Lean Cuisine* Entree), 10 oz.	3.0	1.0
primavera (*Green Giant Pasta Accents*), 2¼ cups	12.0	5.0

	total fat (grams)	saturated fat (grams)
and tuna casserole (*Lean Cuisine Lunch Express*), 9¾ oz.	6.0	2.0
and turkey Dijon (*Lean Cuisine Lunch Express*), 9⅞ oz.	6.0	1.5
Pasta dishes, mix (see also "Macaroni entree, mix" and specific pasta listings):		
(*Buckeye* Oceans of Pasta), ¹⁄₁₆ pkg.	1.0	0
broccoli white cheddar (*Country Inn Recipes*), 2 oz.	4.5	2.0
cheddar broccoli (*Lipton* Pasta & Sauce), ⅔ cup	6.0	2.0
cheese, three (*Lipton* Pasta & Sauce), ½ cup	5.0	3.0
cheese sauce, elbow or shells (*De Boles*), ¾ cup*	9.5	3.0
cheese sauce, whole wheat elbows (*De Boles*), ¾ cup*	10.0	3.0
chicken herb Parmesan (*Lipton Golden Saute*), ½ cup	3.0	1.5
chicken stir-fry (*Lipton Golden Saute*), ½ cup	2.0	0
garlic, creamy (*Country Inn Recipes*), 2.5 oz.	5.0	2.5
garlic, creamy (*Lipton* Pasta & Sauce), ⅔ cup	5.0	3.0
garlic butter (*Lipton Golden Saute*), ½ cup	3.0	2.0
garlic and herb (*Spice Islands*), 1 pkg.	1.0	0
herb tomato (*Lipton* Pasta & Sauce), ⅔ cup	2.0	.5
primavera (*Lipton Golden Saute*), ½ cup	2.0	.5
primavera (*Spice Islands*), 1 pkg.	2.0	.5
salad:		
(*Buckeye* Hearty), 1 cup*	1.0	0
(*Buckeye* Sunny Day), 1 cup*	2.0	0
Caesar, creamy (*Kraft*), 2.5 oz., about ¾ cup*	22.0	4.0
Italian (*Kraft* Light), 2.5 oz., about ¾ cup	2.0	1.0
Italian herb (*Fantastic*), ⅔ cup	1.5	.5
Oriental, spicy (*Fantastic*), about ⅔ cup	3.0	0

	total fat (grams)	saturated fat (grams)
Pasta dishes, mix, salad *(cont.)*		
Parmesan peppercorn (*Kraft*), 2.5 oz., about ¾ cup*	25.0	4.5
primavera, garden (*Kraft*), 2.5 oz., about ¾ cup*	12.0	2.5
ranch, w/bacon (*Kraft*), 2.5 oz., about ¾ cup*	23.0	4.0
spinach and mushroom (*Spice Islands*), 1 pkg.	1.5	.5
tomato basil, creamy (*Spice Islands*), 1 pkg.	2.0	0
vegetable Alfredo (*Country Inn Recipes*), 2 oz.	4.0	2.0
Pasta entree, canned (see also "Macaroni entree" and specific pasta listings), all varieties (*Health Valley Fat Free*), 1 cup	0	0
Pasta entree, freeze-dried* (see also specific pasta listings):		
(*AlpineAire* Roma), 1⅓ cup	1.0	n.a.
primavera (*Mountain House*), 1 cup	6.0	4.0
stew, whole wheat (*AlpineAire*), 1½ cups	1.0	n.a.
Pasta entree, frozen (see also "Pasta dishes, frozen" and specific pasta listings):		
and chicken:		
cacciatore (*Healthy Choice* Generous Serving), 12.5 oz.	3.0	<1.0
marinara (*Lean Cuisine Lunch Express*), 9⅛ oz.	6.0	1.5
teriyaki (*Healthy Choice* Generous Serving), 12.6 oz.	3.0	<1.0
Italiano (*Healthy Choice* Generous Serving), 12 oz.	5.0	2.0
marinara, and breaded chicken breast cutlet, w/cheese (*Celentano*), 10-oz. tray	19.0	4.0
and shrimp (*Healthy Choice* Generous Serving), 12.5 oz.	4.0	2.0
and sun-dried tomatoes (*Weight Watchers Smart Ones*), 10 oz.	9.0	2.5

	total fat (grams)	saturated fat (grams)

and tuna casserole (*Lean Cuisine Lunch Express*),
9⅝ oz. .... 6.0 .... 2.0

and turkey Dijon (*Lean Cuisine Lunch Express*),
9⅞ oz. .... 6.0 .... 1.5

vegetable, Italiano (*Healthy Choice Quick Meal*),
10 oz. .... 1.0 .... 1.0

wide ribbon, w/ricotta and tomato sauce (*The Budget Gourmet*), 10.25 oz. .... 22.0 .... 8.0

Pasta Flour (*Arrowhead Mills*), ½ cup 1.0 0

Pasta sauce, canned (see also "Tomato sauce," "Pizza sauce," and specific sauce listings), ½ cup, except as noted:

(*Del Monte* Traditional Spaghetti Sauce) 1.0 0

(*Eden*) 2.5 0

(*Healthy Choice* Traditional), 4 oz. .... <1.0 0

(*McCormick* Spaghetti Sauce), ⅛ pkg. 0 0

(*Porino's* Gardina Fresca) .... 7.0 .... 1.0

(*Porino's* Traditional) .... 10.0 .... 1.5

(*Prego* Low Sodium) .... 6.0 .... 1.5

(*Prego* Traditional Spaghetti Sauce), 4 oz. .... 6.0 .... 2.0

(*Pritikin* Original Spaghetti Sauce) 5 0

(*Progresso* Spaghetti Sauce) .... 4.5 .... 1.0

all varieties (*Healthy Choice* Fat Free Chunky),
4 oz. 0 0

beef or beef and pork (*Porino's*) .... 7.0 .... 1.0

cheese, three (*Prego*), 4 oz. 2.0 5

cheese, wine and herbs (*Porino's*) .... 9.0 .... 1.5

garden style (*Del Monte* Chunky) 1.0 0

garden style (*Porino's* Classic Chunky) .... 9.0 .... 1.5

garlic and herb (*Del Monte* Chunky) 1.5 0

garden style (*Prego* Chunky) 1.0 5

garden style (*Pritikin* Chunky) 5 0

garlic and herb (*Healthy Choice*), 4 oz. .... <1.0 0

garlic and onion (*Del Monte* Spaghetti Sauce) 1.0 0

	total fat (grams)	saturated fat (grams)

Pasta sauce, canned *(cont.)*

green pepper and mushroom (*Del Monte* Spaghetti Sauce)	1.0	0
w/green pepper or mushroom (*Healthy Choice*), 4 oz.	<1.0	0
herb, Italian (*Del Monte* Chunky)	1.0	0

marinara:

15½-oz. can	14.7	2.1
½ cup	4.2	.6
(*Prego*), 4 oz.	6.0	1.5
(*Pritikin*)	0	0
(*Progresso*)	4.5	.5
(*Progresso* Authenic)	5.0	1.5
or mushroom (*Hain* Spaghetti Sauce), 4 oz.	1.0	0
w/meat (*Del Monte* Spaghetti Sauce)	1.5	0

meat flavored:

(*Healthy Choice*), 4 oz.	<1.0	0
(*Prego*)	6.0	1.5
or mushroom (*Progresso*)	4.5	1.0

w/mushroom:

(*Del Monte* Spaghetti Sauce)	1.5	0
(*Prego*)	5.0	1.5
(*Prego* Extra Chunky Supreme)	4.5	.5
(*Weight Watchers*)	0	0
mushroom and diced onion (*Prego* Extra Chunky), 4 oz.	4.0	.5
olive, black, and mushrooms (*Parino's*)	6.0	1.0
onion, diced, and garlic (*Prego*), 4 oz.	5.0	1.0
pepper and onion (*Porino's*)	5.0	1.0
sausage and green pepper (*Prego* Extra Chunky)	9.0	2.5
sausage, peppers, and mushroom (*Porino's*)	8.0	1.0
tomato, onion, and garlic (*Prego* Extra Chunky), 4 oz.	6.0	1.5
tomato basil (*Del Monte* Chunky)	1.0	0

	total fat (grams)	saturated fat (grams)
tomato basil (*Porino's*)	6.0	1.0
tomato and basil (*Prego*), 4 oz.	3.0	.5
tomatoes:		
(*Contadina Pasta Ready*)	2.0	0
chunky (*Del Monte* Pasta Style)	0	0
w/crushed red pepper (*Contadina Pasta*		
Ready)	3.0	.5
w/mushrooms (*Contadina Pasta Ready*)	1.5	0
w/olives (*Contadina Pasta Ready*)	3.0	.5
primavera (*Contadina Pasta Ready*)	1.5	0
w/three cheeses (*Contadina Pasta Ready*)	4.0	0
vegetable, supreme (*Prego* Extra Chunky)	3.0	.5
Pasta sauce, refrigerated or frozen (see also		
specific sauce listings):		
w/meatless meats (*Bodin's* Spaghetti Sauce),		
3.4 oz.	0	0
tomato, ½ cup:		
w/basil (*Contadina*)	4.0	4.0
chunky (*Contadina Light*)	.5	0
w/garden vegetables (*Contadina*)	0	0
w/Italian sausage and peppers (*Contadina*)	7.0	5.0
marinara (*Contadina*), ½ cup	5.0	2.0
Pasta sauce mix (see also specific sauce listings):		
(*Lawry's* Original Style Spaghetti Sauce),		
1½ tbsp.	0	0
(*Lawry's* Extra Rich & Thick Spaghetti Sauce),		
1 tbsp.	1.0	0
garlic and herb (*Spice Isands*), ¼ pkg., 1 tbsp.	0	0
primavera (*Spice Islands*), ⅕ pkg., 1 tbsp.	1.5	0
Pasta salad mix, see "Pasta dishes, mix"		
Pasta seasoning mix (see also "Spaghetti		
seasoning mix"):		
salad (*Durkee*), ⅙ pkg.	0	0
zesty (*French's*), ⅕ pkg.	0	0
Pasta shells or spirals, see "Pasta"		

	total fat (grams)	saturated fat (grams)

Pasta shells dishes, mix:

w/cheddar, white (*Golden Grain Noodle Roni*),
1 cup* .... 17.0 .... 5.0

and cheese (*Kraft Velveeta*), 4 oz.,
about 1 cup* .... 13.0 .... 8.0

and cheese and bacon (*Kraft Velveeta*), 4 oz., about
1 cup* .... 14.0 .... 8.0

and cheese, salsa (*Kraft Velveeta*), 4.5 oz., about
1 cup* .... 14.0 .... 9.0

Pasta shells entree, frozen, stuffed:

(*Celentano*), 10-oz. pkg., 3 pieces .... 20.0 .... 9.0

(*Celentano* 14 oz.), 7 oz., 2 pieces .... 14.0 .... 7.0

(*Celentano* Great Choice), 10 oz., 3 pieces .... 2.5 .... 1.0

(*Schwan's*), 6 oz., 3 pieces .... 16.0 .... 9.0

broccoli (*Celentano* Great Choice), 10 oz.,
4 pieces .... 4.0 .... 1.0

cheese, w/tomato sauce (*Stouffer's*), 9¼ oz. ..... 16.0 .... 7.0

Florentine (*Celentano* Selects), 10 oz. .... 6.0 .... 1.5

w/sauce (*Celentano* 24 oz.), 8 oz., 3 pieces ...... 15.0 .... 7.0

w/out sauce (*Celentano* 12.5 oz.), 6.25 oz.,
4 pieces .... 15.0 .... 8.0

w/out sauce (*Celentano* 24 oz.), 4.7 oz.,
3 pieces .... 11.0 .... 6.0

tomato sauce (*Healthy Choice Generous Serving*),
12 oz. .... 3.0 .... 2.0

Pasta spirals entree, canned, and chicken (*Libby's Diner*), 7.75 oz. .... 4.0 .... 1.0

Pastrami:

1 oz. .... 8.3 .... 3.0

(*Healthy Choice* Deli Meats), 1 oz. .... 1.0 .... <1.0

(*Hansel 'n Gretel Healthy Deli*), 2 oz. .... 3.0 .... 1.0

(*Hebrew National* Deli Sliced), 2 oz., 4 slices ..... 3.0 .... 1.0

(*Hebrew National* Rounds), 2 oz. .... 3.0 .... 1.0

(*Hillshire Farm* Deli Select), 1 slice .... <1.0 .... n.a.

(*Hillshire Farm* Flavor Pack), 1 oz. .... <1.0 .... n.a.

	total fat (grams)	saturated fat (grams)
brisket (*Boar's Head* 1st Cut), 2 oz.	4.0	1.5
round (*Boar's Head*), 2 oz.	2.5	.5
turkey, see "Turkey pastrami"		

Pastry, see specific listings

Pastry filling, see specific listings

Pastry pocket, 1 piece:

apple (*Tastykake*)	23.0	6.0
cheese (*Tastykake*)	27.0	8.0
cherry (*Tastykake*)	20.0	5.0

Pastry shell (see also "Pie crust or shell"), frozen or refrigerated:

patty (*Pepperidge Farm*), 1.7-oz. shell	14.0	3.0
puff pastry, mini (*Pepperidge Farm*), .4-oz. shell	4.0	n.a.
sheet (*Pepperidge Farm*), ⅙ sheet, 1.5 oz.	11.0	2.5
tart crust or shell:		
(*Oronoque*), 3" tart	9.0	2.0
(*Pet-Ritz*), ¼ of 6" crust	7.0	1.5
(*Pet-Ritz*), 3" crust	9.0	2.0
(*Stilwell*), 1 piece	7.0	2.0

Pâté (see also "Liverwurst"), canned:

1 oz.	7.9	n.a.
1 tbsp.	3.6	n.a.
chicken liver, 1 tbsp.	1.7	n.a.
goose liver, smoked, 1 tbsp.	5.7	n.a.
liver, spread (*Sells*), 2 oz., ¼ cup	14.0	5.0

Patty shell, see "Pastry shell"

Pea, see "Peas," and specific listings

Pea pod, Chinese, see "Peas, edible-podded"

Peach:

fresh, untrimmed, 1 lb.	.3	<.1
fresh, 1 medium, 2½" diameter, 4 per lb.	.1	0
canned (*Del Monte*), ½ cup	0	0
canned (*Libby* Lite), ½ cup	0	0
dried:		
3–4 pieces	0	0

	total fat (grams)	saturated fat (grams)

Peach, dried *(cont.)*

    (*Del Monte* Sun Dried), ⅓ cup 0 0

    (*Sonoma*), 1.4 oz., 3–4 pieces 0 0

  frozen:

    10-oz. pkg. .... .4 .... <.1

    sliced (*Schwan's*), 1⅓ cups 0 0

    sliced (*Stilwell*), 1 cup 0 0

Peach butter (*Smucker's*), 1 tbsp. 0 0

Peach dumpling, frozen (*Pepperidge Farm*),

  3-oz. piece .... 11.0 .... 2.5

Peach juice cocktail (*Mott's Fruit Basket*), 8 fl. oz. .. 0 0

Peach nectar, canned or bottled:

  6 fl. oz. .... <.1 0

  (*R.W. Knudsen*), 8 fl. oz. 0 0

Peanut, shelled, except as noted:

  (*Eagle* Ballpark/Lightly Salted), 1 oz., 28–29

    pieces .... 15.0 .... 3.0

  (*Frito-Lay* Salted), 1 oz. .... 15.0 .... 5.0

  all varieties:

    raw, in shell, 4 oz. .... 40.8 .... 5.7

    raw, 1 oz. .... 13.8 .... 1.9

    boiled, 1 oz. 6.2 9

    dry-roasted, 1 oz. .... 13.9 .... 1.9

    dry-roasted, ½ cup .... 36.3 .... 5.0

    oil-roasted, 1 oz. .... 13.8 .... 1.9

    oil-roasted, ½ cup .... 35.5 .... 4.9

  dry-roasted (*Planters*), 1 oz. .... 13.0 .... 2.0

  dry-roasted (*Planters* Lightly Salted/Unsalted),

    1 oz. .... 14.0 .... 2.0

  cocktail (*Planters/Planters* Unsalted), 1 oz. .... 14.0 .... 2.0

  cocktail (*Planters* Lightly Salted), 1 oz. .... 15.0 .... 2.0

  honey-roasted (*Eagle*), 1 oz., 35 pieces .... 13.0 .... 3.0

  honey-roasted (*Planters*), 1 oz. .... 13.0 .... 1.5

  honey-roasted (*Weight Watchers Smart Snackers*),

    7 oz. .... 5.0 .... 1.0

	total fat (grams)	saturated fat (grams)
hot (*Frito-Lay*), ¼ cup	21.0	5.0
oil-roasted:		
(*Planters*), 1 oz.	14.5	2.0
(*Planters Fun Size!*), 1 oz.	14.0	2.0
spicy, hot or mild (*Planters Heat*), 1 oz.	14.0	2.0
sweet (*Planters Sweet N Crunchy*), 1 oz.	7.0	1.0
roasted (*Eagle*), 1 oz., 28 pieces	15.0	2.0
Spanish:		
(*Planters*), 1 oz.	14.0	2.5
raw, 1 oz.	13.9	2.1
raw (*Planters*), 1 oz.	13.0	3.0
oil-roasted, 1 oz.	13.7	2.1
oil-roasted, ½ cup	36.0	5.6
Valencia:		
raw, 1 oz.	13.3	2.1
oil-roasted, 1 oz.	14.4	2.2
oil-roasted, ½ cup	36.9	5.7
Virginia:		
raw, 1 oz.	13.7	1.8
oil-roasted, 1 oz.	13.6	1.8
oil-roasted, ½ cup	34.8	4.5
Peanut butter, 2 tbsp., except as noted:		
(*Adams* 100% Natural Creamy or Crunchy)	16.0	3.0
(*Adams No-Stir* Creamy)	17.0	4.0
(*Adams No-Stir* Crunchy)	16.0	4.0
(*Arrowhead Mills* Natural)	15.0	3.0
(*Jif/Simply Jif* Regular or Low Salt)	16.0	3.0
(*Peter Pan Smart Choice* Reduced Fat)	12.0	2.0
(*Planters* Chunky or Creamy)	16.0	3.0
(*Reese's*)	16.0	3.0
(*Roaster Fresh*), 1 oz.	14.0	2.4
(*Skippy* Reduced Fat)	12.0	2.5
(*Smucker's*)	15.0	3.0
(*Smucker's* Natural)	16.0	2.0

	total fat (grams)	saturated fat (grams)
Peanut butter *(cont.)*		
unsalted (*Adams* 100% Natural Chunky)	16.0	3.0
unsalted (*Adams* 100% Natural Creamy)	15.0	3.0
Peanut butter and jelly (*Smucker's Goober*),		
3 tbsp.	13.0	2.0
Peanut butter caramel topping (*Smucker's*),		
2 tbsp.	4.5	5.
Peanut flour:		
defatted, 1 cup	.3	<.1
low-fat, 1 cup	13.1	1.8
Peanut oil:		
1 tbsp.	13.5	2.3
(*Hain*), 1 tbsp.	14.0	2.0
(*Planters*), 1 tbsp.	14.0	2.5
w/vitamin E (*Hain*), 1 tbsp.	14.0	2.0
Peanut sauce, Thai, see "Stir-fry sauce"		
Pear:		
fresh		
untrimmed, 1 lb.	1.7	.1
Bartlett, 1 medium, 2½" diameter,		
2½ per lb.	.7	<.1
w/skin, sliced, ½ cup	.3	<.1
canned:		
(*Libby* Lite), ½ cup	0	0
all varieties (*Del Monte*), ½ cup	0	0
diced (*Del Monte* Snack Cup), 1 can	0	0
dried (*Sonoma*), 1.5 oz., 3–4 pieces	0	0
Pear juice (*R.W. Knudsen* Organic), 8 fl. oz.	0	0
Pear nectar, canned, 6 fl. oz.	<.1	<.1
Peas, see specific listings		
Peas, blackeye, see "Blackeye peas"		
Peas, butter, frozen (*Stilwell*), ½ cup	.5	0
Peas, cream, canned (*Allens/East Texas Fair*),		
½ cup	<1.0	.5

	total fat (grams)	saturated fat (grams)

Peas, crowder:

canned (*Allens/East Texas Fair*), ½ cup	1.0	.5
frozen (*McKenzie's*), ½ cup	1.0	0
frozen (*Stilwell*), ½ cup	1.0	0

Peas, edible-podded:

fresh:

raw, untrimmed, 1 lb.	.9	.2
raw, trimmed, ½ cup	.1	<.1
boiled, drained, ½ cup	.2	<.1

frozen:

10-oz. pkg.	.9	.2
boiled, drained, ½ cup	.3	.1
(*Green Giant Select Sugar Snap*), ½ cup	0	0

Peas, field:

canned, ½ cup:

(*Allens*)	1.0	.5
w/bacon or w/bacon and snaps (*Trappey's*) ...	1.0	.5
w/snaps (*Allens*)	1.0	0
frozen (*Stilwell*), ½ cup	1.0	0

Peas, green or sweet:

fresh:

raw, in pods, 1 lb.	.7	.1
raw, shelled, ½ cup	.3	.1
boiled, drained, ½ cup	.2	<.1

canned, ½ cup:

drained	.3	.1
(*Seneca*)	0	0
(*Stokely*)	0	0
all varieties (*Del Monte*)	0	0
all varieties (*Green Giant LeSueur*)	0	0
dry, early June (*Crest Top*)	.5	0
w/pearl onions (*Green Giant Le Sueur*)	0	0
freeze-dried (*AlpineAire*), ½ cup*	.4	0
freeze-dried (*Mountain House*), ½ cup*	1.0	0

	total fat (grams)	saturated fat (grams)

Peas, green or sweet *(cont.)*

  frozen, ½ cup, except as noted:

10-oz. pkg.	1.1	.2
boiled, drained	.2	<.1
(*Schwan's*), ⅔ cup	.5	0
(*Schwan's* Sugar Snap), ¾ cup	0	0
(*Stilwell*), ⅔ cup	0	0
baby, early (*Green Giant Harvest Fresh Le Sueur*), ⅔ cup	0	0
baby, early (*Green Giant Le Sueur*)	0	0
sweet (*Green Giant/Green Giant Harvest Fresh*), ⅔ cup	0	0

  frozen in butter sauce, ¾ cup:

baby, early (*Green Giant Le Sueur*)	2.0	1.5
sweet (*Green Giant*)	2.0	1.5

Peas, lady, canned, w/ or w/out snaps (*Allens/ Sunshine*), ½ cup 1.0 5

Peas, pepper, canned (*Allens/East Texas Fair*), ½ cup 1.0 5

Peas, pigeon:

  fresh:

raw, in pods, 1 lb.	3.6	.8
raw, ½ cup	1.3	.3
boiled, drained, ½ cup	1.1	.1
mature, dried, raw, ½ cup	1.5	.3
mature, dried, boiled, ½ cup	.3	.1

Peas, purple hull:

canned (*Allens/East Texas Fair*), ½ cup	1.0	.5
frozen (*McKenzie's*), ½ cup	.5	0
frozen (*Stilwell*), ½ cup	1.0	0

Peas, snow or Oriental, see "Peas, edible-podded"

Peas, split, dry:

raw, ½ cup	1.1	.2
boiled, ½ cup	.4	.1
green (*Arrowhead Mills*), ¼ cup	.5	0

	total fat (grams)	saturated fat (grams)
Peas, sugar snap, see "Peas, edible-podded"		
Peas, white acre, canned (*Allens/East Texas Fair*),		
½ cup	1.0	.5
Peas and carrots:		
canned, ½ cup:		
w/liquid	.4	.1
(*Del Monte*)	0	0
(*Seneca*)	0	0
(*Stokely/Stokely* No Sugar)	0	0
frozen:		
10-oz. pkg.	1.3	.2
boiled, drained, ½ cup	.3	.1
(*Stilwell*), ½ cup	0	0
Peas and onions:		
canned, w/liquid, ½ cup	.2	<.1
frozen:		
10-oz. pkg.	.9	.2
boiled, drained, ½ cup	.2	<.1
Pecan, shelled, except as noted:		
dried:		
in shell, 4 oz.	40.7	3.3
1 oz., 31 large or 20 jumbo	19.2	1.5
halves, 1 cup	73.1	5.9
chopped, 1 cup	80.5	6.4
dry-roasted, 1 oz.	18.4	1.5
oil-roasted, 1 oz., 15 halves	20.2	1.6
oil-roasted, 1 cup	78.3	6.3
Pecan pastry filling (*Solo*), 2 tbsp.	4.0	0
Pecan flour, 1 oz.	.4	<.1
Pecan topping, in syrup (*Smucker's*), 2 tbsp.	11.0	1.0
Penne, plain, see "Pasta"		
Penne dishes, mix, savory herb and garlic (*Lipton Golden Saute*), ⅓ cup	3.0	2.0
Penne entree, frozen, w/tomato sauce and sausage (*The Budget Gourmet* Light & Healthy), 10 oz.	8.0	2.5

	total fat (grams)	saturated fat (grams)
Pepper, ground (see also specific listings):		
all varieties (*Durkee/Spice Islands*), ¼ tsp.	0	0
black, 1 tbsp.	.2	.1
black, 1 tsp.	.1	<.1
red or cayenne, 1 tbsp.	.9	.2
red or cayenne, 1 tsp.	.3	<.1
seasoned, all varieties (*Durkee/Spice Islands*), ¼ tsp.	0	0
seasoned, coarse (*Lawry's* Colorful), ¼ tsp.	0	0
white, 1 tbsp.	.2	<.1
Pepper, banana:		
(*Nalley*), 1 oz.	0	0
hot or mild (*Trappey's*), 1 oz., 3 pieces	0	0
Pepper, bell, see "Pepper, sweet"		
Pepper, cherry:		
(*Nalley*), 1 oz.	0	0
drained (*Progresso*), 2 tbsp.	2.0	0
hot (*Hebrew National*), 1 oz., about 1⅓ pieces	0	0
hot (*Progresso*), 1 piece	0	0
hot or mild (*Trappey's*), 1 oz., 2 pieces	0	0
Pepper, chili (see also specific listings):		
green and red, hot:		
untrimmed, 1 lb.	.7	.1
1 medium, about 1.6 oz.	.1	tr.
chopped, ½ cup	.2	<.1
canned or in jars:		
green and red, seeded, w/liquid, 4 oz.	.1	<.1
green (*Chi-Chi's*), ¾ piece or 2 tbsp.	0	0
green (*Old El Paso*), 2 tbsp. or 1 piece	0	0
hot (*Del Monte*), 1 oz., 4 pieces	0	0
tomatoes, diced, and, see "Tomatoes, canned"		
Pepper, chilpotle, in spice sauce (*Del Monte*), 2 tbsp.	.5	0

	total fat (grams)	saturated fat (grams)
Pepper, filet (*Hebrew National*), 1 oz., ¼ piece	0	0
Pepper, hot (see also specific pepper listings):		
(*Nalley*), 1 oz.	0	0
(*Tabasco/Trappey's* Torrido Sante Fe), 1-oz. piece ..	0	0
in vinegar (*Tabasco/Trappey's*), 1 oz., 15 pieces ..	0	0
Pepper, jalapeño, canned or in jars:		
w/liquid, 4 oz.	.7	.1
w/liquid, chopped, ½ cup	.4	<.1
all cuts:		
(*La Victoria*), 1.1 oz.	0	0
(*Nalley*), 1 oz.	0	0
green or red (*Chi-Chi's*), 1 oz.	0	0
hot, sliced (*Tabasco/Trappey's*), 1 oz.,		
21 slices	0	0
peeled, pickled or sliced (*Old El Paso*), 1 oz.	0	0
sliced, regular or pickled (*Del Monte*), 2 tbsp.	0	0
whole, regular or pickled (*Del Monte*), 2 pieces ...	0	0
Pepper, jalapeño, frozen, stuffed (*Schwan's*),		
3.1 oz., 3 pieces	13.0	8.0
Pepper, pepperoncini:		
(*Krinos* Imported), ¼ cup	0	0
(*Nalley* Greek), 1 oz.	0	0
(*Progresso* Tuscan), 3 pieces	0	0
(*Zorba*), 5 pieces	0	0
hot (*Tabasco/Trappey's Tempero*), 1-oz. piece	0	0
mild (*Tabasco/Trappey's* Dulcito Italian), 1 oz.,		
3 pieces	0	0
Pepper, pizza, w/Italian herbs (*Lawry's*), ¼ tsp.	0	0
Pepper, roasted, see "Pepper, sweet"		
Pepper, serrano, hot (*Tabasco/Trappey's*), 1 oz.,		
3 peppers	0	0
Pepper, stuffed, entree, frozen:		
(*Stouffer's*), 10 oz.	8.0	1.5
(*Stouffer's*), ½ of 15½-oz. pkg.	7.0	1.0

	total fat (grams)	saturated fat (grams)
Pepper, sweet, green and red, except as noted:		
fresh:		
raw, untrimmed, 1 lb.	.7	.1
raw, 1 medium or ½ cup chopped	.1	<.1
boiled, drained, 1 medium or ½ cup chopped	.1	<.1
in jars (see also "Pimiento"), red:		
w/liquid, 4 oz.	.3	.1
w/liquid, halves, ½ cup	.2	<.1
(*Rosoff*), 1 oz., ¼ piece	0	0
fried, drained (*Progresso*), 2 tbsp.	5.0	.5
roasted (*Krinos*), 1 piece	0	0
roasted (*Progresso*), 1 oz., about ½ piece	0	0
freeze-dried, ¼ cup	.1	tr.
frozen, 10-oz. pkg.	.6	.1
frozen, boiled, drained, chopped, 4 oz.	.2	<.1
Pepper salad, drained (*Progresso*), 2 tbsp.	2.0	0
Pepper sauce, hot:		
(*Tabasco* Brand), 1 tsp.	0	0
jalapeño (*Trappey's* Chef Magic), 1 tsp.	0	0
Pepper seasoning, see "Pepper" and specific listings		
Pepper steak, see "Beef entree"		
Peppered loaf, pork and beef, 1 oz.	1.8	.7
Peppercorn sauce mix:		
(*Knorr* Classic), ⅕ pkg.	1.0	0
green (*McCormick Collection*), ⅙ pkg.	0	0
Pepperoncini, see "Pepper, pepperoncini"		
Pepperoni:		
(*Boar's Head*), 1 oz.	13.0	4.0
(*Hillshire Farm*), 1 oz.	10.0	n.a.
(*Hormel/Rosa Grande*), 1 oz.	13.0	5.0
(*Oscar Mayer*), 1.1 oz., 15 slices	13.0	5.0
pork and beef, 1 oz.	12.5	4.6
pork and beef, 1 sausage, 10¼" × 1⅜", 9 oz.	110.4	40.5
sliced (*Hormel* Deli/*Pillow Pack*), 1 oz.	13.0	6.0

	total fat (grams)	saturated fat (grams)
Pepperoni sandwich, frozen, bagel (*Hormel Quick Meal*), 1 piece	15.0	6.0
Perch, mixed species, meat only:		
raw, 4 oz.	1.1	.2
baked, broiled, or microwaved, 4 oz.	1.3	.3
Perch, ocean, see "Ocean perch"		
Perch entree, frozen, battered (*Van de Kamp's*), 2 fillets	20.0	2.5
Persimmon:		
fresh:		
Japanese, untrimmed, 1 lb.	.7	<.1
Japanese, 1 medium, about 7.1 oz.	.3	<.1
native, untrimmed, 1 lb.	1.5	n.a.
native, 1 medium, about 1.1 oz.	.1	tr.
dried (*Sonoma*), 1.4 oz., 6–8 pieces	0	0
dried, Japanese, 1 oz.	.1	tr.
Pesto sauce, ¼ cup:		
w/basil (*Contadina*)	30.0	5.0
dried tomato (*Sonoma*)	9.0	1.5
w/sun-dried tomatoes (*Contadina*)	24.0	4.0
Pesto sauce mix:		
(*Knorr* Pasta Sauces), ⅓ pkg.	.5	0
(*Spice Islands*), ¼ pkg., 2 tsp.	.5	0
creamy (*Knorr* Pasta Sauces), ⅕ pkg.	1.0	0
tomato (*Spice Islands*), ¼ pkg., 1 tbsp.	0	0
Pheasant, fresh, raw:		
meat w/skin, ½ bird, 14.1 oz. (1 lb. w/bone)	37.2	10.8
meat w/skin, 4 oz.	10.5	3.1
meat only:		
½ bird, 12.4 oz. (1 lb. w/bone and skin)	12.8	4.4
½ breast, about 6.4 oz.	5.9	2.0
1 leg, about 3.8 oz.	4.6	1.6
Picante beans, canned (*Allens/East Texas Fair*), ½ cup	<1.0	0

	total fat (grams)		saturated fat (grams)

Picante sauce (see also "Salsa"), all varieties, 2 tbsp.:

(*Chi-Chi's*)	0	....	0
(*Gracias* Superba)	0	....	0
(*Old El Paso*)	0	....	0
(*Old El Paso* Thick 'n Chunky)	0	....	0
(*Tabasco* Brand)	.2	....	0
(*Taco Bell*)	0	....	0
(*Tostitos* Dip)	0	....	0

Pickles, cucumber:

all varieties (*Claussen*), 1 oz., 4 slices or 1 piece	0	....	0
all varieties, (*Pickle Eater's*), 1 oz.	0	....	0
bread and butter, chunks or slices (*Nalley*), 1 oz.	0	....	0
cucumber chips (*Nalley*), 1 oz.	0	....	0
dill:			
1 lb.	.9	....	.2
1 medium, 3¾" long	.1	....	<.1
all cuts and flavors (*Nalley*), 1 oz.	0	....	0
all cuts and varieties (*Del Monte*), 1 oz.	0	....	0
kosher, all varieties (*Hebrew National*), 1 oz.	0	....	0
kosher, all varieties (*Rosoff*), 1 oz.	0	....	0
kosher, all varieties (*Schorr's*), 1 oz.	0	....	0
sour, 1 medium, 3¾" long	.1	....	<.1
sweet:			
1 lb.	1.2	....	.3
l large, 3" long	.1	....	<.1
all cuts and varieties (*Del Monte*), 1 oz.	0	....	0
all cuts and varieties (*Nalley*), 1 oz.	0	....	0

Pickle dip, dill (*Nalley*), 2 tbsp.	5.0	....	1.0
Pickle and pepper loaf (*Boar's Head*), 2 oz.	13.0	....	7.0

Pickle and pimiento loaf:

(*Oscar Mayer*), 1-oz. slice	6.0	....	2.0
pork, 1 oz.	6.0	....	2.2

	total fat (grams)	saturated fat (grams)
Pickle relish, see "Relish"		
Pickled vegetables, see specific listings		
Pickling spices, 1 tsp.	.6	.1
Picnic loaf, pork and beef, 1 oz.	4.7	1.7
Pico de gallo, 2 tbsp.:		
(*Chi-Chi's*)	0	0
(*Old El Paso*)	0	0
Pie, frozen or refrigerated (see also "Pie, snack" and "Cobbler, frozen"):		
apple:		
(*Banquet*), ⅕ pie	13.0	6.0
(*Entenmann's* Homestyle), ⅙ pie	14.0	3.5
(*Mrs. Smith's,* 10"), ⅒ pie	12.0	2.5
(*Mrs. Smith's,* 9"), ⅛ pie	14.0	2.5
(*Mrs. Smith's,* 8"), ⅙ pie	11.0	2.0
(*Mrs. Smith's Old Fashioned,* 9"), ⅛ pie	16.0	3.0
(*Schwan's*), 1/12 pie	13.0	3.0
Dutch (*Mrs. Smith's,* 10"), ⅒ pie	12.0	2.5
Dutch (*Mrs. Smith's,* 9"), ⅛ pie	12.0	2.5
Dutch (*Mrs. Smith's,* 8"), ⅙ pie	13.0	2.5
Dutch (*Mrs. Smith's Old Fashioned,* 9"), ⅑ pie	14.0	3.0
lattice (*Mrs. Smith's* Ready-to-Serve, 8"), ⅕ pie	13.0	2.5
apple or cherry beehive (*Entenmann's* Fat Free), ⅕ pie	0	0
apple cranberry (*Mrs. Smith's,* 8"), ⅙ pie	11.0	2.0
banana cream:		
(*Banquet*), ⅙ pie	10.5	3.0
(*Mrs. Smith's*), ¼ pie	14.0	4.0
(*Pet-Ritz*), ¼ pie	13.0	8.0
berry (*Mrs. Smith's,* 8"), ⅙ pie	11.0	2.0
blackberry (*Mrs. Smith's,* 8"), ⅙ pie	11.0	2.0
blackberry or blueberry (*Banquet*), ⅕ pie	12.0	5.0

	total fat (grams)	saturated fat (grams)

Pie *(cont.)*

blueberry (Mrs. Smith's, 8"), ⅙ pie .... 11.0 .... 2.0
Boston cream, see "Cake, frozen"
cherry:
    (*Banquet*), ⅕ pie .... 14.0 .... 6.0
    (*Mrs. Smith's*, 10"), ¹⁄₁₀ pie .... 11.0 .... 2.0
    (*Mrs. Smith's*, 9"), ⅛ pie .... 13.0 .... 2.5
    (*Mrs. Smith's*, 8"), ⅙ pie .... 11.0 .... 2.0
    (*Mrs. Smith's Old Fashioned*, 9"), ⅛ pie .... 13.0 .... 2.5
    (*Schwan's*), ¹⁄₁₀ pie .... 15.0 .... 3.0
    lattice (*Mrs. Smith's* Ready-to-Serve, 8"),
      ⅕ pie .... 13.0 .... 2.5
chocolate:
    cream (*Banquet*), ⅙ pie .... 10.0 .... 2.5
    cream (*Mrs. Smith's*), ¼ pie .... 17.0 .... 4.0
    cream (*Pet-Ritz*), ¼ pie .... 13.0 .... 8.0
    French silk (*Mrs. Smith's*), ⅕ pie .... 21.0 .... 6.0
    mocha (*Weight Watchers Sweet Celebrations*),
      2.75 oz. .... 4.0 .... 1.0
coconut:
    cream (*Banquet*), ⅙ pie .... 10.0 .... 3.0
    cream (*Mrs. Smith's*), ¼ pie .... 19.0 .... 5.0
    cream (*Pet-Ritz*), ¼ pie .... 13.0 .... 8.0
    custard (*Entenmann's*), ⅕ pie .... 19.0 .... 8.0
    custard (*Mrs. Smith's*), ⅕ pie .... 12.0 .... 5.0
fudge vanilla cream (*Pet-Ritz*), ¼ pie .... 15.0 .... 9.0
lemon:
    (*Entenmann's*), ⅙ pie .... 17.0 .... 4.5
    cream (*Banquet*), ⅙ pie .... 10.0 .... 2.5
    cream (*Mrs. Smith's*), ¼ pie .... 15.0 .... 4.0
    cream (*Pet-Ritz*), ¼ pie .... 13.0 .... 8.0
    meringue (*Mrs. Smith's*), ⅕ pie .... 8.0 .... 2.0
mince (*Mrs. Smith's*), ⅙ pie .... 11.0 .... 2.0
mincemeat (*Banquet*), ⅕ pie .... 13.0 .... 6.0

	total fat (grams)	saturated fat (grams)
Mississippi mud (*Weight Watchers Sweet Celebrations*), 5.04 oz.	5.0	1.5
peach:		
(*Banquet*), 1/5 pie	12.0	5.0
(*Mrs. Smith's*, 8"), 1/6 pie	11.0	2.0
(*Mrs. Smith's Old Fashioned*, 9"), 1/8 pie	13.0	2.5
peanut butter chocolate (*Pet-Ritz*), 1/4 pie	15.0	8.0
pecan (*Mrs. Smith's*, 10"), 1/10 pie	23.0	4.0
pecan (*Mrs. Smith's*, 8"), 1/6 pie	23.0	4.0
pumpkin:		
(*Banquet*), 1/5 pie	8.0	3.0
(*Schwan's*), 1/10 pie	10.0	2.5
cream (*Pet-Ritz*), 1/4 pie	13.0	8.0
custard (*Mrs. Smith's*, 10"), 1/9 pie	8.0	2.0
custard (*Mrs. Smith's*, 9"), 1/8 pie	8.0	2.0
custard (*Mrs. Smith's*, 8"), 1/5 pie	8.0	2.0
hearty (*Mrs. Smith's*, 9"), 1/8 pie	7.0	1.5
hearty (*Mrs. Smith's*, 8"), 1/5 pie	8.0	1.5
raspberry, red (*Mrs. Smith's*, 8"), 1/6 pie	11.0	2.0
strawberry cream (*Banquet*), 1/6 pie	8.5	2.0
strawberry rhubarb (*Mrs. Smith's*, 8"), 1/5 pie	11.0	2.0
Pie, snack, individual (see also "Cobbler" and "Pastry Pocket"):		
apple:		
(*Aunt Fanny's*), 4-oz. pie	23.0	10.0
(*Aunt Fanny's*), 3.5-oz. pie	20.0	9.0
(*Drake's*), 4 oz., 2 pies	16.0	4.0
(*McMillin's*), 4-oz. pie	23.0	10.0
(*McMillin's*), 3.5-oz. pie	21.0	9.0
(*Pet-Ritz*), 4.25-oz. pie	20.0	10.0
(*Tastykake*), 4-oz. pie	12.0	2.5
French (*Tastykake*), 4.2-oz. pie	12.0	3.0
apple or French apple (*Hostess*), 4.3 oz.	19.0	9.0
banana creme (*Aunt Fanny's*), 4-oz. pie	21.0	10.0

	total fat (grams)	saturated fat (grams)

Pie, snack *(cont.)*

banana or chocolate marshmallow (*Little Debbie*),

   1 pie .... 5.0 .... 3.0

berry:

   (*Aunt Fanny's*), 4-oz. pie .... 22.0 .... 10.0

   (*Aunt Fanny's*), 3.5-oz. pie .... 19.0 .... 9.0

   (*McMillin's*), 4-oz. pie .... 23.0 .... 10.0

   (*McMillin's*), 3.5-oz. pie .... 20.0 .... 9.0

blackberry or blueberry (*Hostess*), 4.3 oz. .... 17.0 .... 8.0

blueberry:

   (*Drake's*), 4 oz., 2 pies .... 16.0 .... 4.0

   (*Pet-Ritz*), 4.25-oz. pie .... 21.0 .... 9.0

   (*Tastykake*), 4-oz. pie .... 11.0 .... 2.5

Boston cream:

   (*Aunt Fanny's*), 4-oz. pie .... 22.0 .... 11.0

   (*Aunt Fanny's*), 3.5-oz. pie .... 19.0 .... 8.0

   (*McMillin's*), 4-oz. pie .... 22.0 .... 11.0

   (*McMillin's*), 3.5-oz. pie .... 19.0 .... 8.0

cherry:

   (*Aunt Fanny's*), 4-oz. pie .... 22.0 .... 10.0

   (*Aunt Fanny's*), 3.5-oz. pie .... 19.0 .... 9.0

   (*Drake's*), 4 oz., 2 pies .... 18.0 .... 5.0

   (*Hostess*), 4.3 oz. .... 19.0 .... 9.0

   (*McMillin's*), 4-oz. pie .... 25.0 .... 11.0

   (*McMillin's*), 3.5-oz. pie .... 22.0 .... 10.0

   (*Pet-Ritz*), 4.25-oz. pie .... 23.0 .... 11.0

   (*Tastykake*), 4-oz. pie .... 12.0 .... 3.0

chocolate creme (*Aunt Fanny's*), 4-oz. pie .... 26.0 .... 11.0

chocolate creme (*Aunt Fanny's*), 3.5-oz. pie ...... 23.0 .... 10.0

chocolate pudding (*McMillin's*), 4-oz. pie .... 26.0 .... 11.0

chocolate pudding (*McMillin's*), 3.5-oz. pie ...... 21.0 .... 9.0

coconut creme:

   (*Aunt Fanny's*), 4-oz. pie .... 23.0 .... 11.0

   (*Aunt Fanny's*), 3.5-oz. pie .... 20.0 .... 10.0

   (*Tastykake*), 4-oz. pie .... 20.0 .... 5.0

	total fat (grams)	saturated fat (grams)
coconut pudding (*McMillin's*), 4-oz. pie	22.0	11.0
coconut pudding (*McMillin's*), 3.5-oz. pie	21.0	10.0
eclair (*Tastykake Tastyklair*), 4-oz. pie	20.0	5.0
lemon:		
(*Drake's*), 4 oz., 2 pies	20.0	6.0
(*Hostess*), 4.3 oz.	20.0	9.0
(*McMillin's*), 4-oz. pie	22.0	10.0
(*McMillin's*), 3.5-oz. pie	19.0	9.0
(*Pet-Ritz*), 4.25-oz. pie	21.0	10.0
(*Tastykake*), 4-oz. pie	12.0	3.0
lemon creme (*Aunt Fanny's*), 4-oz. pie	22.0	10.0
lemon creme (*Aunt Fanny's*), 3.5-oz. pie	19.0	9.0
oatmeal creme (*Little Debbie*)	8.0	1.5
peach:		
(*Aunt Fanny's*), 4-oz. pie	22.0	10.0
(*Aunt Fanny's*), 3.5-oz. pie	19.0	9.0
(*Hostess*), 4.3 oz.	18.0	9.0
(*McMillin's*), 4-oz. pie	22.0	10.0
(*McMillin's*), 3.5-oz. pie	19.0	9.0
(*Tastykake*), 4-oz. pie	11.0	2.5
peanut butter creme (*McMillin's*), 4-oz. pie	26.0	11.0
pineapple (*Hostess*), 4.3 oz.	16.0	6.0
pineapple (*Tastykake*), 4-oz. pie	12.0	1.0
pineapple cheese (*Tastykake*), 4-oz. pie	12.0	2.5
pumpkin:		
(*Aunt Fanny's*), 4-oz. pie	21.0	8.0
(*McMillin's*), 4-oz. pie	21.0	8.0
(*Tastykake*), 4-oz. pie	14.0	4.0
raisin creme (*Little Debbie*)	5.0	1.0
strawberry:		
(*Aunt Fanny's*), 4-oz. pie	21.0	9.0
(*Aunt Fanny's*), 3.5-oz. pie	18.0	8.0
(*Hostess*), 4.3 oz.	18.0	9.0
(*McMillin's*), 4-oz. pie	20.0	9.0
(*McMillin's*), 3.5-oz. pie	18.0	8.0

	total fat (grams)	saturated fat (grams)

Pie, snack, strawberry *(cont.)*

(*Tastykake*), 3.7-oz. pie	12.0	.... 3.0
vanilla creme (*Aunt Fanny's*), 4-oz. pie	21.0	.... 10.0
vanilla creme (*Aunt Fanny's*), 3.5-oz. pie	18.0	.... 9.0
vanilla pudding (*McMillin's*), 4-oz. pie	21.0	.... 10.0
vanilla pudding (*McMillin's*), 3.5-oz. pie	21.0	.... 10.0

Pie, mix*:

banana cream (*Betty Crocker* No-Bake), ⅑ pie	10.0	.... 3.0
cheesecake:		
(*Jell-O* Homestyle No Bake), ⅛ pie	15.0	.... 4.0
blueberry (*Jell-O* No Bake), ⅛ pie	12.0	.... 4.0
cherry (*Jell-O* No Bake), ⅛ pie	12.0	.... 4.0
real (*Jell-O* No Bake), ⅛ pie	16.0	.... 5.0
strawberry (*Jell-O* No Bake), ⅛ pie	12.0	.... 4.0
chocolate silk (*Jell-O* No Bake), ⅙ pie	16.0	.... 6.0
coconut cream (*Betty Crocker* No-Bake), ⅑ pie	13.0	.... 6.0
coconut cream (*Jell-O* No Bake), ⅙ pie	19.0	.... 9.0
cookies 'n cream (*Betty Crocker* No-Bake), ⅙ pie	16.0	.... 4.0
lemon supreme (*Betty Crocker* No-Bake), ⅑ pie	13.0	.... 3.5

Pie crust or shell (see also "Pastry shell"):

butter flavor (*Keebler*), ⅛ crust	5.0	.... 1.0
chocolate cookie:		
(*Keebler Hershey*), ⅛ crust	5.0	.... 1.0
(*Oreo*), .6 oz., 2 tbsp.	3.0	5
(*Oreo*), ⅙ crust	7.0	.... 1.5
graham cracker:		
(*Honey Maid*), .6 oz., for ⅛ crust	1.5	 0
(*Honey Maid*), ⅙ crust	7.0	.... 1.5
(*Keebler*), ⅛ crust	6.0	.... 1.0
crumbs (*Sunshine*), 3 tbsp.	2.0	5
vanilla cookie (*Nilla*), .6 oz., 2 tbsp.	2.5	5
vanilla cookie (*Nilla*), ⅙ crust	8.0	.... 1.5

	total fat (grams)		saturated fat (grams)

Pie crust or shell, refrigerated or frozen,
⅛ of 9" crust, except as noted:

(*Oronoque*)	6.0	....	1.5
(*Oronoque*), 6" crust	7.0	....	1.5
(*Pet-Ritz*)	5.0	....	2.0
(*Pet-Ritz*), ⅛ of 9⅝" shell	7.0	....	3.0
(*Pillsbury* All Ready)	7.0	....	3.0
(*Stilwell*)	5.0	....	1.5
all vegetable shortening (*Pet-Ritz*)	6.0	....	1.5
deep dish:			
(*Oronoque*)	7.0	....	1.5
(*Oronoque*), ⅛ of 10" crust	8.0	....	2.0
(*Pet-Ritz*)	6.0	....	2.0
(*Stilwell*)	6.0	....	3.0
all vegetable shortening (*Pet-Ritz*)	7.0	....	2.0
graham cracker:			
(*Oronoque*)	6.0	....	1.5
(*Pet-Ritz*)	6.0	....	1.5
(*Stilwell*), ⅙ shell	9.0	....	2.0

Pie crust or shell mix:

(*Betty Crocker*), ⅛ of 9" crust	8.0	....	2.0
(*Flako*), ¼ cup	8.0	....	3.0
(*Pillsbury*), 2 tbsp.	6.0	....	1.5

Pie filling, ⅓ cup, except as noted:

apple (*Comstock*)	0	....	0
apple (*Musselmans*)	0	....	0
banana cream (*Comstock*)	1.5	....	0
blueberry (*Comstock*)	0	....	0
blueberry (*Lucky Leaf*)	0	....	0
cherry:			
dark, sweet (*Comstock*)	0	....	0
lite (*Comstock*)	0	....	0
lite (*Comstock* 25% More Fruit)	0	....	0
lite (*Lucky Leaf*)	0	....	0
red ruby (*Comstock/Thank You*)	0	....	0

	total fat (grams)		saturated fat (grams)
Pie filling *(cont.)*			
chocolate cream (*Comstock*)	1.5	....	1.0
coconut cream (*Comstock*)	3.0	....	1.0
lemon (*Comstock*)	1.5	....	0
mincemeat (*Comstock*)	0	....	0
peach (*Comstock* 25% More Fruit)	0	....	0
peach (*Lucky Leaf*)	0	....	0
pineapple (*Comstock*)	0	....	0
pumpkin (*Comstock*)	0	....	0
raisin (*Cormtock*)	0	....	0
raspberry (*Comstock*)	0	....	0
strawberry (*Comstock*)	0	....	0
strawberry (*Lucky Leaf*)	0	....	0
Pie filling mix, see "Pudding mix"			
Pierogies, frozen, 3 pieces:			
(*Schwan's*), 4.2 oz.	2.5	....	1.0
potato and cheddar (*Mrs. T's*), 4.2 oz.	2.5	....	1.0
potato cheese (*Empire* Kosher), 4.6 oz.	6.0	....	2.5
potato onion (*Empire* Kosher), 4.6 oz.	4.5	....	1.0
Pig, see "Ham" and "Pork"			
Pig's ear, frozen, simmered, 4 oz.	12.2	....	n.a.
Pig's feet:			
simmered, 4 oz.	14.1	....	4.9
pickled, 4 oz.	18.3	....	6.3
pickled (*Hormel*), 2 oz.	6.0	....	2.0
Pig's tail, simmered, 4 oz.	40.6	....	14.1
Pigeon peas, see "Peas, pigeon"			
Pignolia, see "Pine nuts"			
Pike, meat only, 4 oz.:			
northern, raw	.8	....	.1
northern, baked, broiled, or microwaved	1.0	....	.2
walleye, raw	1.4	....	.3
walleye, baked, broiled, or microwaved	1.8	....	.4
Pili nut, canary tree:			
dried, in shell, 4 oz.	17.1	....	6.7

	total fat (grams)	saturated fat (grams)
dried, shelled, 1 oz., about 15 kernels	22.6	8.9
Pimiento (see also "Pepper, sweet, in jars"):		
2 oz.	.2	<.1
1 tbsp.	<.1	0
all varieties (*Dromedary*), 2 oz.	0	0
Piña colada, 1 fl. oz.	.6	.3
Piña colada mixer:		
(*Holland House*), 4.5 fl. oz.	0	0
(*Mr. & Mrs. "T"*), 4.5 fl. oz.	0	0
canned, 1 fl. oz.	2.5	2.1
frozen* (*Bacardi*), 8 fl. oz.	6.0	5.0
Pine nuts, shelled, except as noted:		
pignolia:		
in shell, 4 oz.	44.3	6.8
1 oz.	14.4	2.2
(*Krinos*), 2 tbsp.	15.0	1.5
(*Progresso*), 1-oz. jar	13.0	1.0
piñon:		
in shell, 4 oz.	39.4	6.1
1 oz.	17.3	2.7
10 kernels	.6	.1
Pineapple:		
fresh:		
untrimmed, 1 lb.	1.0	.1
sliced, 3-oz. slice, 3½" diameter	.4	<.1
(*Dole*), 1 slice	.5	0
canned:		
all varieties (*Del Monte*), ½ cup, 2 slices	0	0
in water, juice, or syrup, 1 slice, ½ cup tidbits	.1	<.1
in juice (*Dole*), ½ cup	<1.0	0
in syrup (*Dole*), ½ cup	0	0
w/mandarin orange (*Dole*), ½ cup	<1.0	0
dried (*Sonoma*), 1.4 oz., 2 pieces	2.0	0
frozen, sweetened, 4 oz., ½ cup chunks	.1	tr.

	total fat (grams)	saturated fat (grams)
Pineapple juice or drink, all varieties, all brands, 8 fl. oz.	0	0
Pineapple juice float (*R.W. Knudsen*), 8 fl. oz.	0	0
Pineapple pastry filling (*Solo*), 2 tbsp.	0	0
Pineapple topping:		
(*Kraft*), 2 tbsp.	0	0
(*Smucker's*), 2 tbsp.	0	0
Pineapple-coconut juice (*R.W. Knudsen* Tropical Blend), 8 fl. oz.	0	0
Pink beans, dried:		
raw, ½ cup	1.2	.3
boiled, ½ cup	.4	.1
Piñon, see "Pine nuts"		
Pinto beans:		
dried:		
raw, ½ cup	1.1	.2
raw (*Arrowhead Mills*), ¼ cup	.5	0
boiled, ½ cup	.4	.1
canned, ½ cup		
w/liquid	.4	.1
(*Eden*)	.5	0
(*Green Giant/Joan of Arc*)	.5	0
(*Old El Paso*)	.5	0
(*Progresso*)	1.0	0
regular or chili style (*Stokely*)	.5	0
regular or red (*Allens/East Texas Fair*)	.5	0
w/bacon (*Trappey's*)	1.0	.5
w/tamari (*Eden*)	0	0
freeze-dried (*AlpineAire*), ½ cup*	.4	0
frozen, 10-oz. pkg.	1.4	.2
frozen, boiled, drained, 4 oz.	.5	.1
Pinto beans, sprouted:		
raw, 4 oz.	1.0	.1
boiled, drained, 4 oz.	.4	<.1

	total fat (grams)	saturated fat (grams)

Pistachio nuts, shelled, except as noted:

in shell (*Planters*), 1 oz.	7.0	n.a.

dried:

in shell, 4 oz.	27.4	3.5
1 oz., about 47 kernels	13.7	1.7
1 cup	61.9	7.8
(*Dole*), 1 oz.	14.0	n.a.
(*Sonoma*), 1.1 oz., ¼ cup	14.0	2.0

dry-roasted:

in shell, 4 oz.	31.1	4.0
1 oz.	15.0	1.9
1 cup	67.6	8.6
natural or red (*Planters*), 1 oz.	14.0	2.0

Pita, see "Bread"

Pitanga:

untrimmed, 1 lb.	1.6	n.a.
trimmed, ½ cup	.3	0

Pizza, fresh, see specific restaurant listings

Pizza, frozen (see also "Pizza, bagel," "Pizza, French bread," etc.):

(*Celentano*, 9 slice), ¼ of 22.5 oz. pkg.	11.0	5.0
(*Celentano* Thick Crust), ½ pie, 7 oz.	12.0	8.0
bacon burger (*Totino's Party*), ½ pie	20.0	4.5

Canadian bacon:

(*Jeno's Crisp 'N Tasty*), ½ pie	10.0	2.0
(*Schwan's Special Recipe*), ⅓ pie	23.0	9.0
(*Tombstone* Original), ¼ of 12" pie	16.0	7.0
(*Totino's Party*), ½ pie	15.0	2.5

cheese:

(*Celeste*), ¼ pie	16.0	8.0
(*Celeste* Pizza For One), 1 pie	25.0	13.0
(*Empire* Kosher), 3-oz. pie	9.0	4.0
(*Empire* Kosher), ½ of 10-oz. pie	13.0	7.0
(*Jeno's Crisp 'N Tasty*), ½ pie	10.0	3.0

	total fat (grams)	saturated fat (grams)
Pizza, cheese *(cont.)*		
(*Jeno's* Microwave For One), 1 pie	11.0	3.5
(*Pillsbury Oven Lovin'*), ½ pie	12.0	4.0
(*Schwan's Special Recipe*), ⅓ pie	24.0	10.0
(*Schwan's* Single Serve Deep Dish), 1 pie	26.0	10.0
(*Tombstone For One* ½ Less Fat), 1 pie	10.0	4.5
(*Totino's* Microwave), 1 pie	11.0	3.5
(*Totino's Pan Pizza*), ⅙ pie	10.0	4.0
(*Totino's Party*), ½ pie	14.0	5.0
(*Totino's Party* Family Size), ⅓ pie	16.0	6.0
extra (*Tombstone* Original), ½ of 9" pie	19.0	9.0
extra (*Tombstone* Original), ¼ of 12" pie	17.0	9.0
extra (*Tombstone For One*), 1 pie	30.0	14.0
extra (*Weight Watchers*), 5.7 oz.	12.0	4.0
four (*Celeste* Pizza For One), 1 pie	30.0	12.0
four (*Tombstone* Special Order), ⅕ of 12" pie	18.0	10.0
four, hot and zesty (*Celeste* Pizza For One), 1 pie	27.0	13.0
three (*Pappalo's*), ½ of 9" pie	15.0	8.0
three (*Pappalo's*), ¼ of 12" pie	12.0	6.0
three (*Pappalo's* Deep Dish), ⅕ pie	12.0	6.0
three (*Pappalo's* Pizza For One/Deep Dish For One), 1 pie	20.0	10.0
three (*Tombstone ThinCrust*), ¼ of 12" pie	22.0	12.0
three (*Totino's Select*), ⅓ pie	14.0	6.0
two, and Canadian bacon (*Totino's Select*), ⅓ pie	14.0	5.0
two, and pepperoni (*Totino's Select*), ⅓ pie	20.0	8.0
two, and sausage (*Totino's Select*), ⅓ pie	19.0	7.0
combination:		
(*Jeno's Crisp 'N Tasty*), ½ pie	15.0	4.0
(*Jeno's* Microwave For One), 1 pie	18.0	4.5
(*Pillsbury Oven Lovin'*), ½ pie	18.0	7.0
(*Totino's* Microwave), 1 pie	18.0	4.5

	total fat (grams)	saturated fat (grams)
(*Totino's Party*), ½ pie	21.0	4.5
(*Totino's Party* Family Size), ¼ pie	16.0	3.5
(*Weight Watchers*), 6.6 oz.	11.0	3.5
deluxe:		
(*Celeste*), ¼ pie	18.0	6.0
(*Celeste* Pizza For One), 1 pie	29.0	10.0
(*Stouffer's Lunch Express*), 6⅝-oz. pkg.	25.0	8.0
(*Tombstone* Original), ⅓ of 9" pie	16.0	7.0
(*Tombstone* Original), ⅕ of 12" pie	16.0	7.0
hamburger:		
(*Jeno's Crisp 'N Tasty*), ½ pie	14.0	4.0
(*Schwan's Special Recipe*), ¼ pie	20.0	8.0
(*Tombstone* Original), ⅕ of 12" pie	16.0	8.0
(*Totino's Party*), ½ pie	18.0	4.0
hamburger or sausage (*Tombstone* Original),		
⅓ of 9" pie	16.0	7.0
Italiano, zesty (*Totino's Party*), ½ pie	21.0	4.5
meat, four:		
(*Tombstone* Special Order), ⅓ of 9" pie	19.0	9.0
(*Tombstone* Special Order), ⅙ of 12" pie	17.0	8.0
(*Tombstone ThinCrust*), ¼ of 12" pie	25.0	12.0
meat, three (*Totino's Party*), ½ pie	19.0	4.0
Mexican style:		
(*Schwan's* Single Serve Deep Dish), 1 pie	25.0	10.0
(*Schwan's Barquito Meat Trio*), 4.9 oz.	22.0	8.0
beef (*Schwan's Barquito*), 4.9 oz.	18.0	7.0
zesty (*Totino's* Microwave), 1 pie	16.0	4.0
zesty (*Totino's Party*), ½ pie	19.0	4.5
pepperoni:		
(*Celeste*), ¼ pie	20.0	7.0
(*Celeste* Pizza For One), 1 pie	27.0	10.0
(*Jeno's Crisp 'N Tasty*), ½ pie	15.0	4.0
(*Jeno's* Microwave For One), 1 pie	16.0	3.5
(*Pappalo's*), ½ of 9" pie	19.0	9.0
(*Pappalo's*), ¼ of 12" pie	17.0	8.0

	total fat (grams)	saturated fat (grams)

Pizza, pepperoni *(cont.)*

(*Pappalo's Deep Dish*), ⅕ pie	14.0	.... 6.0
(*Pappalo's* Pizza For One), 1 pie	27.0	.... 13.0
(*Pappalo's* Pizza For One Deep Dish), 1 pie ...	26.0	.... 12.0
(*Pillsbury Oven Lovin'*), ½ pie	17.0	.... 6.0
(*Schwan's* Single Serve Deep Dish), 1 pie	31.0	.... 11.0
(*Schwan's Special Recipe*), ⅓ pie	28.0	.... 11.0
(*Stouffer's Lunch Express*), 5¾-oz. pkg.	23.0	.... 8.0
(*Tombstone* Original), ⅓ of 9" pie	19.0	.... 8.0
(*Tombstone* Original), ⅕ of 12" pie	18.0	.... 8.0
(*Tombstone* Special Order), ⅓ of 9" pie	20.0	.... 10.0
(*Tombstone* Special Order), ⅕ of 12" pie	21.0	.... 10.0
(*Tombstone* For One), 1 pie	35.0	.... 15.0
(*Tombstone* For One ½ Less Fat), 1 pie	13.0	.... 5.0
(*Tombstone ThinCrust*), ¼ of 12" pie	27.0	.... 13.0
(*Totino's Microwave*), 1 pie	16.0	.... 3.5
(*Totino's Pan Pizza*), ⅙ pie	10.0	.... 4.0
(*Totino's Party*), ½ pie	21.0	.... 5.0
(*Totino's Party* Family Size), ⅓ pie	22.0	.... 5.0
(*Weight Watchers*), 5.6 oz.	12.0	.... 4.0
w/double cheese (*Tombstone* Double Top), ⅙ pie	20.0	.... 10.0
pepperoni and sausage (*Tombstone* Original), ⅓ of 9" pie	21.0	.... 9.0

sausage:

(*Celeste* Pizza For One), 1 pie	27.0	.... 9.0
(*Jeno's Crisp 'N Tasty*), ½ pie	15.0	.... 3.0
(*Jeno's* Microwave For One), 1 pie	16.0	.... 4.0
(*Pappalo's*), ½ of 9" pie	18.0	.... 11.0
(*Pappalo's*), ¼ of 12" pie	16.0	.... 10.0
(*Pappalo's Deep Dish*), ⅕ pie	13.0	.... 8.0
(*Pillsbury Oven Lovin'*), ½ pie	16.0	.... 7.0
(*Schwan's* Single Serve Deep Dish), 1 pie	29.0	.... 10.0
(*Schwan's Special Recipe*), ¼ pie	23.0	.... 9.0
(*Tombstone* Original), ⅕ of 12" pie	16.0	.... 8.0

	total fat (grams)	saturated fat (grams)
(*Totino's* Microwave), 1 pie	16.0	4.0
(*Totino's Pan Pizza*), ⅙ pie	13.0	7.0
(*Totino's Party*), ½ pie	20.0	4.5
(*Totino's Party* Family Size), ¼ pie	16.0	3.5
w/double cheese (*Tombstone* Double Top), ⅙ pie	19.0	10.0
Italian (*Tombstone For One*), 1 pie	33.0	14.0
Italian (*Tombstone ThinCrust*), ¼ of 12" pie	24.0	11.0
three (*Tombstone* Special Order), ⅓ of 9" pie	18.0	9.0
three (*Tombstone* Special Order), ⅙ of 12" pie	16.0	8.0
sausage and mushroom (*Tombstone* Original), ⅕ of 12" pie	16.0	7.0
sausage and pepperoni:		
(*Pappalo's*), ½ of 9" pie	19.0	11.0
(*Pappalo's*), ¼ of 12" pie	17.0	9.0
(*Pappalo's Deep Dish*), ⅕ pie	14.0	8.0
(*Pappalo's* Pizza For One), 1 pie	27.0	16.0
(*Pappalo's* Pizza For One Deep Dish), 1 pie	27.0	15.0
(*Schwan's Special Recipe*), ¼ pie	23.0	9.0
(*Stouffer's Lunch Express*), 6⅜-oz. pkg.	27.0	9.0
(*Tombstone For One*), 1 pie	37.0	15.0
(*Tombstone* Original), ⅕ of 12" pie	18.0	8.0
(*Totino's Select*), ⅓ pie	19.0	7.0
w/double cheese (*Tombstone* Double Top), ⅙ pie	20.0	10.0
supreme:		
(*Pappalo's*), ⅓ of 9" pie	13.0	7.0
(*Pappalo's*), ¼ of 12" pie	16.0	9.0
(*Pappalo's Deep Dish*), ⅕ pie	14.0	8.0
(*Pappalo's* Pizza For One/Pizza For One Deep Dish), 1 pie	27.0	16.0
(*Pillsbury Oven Lovin'*), ½ pie	18.0	7.0
(*Schwan's* Single Serve Deep Dish), 1 pie	28.0	10.0

	total fat (grams)	saturated fat (grams)

Pizza, supreme *(cont.)*

(*Schwan's Special Recipe*), ¼ pizza	24.0	9.0
(*Tombstone For One*), 1 pie	34.0	14.0
(*Tombstone For One* ½ Less Fat), 1 pie	13.0	5.0
(*Tombstone* Original), ⅕ of 12" pie	17.0	8.0
(*Tombstone ThinCrust*), ¼ of 12" pie	24.0	11.0
(*Tombstone* Light), ⅕ of 12" pie	9.0	3.5
(*Totino's* Microwave Pizza For One), 1 pie	17.0	4.0
(*Totino's* Party), ½ pie	20.0	4.5
(*Totino's Select*), ⅓ pie	18.0	7.0
with meat (*Celeste*), ⅕ pie	16.0	5.0
with meat (*Celeste* Pizza For One), 1 pie	31.0	10.0
super (*Tombstone* Special Order), ⅓ of 9" pie	20.0	9.0
super (*Tombstone* Special Order), ⅙ of 12" pie	17.0	8.0
taco (*Tombstone ThinCrust*), ¼ of 12" pie	23.0	11.0

vegetable:

(*Celeste* Pizza For One), 1 pie	23.0	8.0
(*Tombstone For One* ½ Less Fat), 1 pie	10.0	4.0
(*Tombstone* Light), ⅕ of 12" pie	7.0	2.5

Pizza, bagel, frozen (*Empire* Kosher), 2-oz. piece — 5.0 — 2.5

Pizza, breakfast, frozen, 1 pie:

bacon (*Schwan's Bright Starts*)	25.0	9.0
Western (*Schwan's Bright Starts*)	24.0	9.0

Pizza, croissant crust, frozen, 1 piece:

cheese (*Pepperidge Farm*)	20.0	7.0
deluxe (*Pepperidge Farm*)	27.0	10.0
pepperoni (*Pepperidge Farm*)	23.0	9.0

Pizza, English muffin, frozen (*Empire* Kosher), 2-oz. piece — 5.0 — 2.5

Pizza, French bread, frozen:

bacon cheddar (*Stouffer's*), ½ of 11⅜-oz. pkg.	22.0	7.0

cheese:

(*Healthy Choice*), 5.6 oz.	4.0	2.0

	total fat (grams)	saturated fat (grams)
(*Lean Cuisine*), 6-oz. pkg.	8.0	4.0
(*Pillsbury Oven Lovin'*), 1 piece	14.0	5.0
(*Stouffer's*), ½ of 10⅜-oz. pkg.	14.0	5.0
double (*Stouffer's*), ½ of 11¾-oz. pkg.	19.0	7.0
cheeseburger (*Stouffer's*), ½ of 11⅞-oz. pkg.	26.0	9.0
combination (*Pillsbury Oven Lovin'*), 1 piece	21.0	10.0
deluxe:		
(*Healthy Choice*), 6.35 oz.	7.0	3.0
(*Lean Cuisine*), 6⅛-oz. pkg.	6.0	2.5
(*Stouffer's*), ½ of 12⅜-oz. pkg.	22.0	7.0
pepperoni:		
(*Healthy Choice*), 6 oz.	7.0	3.0
(*Lean Cuisine*), 5¼-oz. pkg.	7.0	3.0
(Pillsbury Oven Lovin'), 1 piece	21.0	8.0
(*Stouffer's*), ½ of 11¼-oz. pkg.	20.0	6.0
and mushroom (*Stouffer's*), ½ of 12¼-oz. pkg.	21.0	6.0
sausage:		
(*Pillsbury Oven Lovin'*), 1 piece	20.0	10.0
(*Stouffer's*), ½ of 12-oz. pkg.	20.0	5.0
Italian turkey (*Healthy Choice*), 6.35 oz.	5.0	2.0
and pepperoni (*Stouffer's*), ½ of 12½-oz. pkg.	25.0	7.0
vegetable, garden (*Stouffer's*), ½ of 12⅝-oz. pkg.	14.0	5.0
vegetable deluxe (*Stouffer's*), ½ of 12¾-oz. pkg.	17.0	6.0
white (*Stouffer's*), ½ of 10⅛-oz. pkg.	28.0	8.0
Pizza, Italian bread, frozen, 1 piece:		
deluxe (*Celeste*)	11.0	3.0
garlic and herb (*Celeste*)	8.0	2.0
pepperoni (*Celeste*)	13.0	4.0
Pizza crust, prepared (see also "Bread shell"):		
(*Contadina*), ⅕ crust	2.5	.5
(*Pillsbury*), ¼ crust	2.5	.5
(*Totino's*), ¼ crust	7.0	1.0
Pizza entree, frozen:		
w/cheese (*Kid Cuisine*), 6.85 oz.	8.0	3.0

	total fat (grams)	saturated fat (grams)
Pizza entree *(cont.)*		
w/hamburger (*Kid Cuisine*), 6.85 oz.	9.0	2.5
Pizza Hut:		
Bigfoot, 1 slice:		
cheese	6.0	3.0
pepperoni	7.0	3.0
pepperoni, mushroom, and sausage	8.0	4.0
breadsticks, 5 pieces	15.0	4.0
hand-tossed pizza, 1 slice of medium pie:		
beef	9.0	4.0
cheese	7.0	4.0
ham	5.0	3.0
Meat Lovers	11.0	6.0
pepperoni	8.0	4.0
Pepperoni Lovers	14.0	6.0
pork	10.0	5.0
sausage, Italian	11.0	5.0
supreme	12.0	5.0
supreme, super	13.0	5.0
Veggie Lovers	6.0	3.0
Pan Pizza, 1 slice of medium pie:		
beef	13.0	5.0
cheese	11.0	5.0
ham	9.0	3.0
Meat Lovers	18.0	7.0
pepperoni	12.0	4.0
Pepperoni Lovers	17.0	7.0
pork	14.0	5.0
sausage, Italian	15.0	5.0
supreme	15.0	6.0
supreme, super	17.0	6.0
Veggie Lovers	10.0	3.0
Thin 'N Crispy pizza, 1 slice of medium pie:		
beef	11.0	5.0
cheese	8.0	4.0

	total fat (grams)	saturated fat (grams)
ham	7.0	3.0
Meat Lovers	13.0	6.0
pepperoni	10.0	4.0
Pepperoni Lovers	16.0	7.0
pork	12.0	5.0
sausage, Italian	12.0	5.0
supreme	13.0	5.0
supreme, super	14.0	6.0
Veggie Lovers	7.0	3.0
Pizza mix, ¼ pie*:		
cheese (*Contadina* Pizza Kit)	11.0	5.0
pepperoni (*Contadina* Pizza Kit)	18.0	7.0
Pizza pocket, frozen, 1 piece:		
(*Weight Watchers*), 5 oz.	7.0	2.5
pepperoni (*Jeno's*)	20.0	6.0
sausage (*Jeno's*)	19.0	7.0
sausage and pepperoni (*Jeno's*)	20.0	7.0
supreme (*Jeno's*)	19.0	7.0
supreme (*Mrs. Peterson's Aussie Pie*)	26.0	9.0
Pizza pops, 1 piece:		
pepperoni (*Totino's*)	16.0	6.0
sausage (*Totino's*)	15.0	6.0
sausage and pepperoni (*Totino's*)	17.0	6.0
supreme (*Totino's*)	15.0	5.0
Pizza roll, frozen:		
Canadian bacon (*Jeno's Crisp 'N Tasty*), 1 roll	18.0	3.5
cheese (*Jeno's Crisp 'N Tasty*), 1 roll	19.0	6.0
cheese, three (*Totino's*), 10 rolls	15.0	6.0
combination or supreme (*Jeno's Crisp 'N Tasty*), 1 roll	28.0	7.0
combination or pepperoni (*Totino's*), 10 rolls	17.0	5.0
hamburger (*Jeno's Crisp 'N Tasty*), 1 roll	23.0	5.0
hamburger and cheese (*Totino's*), 10 rolls	14.0	4.5
meat, three (*Jeno's Crisp 'N Tasty*), 1 roll	26.0	6.0

	total fat (grams)	saturated fat (grams)

Pizza roll *(cont.)*

meat, three (*Totino's*), 10 rolls .... 15.0 .... 4.5
nacho cheese and beef (*Totino's*), 10 rolls .... 16.0 .... 6.0
pepperoni (*Jeno's Crisp 'N Tasty*), 1 roll .... 26.0 .... 6.0
sausage (*Jeno's Crisp 'N Tasty*), 1 roll .... 27.0 .... 6.0
sausage and cheese (*Totino's*), 10 rolls .... 15.0 .... 4.0
sausage and mushroom (*Totino's*), 10 rolls ...... 14.0 .... 4.0
spicy, Italian style (*Totino's*), 10 rolls .... 18.0 .... 5.0

Pizza sauce, ¼ cup:

(*Boboli*) 0 0
(*Contadina Pizza Squeeze*) 1.5 0
(*Progresso*) 1.0 0
basic or w/mushroom (*Contadina* Chunky) 0 0
cheese, three (*Contadina* Chunky) 5 0
w/Italian cheeses (*Contadina*) 1.5 0
w/Italian cheeses (*Contadina* Pizza Squeeze) 1.5 0
w/pepperoni (*Contadina*) 2.0 5

Plantain:

raw:

untrimmed, 1 lb. .... 1.1 .... n.a.
1 medium, about 9.7 oz. .... .7 .... n.a.
sliced, ½ cup .... .3 .... n.a.
cooked, sliced, ½ cup .... .1 .... <.1

Plum:

fresh:

untrimmed, 1 lb. 2.6 2
pitted, sliced, ½ cup 5 4
Japanese or hybrid, 1 medium, 2.5 oz. ...... .4 .... <.1

canned:

halves or whole, in water, juice, or syrup,
4 oz. .... .1 .... tr.
whole, 3 plums and 2 tbsp. liquid .... .1 .... <.1
whole, in syrup (*Wilderness*), ½ cup 0 0

Plum, Java, see "Java plum"

Poi, ½ cup .... .2 .... <.1

	total fat (grams)	saturated fat (grams)
Poke greens, canned (*Allens*), ½ cup	1.0	0
Pokeberry shoots, raw or boiled and drained, ½ cup ...	.3	<.1
Polenta, see "Cornmeal"		
Polenta mix (*Fantasic Foods* Polenta Fantastica), ⅜ cup	5.0	1.5
Polish sausage (see also "Kielbasa"):		
1 large link, 10" long, about 8 oz.	65.2	23.4
(*Hillshire Farm* Links), 2 oz.	17.0	n.a.
(*Schwan's*), 1 link, 2.7 oz.	24.0	8.0
beef, smoke flavor (*Hebrew National*), 4-oz. link ..	29.0	12.0
beef, smoke flavor (*Hebrew National*), 3-oz. link ..	22.0	9.0
turkey, see "Turkey sausage"		
Pollock, meat only, 4 oz.:		
Atlantic or Alaska, raw	1.1	.2
Atlantic or Alaska, baked, broiled, or microwaved ...	1.4	.2
walleye, raw	.9	.2
walleye, baked, broiled, or microwaved	1.3	.3
Pomegranate:		
untrimmed, 1 lb.	.8	n.a.
1 medium, about 9.7 oz.	.5	n.a.
Pomegranate juice (*R.W. Knudsen* Organic), 8 fl. oz.	0	0
Pompano, Florida, meat only:		
raw, 4 oz.	10.7	4.0
baked, broiled, or microwaved, 4 oz.	13.8	5.1
Popcorn, popped, except as noted:		
(*Cape Cod*), 1.1 oz., 3½ cup	9.0	2.0
(*Kettle Poppins* Lightly Salted), .5 oz.	2.5	.3
(*Old Dutch* Gourmet White), 1.5-oz. bag	13.0	1.5
(*Old Dutch* Gourmet White), ⅝-oz. bag	5.0	.5
(*Old Dutch* Gourmet White), 1.1 oz., 2¾ cups	9.0	1.0
(*Smartfood* Plain & Simple), 3 cups	11.0	1.5
(*Tom's* Natural), .75-oz. pkg.	4.0	.5
(*Tom's* Natural), 1 oz.	5.0	.5
air-popped, white (*Jolly Time*), 1.2 oz., 5 cups ...	.5	0

	total fat (grams)	saturated fat (grams)

Popcorn *(cont.)*

air-popped, yellow (*Jolly Time*), 1.2 oz., 5 cups .. | 1.0 | 0

butter/butter flavor:

(*Cape Cod*), 1.1 oz., 3 cups .... | 10.0 | 3.0
(*Chester's*), 3 cups .... | 12.0 | 1.5
(*Smartfood*), 3 cups .... | 9.0 | 2.0
(*Tom's*), .75-oz. pkg. .... | 4.0 | .5
(*Tom's*), 1 oz. .... | 5.0 | 1.5
(*Weight Watchers Smart Snackers*), .66 oz. ... | 2.5 | 0
toffee (*Weight Watchers Smart Snackers*),
.9 oz. .... | 2.5 | 1.0

caramel:

(*Tom's*), 1 oz. pkg. .... | 2.0 | .5
(*Weight Watchers Smart Snackers*), .9 oz. .... | 1.0 | 0
regular or w/peanuts (*Nature's Choice*), 1 oz. ... | 1.0 | n.a.

cheddar:

(*Smartfood*), 2 cups .... | 12.0 | 2.5
white (*Cape Cod*), 1.1 oz., 2⅓ cups .... | 12.0 | 2.5
white (*Kettle Poppins*), .5 oz. .... | 2.5 | .3
white (*Old Dutch* Premium), 1.1 oz., 2⅓ cups ... | 10.0 | 1.5
white (*Weight Watchers Smart Snackers*),
.6 oz. .... | 4.0 | 1.0
yellow (*Old Dutch*), 1.5-oz. bag .... | 13.0 | 2.5
yellow (*Old Dutch*) ⅝-oz. bag .... | 6.0 | 1.0
yellow (*Old Dutch*), 1.1 oz., 2½ cups .... | 9.0 | 1.5

cheese:

(*Chester's*), 3 cups .... | 13.0 | 2.5
(*Tom's*), .75-oz. pkg. .... | 4.0 | 1.0
(*Tom's*), 1 oz. .... | 5.0 | 1.5

hot (*Chester's* Flamin' Hot), 3 cups .... | 9.0 | 1.5

microwave:

(*Chester's* Natural), 5 cups .... | 12.0 | 1.5
(*Jiffy Pop*), 3 cups .... | 10.0 | 1.5
(*Jiffy Pop* Lite), 3 cups .... | 5.0 | .5
(*Jolly Time* Natural), 4 cups .... | 10.0 | 2.0
(*Jolly Time* Light), 5 cups .... | 5.0 | 1.0

	total fat (grams)	saturated fat (grams)
(*Pop Weaver* Small Kernel), 3 tbsp. unpopped	1.5	0
(*Pop Weaver* Natural), ⅓ bag unpopped	7.0	1.5
(*Pop Weaver* Natural), 4 cups	6.0	1.5
(*Pop Weaver* Natural Light), ½ bag unpopped	3.5	.5
(*Pop Weaver* Natural Light), 6 cups	3.0	.5
(*Weight Watchers Smart Snackers*), 1 oz.	1.0	0
microwave, butter/butter flavor:		
(*America's Best*), 5 cups	2.5	.5
(*Betty Crocker*), 1 cup	2.5	0
(*Betty Crocker* Light), 1 cup	1.0	0
(*Chester's*), 5 cups	12.0	1.5
(*Jolly Time*), 4 cups	9.0	1.5
(*Jolly Time* Light), 5 cups	5.0	1.0
(*Pop Weaver* Butter), ⅓ bag unpopped	7.0	1.5
(*Pop Weaver* Butter), 4 cups	6.0	1.5
(*Pop Weaver* Butter Light), ½ bag unpopped	3.5	.5
(*Pop Weaver* Butter Light), 6 cups	3.0	.5
(*Pop Weaver* Extra Butter), ⅓ bag unpopped	11.0	2.0
(*Pop Weaver* Extra Butter), 3 cups	9.0	2.0
(*Pop Weaver* Extra Butter Light), ⅓ bag unpopped	5.0	1.0
(*Pop Weaver* Extra Butter Light), 4 cups	5.0	1.5
(*Pop Weaver* 96% Fat Free) 3 tbsp. unpopped, 3 cups popped	1.5	0
(*Schwan's*), 3 tbsp. unpopped	12.0	2.5
(*Schwan's* Light), 3 tbsp. unpopped	5.0	1.0
cheddar (*Jolly Time*), 3 cups	10.0	1.5
mix, triple (*Chester's*), 1½ cups	7.0	1.0
yellow (*Arrowhead Mills*), ¼ cup unpopped	2.5	0
Popcorn oil (*Planters*), 1 tbsp.	14.0	2.5
Popcorn seasoning, cheese (*Spice Islands*), ½ tsp.	0	0
Poppy seed pastry filling (*Solo*), 2 tbsp.	4.0	0
Poppy seeds:		
1 tbsp.	3.9	.4

	total fat (grams)	saturated fat (grams)

Poppy seeds *(cont.)*

1 tsp.	1.3	.1

Pork, fresh, 4 oz., except as noted:

leg, see "Ham"

loin, whole:

braised, lean and fat	31.6	11.4
braised, lean only	16.6	5.7
broiled, lean and fat	30.9	11.1
broiled, lean only	17.3	6.0
broiled, lean and fat, 1 chop, 2.9 oz. (3.7 oz. raw w/bone)	22.3	8.1
broiled, lean only, 1 chop, 2.3 oz. (3.7 oz. raw w/bone and fat)	10.1	3.5
roasted, lean and fat	27.5	10.0
roasted, lean only	15.8	5.4

loin, blade:

braised, lean and fat	38.7	13.9
braised, lean only	23.3	8.1
broiled, lean and fat	38.4	14.2
broiled, lean only	24.3	8.4
broiled, lean and fat, 1 chop, 2.1 oz. (3.7 oz. raw w/bone)	26.1	9.4
broiled, lean only, 1 chop, 2.1 oz. (3.7 oz. raw w/bone and fat)	12.7	4.4
roasted, lean and fat	34.5	12.4
roasted, lean only	21.9	7.5

loin, center:

braised, lean and fat	28.7	10.4
braised, lean only	15.5	5.4
broiled, lean and fat	25.1	9.1
broiled, lean only	11.9	4.1
broiled, lean and fat, 1 chop, 3.1 oz. (3.7 oz. raw w/bone)	19.2	7.0
broiled, lean only, 1 chop, 2.5 oz. (3.7 oz. raw w/bone and fat)	7.5	2.6

	total fat (grams)	saturated fat (grams)
roasted, lean and fat	24.7	8.9
roasted, lean only	14.8	5.1
loin, center rib:		
braised, lean and fat	30.8	11.1
braised, lean only	16.4	5.6
broiled, lean and fat	29.9	10.8
broiled, lean only	16.9	5.8
broiled, lean and fat, 1 chop, 2.7 oz. (3.7 oz. raw w/bone)	20.3	7.3
broiled, lean only, 1 chop, 2.2 oz. (3.7 oz. raw w/bone and fat)	9.4	3.2
roasted, lean and fat	26.8	9.7
roasted, lean only	15.6	5.4
loin, sirloin:		
braised, lean and fat	29.2	10.6
braised, lean only	14.8	5.1
broiled, lean and fat	28.6	10.4
broiled, lean only	15.4	5.3
broiled, lean and fat, 1 chop, 3 oz. (3.7 oz. raw w/bone)	21.2	7.7
broiled, lean only, 1 chop, 2.4 oz. (3.7 oz. raw w/bone and fat)	9.2	3.2
roasted, lean and fat	23.1	8.4
roasted, lean only	14.9	5.2
loin, top:		
braised, lean and fat	33.1	12.0
braised, lean only	16.4	5.6
broiled, lean and fat	32.5	11.7
broiled, lean only	16.9	5.8
broiled, lean and fat, 1 chop, 3 oz. (3.7 oz. raw w/bone)	23.5	8.5
broiled, lean only, 1 chop, 2.3 oz. (3.7 oz. raw w/bone and fat)	9.6	3.3
roasted, lean and fat	28.5	10.3

	total fat (grams)	saturated fat (grams)

Pork, loin, top *(cont.)*

roasted, lean only	15.6	5.4
shoulder, whole:		
roasted, lean and fat	29.1	10.5
roasted, lean only	17.0	5.9
shoulder, arm (picnic):		
braised, lean and fat	29.0	10.5
braised, lean only	13.8	4.8
roasted, lean and fat	29.6	10.7
roasted, lean only	14.3	4.9
shoulder, Boston blade:		
braised, lean and fat	32.5	11.7
braised, lean only	19.9	6.9
broiled, lean and fat	32.3	11.6
broiled, lean only	20.9	7.2
spareribs, braised, lean and fat, 6.3 oz. (1 lb. raw w/bone)	53.6	20.8
tenderloin, roasted, lean only	5.5	1.9
tenderloin, roasted, chopped or diced, 1 cup	6.7	2.3
Pork, canned, 4 oz.	34.4	12.4

Pork, cured, 4 oz.:

arm (picnic), roasted, lean and fat	24.2	8.7
arm (picnic), roasted, lean only	8.0	2.7
blade roll, unheated, lean and fat	24.8	9.2
blade roll, roasted, lean and fat	26.6	9.5

Pork, frozen or refrigerated:

(*Schwan's Haugin's Farm*), 2 oz.	2.0	.5
fritter (*Schwan's*), 2.7-oz. piece	10.0	5.0
loin chops (*Schwan's*), 4.2-oz. chop	5.0	1.5
loin roast (*Thorn Apple Valley*), 3 oz.	3.0	n.a.
shoulder, fresh (*Thorn Apple Valley*), 3 oz.	12.0	n.a.
shoulder butt, smoked (*Oscar Mayer Sweet Morsel*), 3 oz.	15.0	5.0
spareribs (*Schwan's*), 5 oz.	18.0	7.0
spareribs, barbecued (*Schwan's*), 6-oz. piece	28.0	9.0

	total fat (grams)	saturated fat (grams)
Pork backfat, raw, 1 oz.	25.1	9.1
Pork dinner, frozen:		
ribs, boneless (*Swanson's*), 10 oz.	23.0	8.0
ribs, boneless (*Swanson's Hungry-Man*),		
14.1 oz.	38.0	13.0
sweet and sour (*Chun King*), 13 oz.	6.0	2.5
Pork entree, freeze-dried, sweet and sour, w/rice		
(*Mountain-House*), 1 cup*	8.0	2.0
Pork entree, frozen, see "Pork, frozen or refrigerated"		
Pork fat, 1 oz.	17.5	6.4
Pork gravy, canned (*Swanson's*), ¼ cup	4.0	1.5
Pork gravy mix:		
¼ cup*	.5	.2
(*Durkee*), ¼ pkg.	0	0
(*French's*), ¼ pkg.	.5	0
Pork luncheon meat, see "Ham luncheon meat"		
Pork sandwich, frozen, barbecue (*Hormel Quick Meal*		
BBQ), 1 piece	15.0	6.0
Pork sausage, see "Sausage" and specific listings		
Pork seasoning mix:		
(*Durkee/French's* Roasting Bag), ⅙ pkg.	0	0
(*Shake 'N Bake* Original), ⅛ pkg.	0	0
barbecue (*Shake 'N Bake*), ⅛ pkg.	0	0
chop (*McCormick Bag'n Season*), ⅙ pkg.	0	0
crispy (*Oven Fry*), ⅛ pkg.	1.5	0
frying batter (*House of Tsang*), 4 tbsp.	4.0	0
hot and spicy (*Shake 'N Bake*), ⅛ pkg.	.5	0
Pot roast entree, see "Beef entree"		
Pot roast seasoning mix:		
(*Lawry's*), 1 tsp.	0	0
(*McCormick Bag'n Season*), ⅛ pkg.	0	0
regular or onion (*Durkee* Roasting Bag), ⅙ pkg.	0	0
regular or onion (*French's*), ⅙ pkg.	0	0

	total fat (grams)	saturated fat (grams)

Potato (see also "Sweet potato"):

raw, unpeeled, 1 lb.	.3	.1
raw, 1 medium 2½" diameter, 5.3 oz.	.1	<.1
baked or microwaved in skin, 7-oz. potato	.2	.1
baked, boiled, or microwaved in skin, pulp only, ½ cup	.1	<.1
baked in skin, skin from 7-oz. potato	.1	<.1
boiled, w/out skin, 1 potato or ½ cup	.1	<.1

Potato, canned:

w/liquid, 4 oz. or ½ cup drained	.2	<.1
(*Seneca*), ½ cup	0	0
all styles (*Allens/Butterfield*), 5.6 oz.	0	0
all styles (*Del Monte*), ½ cup	0	0
whole (*Stokely*), 5.5 oz.	0	0

Potato, freeze-dried*, mashed:

(*AlpineAire*), ¾ cup	.3	0
and cheddar, w/chives (*AlpineAire*), 1½ cups	7.0	n.a.
and gravy, w/turkey (*AlpineAire*), 1½ cups	1.0	n.a.

Potato, frozen (see also "Potato dishes, frozen"):

whole:

(*Stilwell*), 3 pieces	0	0
peeled, 10-oz. pkg.	.5	.1
boiled, drained, 4 oz.	.1	<.1

fried or french fried:

9-oz. pkg.	16.5	7.8
heated in oven, 10 strips, about 1.75 oz.	4.4	2.1
(*Empire* Kosher Crinkle Cut), ½ cup, 3 oz.	1.5	1.0
(*Ore-Ida* Cottage Fries) 3 oz., 14 pieces	4.0	1.0
(*Ore-Ida* Country Style *Dinner Fries*), 3 oz., 8 pieces	3.0	1.0
(*Ore-Ida* Crispier!), 3 oz., 17 pieces	13.0	2.0
(*Ore-Ida* Crispy Crunchies!), 3 oz., 12 pieces	9.0	1.5
(*Ore-Ida* Deep Fries Crinkle Cuts), 3 oz., 18 pieces	7.0	1.0

	total fat (grams)	saturated fat (grams)
(*Ore-Ida* Deep Fries French Fries), 3 oz., 22 pieces	7.0	1.0
(*Ore-Ida Fast Fries*), 3 oz., 23 pieces	6.0	2.0
(*Ore-Ida Golden Crinkles*), 3 oz., 16 pieces	3.5	1.0
(*Ore-Ida Golden Fries*), 3 oz. 16 pieces	4.0	.5
(*Ore-Ida Golden Twirls*), 3 oz., 28 pieces	7.0	1.0
(*Ore-Ida* Microwave Crinkle Cuts), 3.5-oz. pkg.	8.0	1.5
(*Ore-Ida* Nacho *Crispers!*), 3 oz., 10 pieces	9.0	3.0
(*Ore-Ida Pixie Crinkles*), 3 oz., 33 pieces	5.0	1.0
(*Ore-Ida Potato Wedges* w/Skin), 3 oz., 9 pieces	2.5	1.0
(*Ore-Ida* Shoestrings), 3 oz., 38 pieces	5.0	1.0
(*Ore-Ida* Texas *Crispers!*)	10.0	2.5
(*Ore-Ida Waffle Fries*), 3 oz., 15 pieces	5.0	1.5
(*Ore-Ida Zesties*), 3 oz., 12 pieces	9.0	1.5
(*Schwan's*), 3 oz.	5.0	1.5
(*Schwan's* Crinkle Cuts), 3 oz.	4.0	1.0
(*Schwan's* Seasoned Curls), 3 oz.	9.0	2.0
hash browns:		
12-oz. pkg.	2.1	.6
prepared in vegetable oil, ½ cup	13.0	5.1
(*Ore-Ida* Microwave), 1 patty	6.0	1.5
(*Ore-Ida* Shredded), 1 patty	0	0
(*Schwan's*), 1 patty	0	0
cheddar (*Ore-Ida Cheddar Browns!*), 1 patty	2.5	1.0
country style (*Ore-Ida*), 1 cup	0	0
Southern style (*Ore-Ida*), ¾ cup	0	0
toaster (*Ore-Ida*), 2 patties	12.0	2.0
mashed, natural butter flavor (*Ore-Ida*), ½ cup	2.0	.5
O'Briens (*Ore-Ida*), ¾ cup	0	0
patties (*Ore-Ida Golden Patties*), 1 patty	7.0	1.5
puffs:		
10-oz. pkg.	24.2	11.5
prepared in vegetable oil, 1 puff, about. 2 oz.	.8	.4
(*Ore-Ida Crispy Crowns!*), about 12 pieces	11.0	2.0

	total fat (grams)	saturated fat (grams)

Potato, frozen, puffs *(cont.)*

(*Ore-Ida Tater ABC's*), 3 oz., 10 pieces	11.0	.... 4.5
(*Ore-Ida Tater Tots*), 3 oz., 9 pieces	8.0	.... 1.5
(*Ore-Ida* Microwave *Tater Tots*), 3¾-oz. pkg. ..	10.0	.... 2.5
(*Schwan's Quik Taters*), 13 pieces, 3 oz.	8.0	.... 2.0
bacon or onion (*Ore-Ida Tater Tots*), 3 oz., 9 pieces	7.0	.... 1.5

Potato, mix (see also "Potato dishes, mix"):

au gratin (*Idahoan*), ⅓ cup	1.5	5
cheddar (*Betty Crocker* Homestyle Skin-On), 1 oz.	2.0	5
cheddar and bacon or tangy (*Pillsbury*), ½ cup* ..	6.0	.... 3.0
cheddar and sour cream (*Betty Crocker*), ⅔ cup	1.5	5
cheese, three (*Betty Crocker*), ½ cup	1.5	5
hash browns (*Idahoan Real*), 4 oz.*	10.0	.... 1.5
mashed:		
(*Barbara's*), 4 oz.	1.0	 0
(*Betty Crocker Potato Buds*), ⅓ cup	.5	 0
(*Hungry Jack* Flakes), ½ cup*	6.0	.... 1.0
(*Idahoan/Idahoan Real*), ⅓ cup	0	 0
(*Idahoan* Complete), ⅓ cup	2.0	5
(*Pillsbury Idaho* Granules), ½ cup*	5.0	 0
(*Pillsbury Spuds*), ½ cup*	6.0	.... <1.0
flakes, dry, ½ cup	.1	.... <.1
flakes, ½ cup*	5.9	.... .36
granules, w/milk, dry, ½ cup	1.1	5
granules, w/milk, ½ cup*	2.3	7
ranch (*Idahoan*), ¼ cup	2.0	.... 1.5
scalloped:		
(*Idahoan*), ⅓ cup	1.5	5
cheesy (*Betty Crocker* Homestyle Skin-On), 1 oz.	1.5	5
cheesy or creamy (*Pillsbury*), ½ cup*	6.0	.... 3.0
dry, 5½-oz. pkg.	7.2	.... 1.9

	total fat (grams)	saturated fat (grams)
ranch (*Idahoan*), ¼ cup	2.0	1.5
sour cream and chives (*Betty Crocker*), ½ cup	1.5	.5
sour cream and chives (*Pillsbury*), ½ cup*	6.0	4.0
Western (*Idahoan*), ¼ cup	1.0	0

Potato coating and seasoning mix:

	total fat (grams)	saturated fat (grams)
cheddar, crispy (*Shake 'N Bake Perfect Potatoes*), ⅙ pkg.	2.0	1.5
herb and garlic (*Shake 'N Bake Perfect Potatoes*), ⅙ pkg.	0	0

Potato, stuffed, see "Potato dishes, frozen"
Potato, sweet, see "Sweet potato"
Potato chips and crisps:

	total fat (grams)	saturated fat (grams)
1 oz.	10.1	2.6
(*Barbara's/Barbara's* Ripple), 1 oz., 1¼ cups	10.0	1.0
(*Cape Cod*), 1 oz., 19 pieces	8.0	2.0
(*Eagle* Ripples Natural), 1 oz., 17 pieces	10.0	2.5
(*Eagle* Thins), 1 oz., 20 pieces	10.0	2.5
(*Lay's* Original/Unsalted), 1 oz., 18 pieces	10.0	2.5
(*Lay's* Wavy Original), 1 oz., 11 pieces	10.0	2.5
(*Mr. Phipps* Original), 1 oz., 28 pieces	4.5	.5
(*Old Dutch*), 1.75-oz. bag	16.0	2.0
(*Old Dutch/Old Dutch Ripl*), 1 oz., 12–15 pieces	9.0	1.0
(*Old Dutch* Kettle Chips), 1.75-oz. bag	10.0	2.0
(*Old Dutch* Kettle Chips), 1 oz., 15–20 pieces	6.0	1.0
(*Old Dutch Ripl*), 1.75-oz. bag	15.0	2.0
(*Pringles* Original), 1 oz., 14 pieces	11.0	2.5
(*Pringles* Ridges), 1 oz., 12 pieces	10.0	2.5
(*Pringles* Right Crisps), 1 oz., 16 pieces	7.0	2.0
(*Ruffles* Choice), 1 oz., 16 pieces	6.0	1.0
(*Ruffles* Original), 1 oz., 12 pieces	10.0	3.0
(*Wise Ridgies*), 1 oz., 15 pieces	10.0	3.0
all varieties (*Lay's Crunch Tators*), 1 oz.	8.0	2.0
au gratin (*Barbara's*), 1 oz., 1 cup	10.0	1.5
au gratin (*Lay's* Wavy), 1 oz., 13 pieces	10.0	2.5

	total fat (grams)	saturated fat (grams)

Potato chips and crisps *(cont.)*

barbecue:

(*Barbara's*), 1 oz., 1¼ cups	10.0	1.0
(*Lay's*), 1 oz., 15 pieces	10.0	2.0
(*Lay's KC Masterpiece*), 1 oz., 15 pieces	9.0	2.5
(*Mr. Phipps*), 1 oz., 21 pieces	4.0	.5
(*Old Dutch*), 1.75-oz. bag	15.0	2.0
(*Old Dutch*), 1 oz., 12–15 pieces	9.0	1.0
mesquite (*Eagle* BBQ Ripples/Thins), 1 oz., 19 pieces	10.0	2.0
mesquite (*Old Dutch* BBQ Kettle Chips), 1.75-oz. bag	10.0	2.0
mesquite (*Old Dutch* BBQ Kettle Chips), 1 oz., 15–20 pieces	6.0	1.0

cheddar and sour cream:

(*Eagle* Ripples), 1 oz., 16 pieces	11.0	1.0
(*Old Dutch*), 1.75-oz. bag	17.0	2.5
(*Old Dutch*), 1-oz. bag	9.0	1.5
(*Pringles* Ridges), 1 oz., 12 pieces	10.0	2.5
(*Ruffles*), 1 oz., 13 pieces	10.0	2.5
(*Wise Ridgies*), 1 oz., 14 pieces	10.0	3.0
crispy cooked (*Eagle* Thins), 1 oz., 19 pieces	8.0	2.0
crunch, extra (*Eagle* Hawaiian Kettle), 1 oz., 19 pieces	8.0	2.0
dark and crunchy (*Eagle* Idaho Russet), 1 oz., 22 pieces	7.0	1.5
dill flavor (*Old Dutch*), 1.75-oz. bag	14.0	2.0
dill flavor (*Old Dutch*), 1 oz., 12–15 pieces	8.0	1.0
hot, Louisiana spicy, crispy cooked (*Eagle* Thins), 1 oz., 18 pieces	8.0	2.0

jalapeño and cheddar:

(*Old Dutch* Kettle Chips), 1.75-oz. bag	11.0	2.5
(*Old Dutch* Kettle Chips), 1 oz., 15–20 pieces	6.0	1.5
mesquite, see "barbecue," above		
mesquite grille (*Ruffles*), 1 oz., 15 pieces	9.0	3.0
onion and garlic flavor (*Old Dutch*), 1.75-oz. bag	14.0	2.0

	total fat (grams)	saturated fat (grams)
onion and garlic flavor (*Old Dutch*), 1 oz., 12–15 pieces	8.0	1.0
pizza, spicy (*Health Valley* Healthy Hot Potatoes), 1½ cups, 1.1 oz.	0	0
ranch (*Ruffles*), 1 oz., 13 pieces	9.0	2.5
ranch, tangy (*Lay's*), 1 oz., 17 pieces	9.0	2.5
salt and vinegar:		
(*Lay's*), 1 oz., 19 pieces	10.0	2.5
(*Old Dutch* Kettle Chips), 1.75-oz. bag	10.0	2.0
(*Old Dutch* Kettle Chips), 1 oz., 15–20 pieces	6.0	1.0
sea salt (*Cape Cod*), 1 oz., 18 pieces	8.0	2.0
sea salt (*Eagle* Ripples), 1 oz., 16 pieces	8.0	2.0
sour cream and onion:		
(*Eagle* Ripples), 1 oz., 16 pieces	10.0	2.0
(*Eagle* Thins), 1 oz., 19 pieces	10.0	2.0
(*Lay's*), 1 oz., 22 pieces	9.0	2.5
(*Mr. Phipp's*), 1 oz., 22 pieces	4.0	.5
(*Old Dutch*), 1.75-oz. bag	15.0	2.0
(*Old Dutch*), 1 oz., 12–15 pieces	9.0	1.0
(*Pringles*), 1 oz., 14 pieces	10.0	2.5
(*Ruffles*), 1 oz., 13 pieces	10.0	3.0
(*Wise Ridgies*), 1 oz., 13 pieces	10.0	3.0
spicy (*Eagle* Fiesta Thins), 1 oz., 10 pieces	9.0	2.5
sweet potato (*Barbara's*), 1 oz., 1 cup	8.0	1.0
yogurt and green onion (*Barbara's*), 1 oz., 1¼ cups	9.0	1.0
Potato dishes, canned or packaged:		
au gratin (*Green Giant Pantry Express*), ½ cup	5.0	2.0
au gratin, and bacon (*Hormel*), 7.5-oz. can	14.0	5.0
scalloped, and ham (*Hormel*), 7.5-oz. can	16.0	5.0
scalloped, w/ham (*Nalley*), 7.5 oz.	7.0	3.0
sliced, and beef (*Hormel*), 7.5-oz. can	9.0	4.0
Potato dishes, frozen (see also "Potato, frozen"):		
au gratin (*Stouffer's* Side Dish), ½ cup	6.0	2.5

	total fat (grams)	saturated fat (grams)

Potato dishes, frozen *(cont.)*

broccoli w/cheese (*Green Giant* One Serving),
5.5 oz. .... 4.0 .... 2.0

baked, broccoli and cheese:

   (*The Budget Gourmet* Light & Healthy Entree),
10.5 oz. .... 8.0 .... 5.0

   (*Ore-Ida* Twice Baked), ½ pkg. .... 4.0 .... 1.5

   (*Lean Cuisine Lunch Express*), 10¼ oz. ...... 9.0 .... 4.0

   (*Weight Watchers Smart Ones*), 10 oz. .... 7.0 .... 2.0

   cheddar, deluxe (*Lean Cuisine* Entree),
10⅜ oz. .... 10.0 .... 3.5

   wedges (*Healthy Choice*), 9.5 oz. .... 5.0 .... 2.0

baked, butter flavor (*Ore-Ida* Twice Baked),
½ pkg. .... 9.0 .... 3.0

baked, cheddar (*Ore-Ida* Twice Baked), ½ pkg. ... 8.0 .... 2.5

baked, ranch (*Ore-Ida* Twice Baked), ½ pkg. ...... 6.0 .... 2.0

baked, salsa and cheese (*Ore-Ida* Twice Baked),
½ pkg. .... 4.5 .... 1.5

baked, sour cream and chives (*Ore-Ida* Twice
Baked), ½ pkg. .... 6.0 .... 1.5

casserole, garden (*Healthy Choice Quick Meal*),
9.25 oz. .... 4.0 .... 2.0

cheddared (*The Budget Gourmet* Side Dish),
5.5 oz. .... 17.0 .... 9.0

cheddared, and broccoli (*The Budget Gourmet* Side
Dish), 5.25 oz. .... 8.0 .... 6.0

cheese, three (*The Budget Gourmet* Side Dish),
6.125 oz. .... 12.0 .... 7.0

scalloped (*Stouffer's* Side Dish), ½ cup .... 6.0 .... 1.0

scalloped, w/ham (*Swanson's*), 9 oz. .... 12.0 .... 8.0

Potato flour, 1 cup 1.4 4

Potato pancake, frozen:

(*Empire* Kosher Latkes), 2-oz. cake .... 2.0 .... 1.5

mini (*Empire* Kosher Latkes), 2 pieces, 2 oz. ...... 2.5 .... 1.0

	total fat (grams)	saturated fat (grams)
Potato pancake mix:		
(*Knorr*), ¼ pkg.	.5	0
(*Pillsbury*), 3 cakes, 3" each	2.0	0
Potato sticks:		
1 oz.	9.8	2.5
(*Allens/Butterfield*), ⅔ cup	9.0	3.0
(*Planters*), 1 oz.	16.0	2.5
barbecue (*Planters*), 1 oz.	18.0	5.5
Poultry, see specific listings		
Poultry salad spread, chicken and turkey, 1 tbsp.	1.8	.5
Poultry seasoning, 1 tbsp.	.3	n.a.
Pout, ocean, meat only:		
raw, 4 oz.	1.0	.4
baked, broiled, or microwaved, 4 oz.	1.3	.5
Pretzel (see also "Cracker"):		
all varieties:		
(*Mister Pretzel* Fat Free), 1 oz.	0	0
(*Mr. Phipp's* Fat Free), 1 oz.	0	0
(*Rold Gold* Fat Free), 1 oz.	0	0
Bavarian:		
(*Rold Gold*), 1 oz., 3 pieces	2.0	.5
(*Barbara's*), 1 oz., 2 pieces	1.5	0
hard, sourdough (*Eagle* No Fat), 1 oz., 2 pieces	0	0
bits, garlic or honey-mustard (*Rold Gold*), 1 oz., 11 pieces	8.0	1.0
cheddar cheese (*Combos*), 1.8-oz. bag	9.0	1.5
cheddar cheese (*Combos*), 1 oz.	5.0	1.0
chips:		
(*Mr. Phipp's* Original/Lower Sodium), 1 oz., 16 pieces	2.5	0
(*Rold Gold* Original), 1 oz., 10 pieces	1.0	0
cheese (*Rold Gold*), 1 oz., 9 pieces	2.5	.5
Dutch (*Mister Salty*), 1.1 oz., 2 pieces	1.0	0
hard, sourdough (*Rold Gold*), 1-oz. piece	1.5	0

	total fat (grams)	saturated fat (grams)

Pretzel *(cont.)*

honeysweet (*Barbara's*), 1 oz., 2 pieces	1.0	0
grain, nine (*Barbara's*), 1 oz., 2 pieces	1.5	0
mini (*Barbara's*), 1 oz., 18 pieces	1.5	0
mini (*Mister Pretzel*), 1 oz., about 22 pieces	1.0	0
mini bites (*Eagle*), 1 oz., ¾ cup	1.0	0
multigrain (*Cape Cod* No Fat), 1.1 oz., 30 pieces	0	0
mustard (*Combos*), 1.8-oz. bag	8.0	1.0
mustard (*Combos*), 1 oz.	4.0	.5
nacho cheese (*Combos*), 1.7-oz. bag	8.0	1.5
nacho cheese (*Combos*), 1 oz.	5.0	.5
oat bran (*Weight Watchers Smart Snackers*), 1.5 oz.	2.5	0
sourdough (*Tom's*), 1 oz.	0	0
pizzeria (*Combos*), 1.8-oz. bag	8.0	1.5
pizzeria (*Combos*), 1 oz.	4.0	.5
rods (*Rold Gold*), 1 oz., 3 pieces	1.5	.5
(*Pepperidge Farm Goldfish*), 1.1 oz., 45 pieces	2.5	.5
(*Pepperidge Farm* Snack Sticks), 1.1 oz., 9 pieces	3.0	0
soft:		
(*J&J Superpretzel*), 1 piece	0	0
bites (*J&J Superpretzel*), 5 pieces	0	0
sticks, all varieties (*J&J Superpretzel*), 2 pieces	2.0	1.0
sticks:		
(*Bachman*), 1 oz.	1.0	0
(*Eagle*), 1 oz., 46 pieces	1.0	0
(*Rold Gold*), 1 oz., 48 pieces	1.0	0
(*Tom's*), 1 oz.	0	0
(*Sunshine* California), 1 oz.	1.5	0
twists:		
(*Planters*), 1 oz.	.5	0
mini (*Tom's*), 1 oz.	1.0	0
large (*Tom's*), 1 oz.	1.0	0
thin (*Eagle*), 1 oz., 10 pieces	1.0	0

	total fat (grams)	saturated fat (grams)
thin (*Eagle* No Fat), 1 oz., 10 pieces	0	0
thin (*Rold Gold*), 1 oz., 10 pieces	1.0	0
thiy (*Rold Gold*), 1 oz., 18 pieces	1.0	0
Prickly pear:		
untrimmed, 1 lb.	1.7	n.a.
1 medium, about 4.8 oz.	.5	n.a.
Prosciutto (*Hormel Primissimo*), 1 oz.	4.5	1.5
Protein shake, all flavors (*Naturade*), 1 oz.	0	0
Prune:		
canned, pitted (*Sonoma*), 1.4 oz., 3–4 pieces	0	0
dehydrated, 4 oz.	.8	.1
dehydrated, cooked, ½ cup	.3	<.1
dried:		
w/pits, ½ cup	.4	<.1
pitted, 10 prunes, about 3 oz.	.4	<.1
(*Del Monte*), ¼ cup	0	0
(*Dole*), 2 oz.	1.0	n.a.
(*Sonoma*), 1.4 oz., ¼ cup	0	0
(*Sunsweet*), 2 oz.	.2	0
cooked, w/pits, ½ cup	.2	<.1
Prune juice, canned or bottled:		
6 fl. oz.	.1	<.1
(*Del Monte*), 8 fl. oz.	0	0
(*R.W. Knudsen* Organic), 8 fl. oz.	0	0
Prune-plum pastry filling (*Solo* Lekvar), 2 tbsp.	0	0
Pudding, ready-to-eat:		
all varieties (*Jell-O* Fat Free Snacks), 4 oz.	0	0
almond or almond-cinnamon (*Amazake*), 6 oz. ...	3.5	n.a.
banana:		
(*Del Monte*), 4-oz. cup	4.0	1.0
(*Jell-O* Snacks), 4 oz.	7.0	2.0
(*Thank You*), ½ cup	4.0	2.0
butterscotch:		
(*Del Monte*), 4-oz. cup	4.0	1.0
(*Rich's*), 3-oz. container	6.0	6.0

	total fat (grams)	saturated fat (grams)

Pudding, butterscotch *(cont.)*

| (*Thank You*), ½ cup | 5.0 | 2.0 |

chocolate:

(*Amazake*), 6 oz.	1.0	n.a.
(*Del Monte*), 4-oz. cup	4.0	1.0
(*Del Monte* Lite), 4-oz. cup	1.0	0
(*Jell-O* Snacks), 4 oz.	5.0	2.0
(*Rich's*), 3-oz. container	7.0	6.0
(*Thank You*), ½ cup	5.0	2.0

chocolate caramel or vanilla swirl (*Jell-O* Snacks), 4 oz.	5.0	2.0
chocolate fudge (*Del Monte*), 4-oz. cup	4.0	1.0
chocolate fudge (*Thank You*), ½ cup	5.0	2.5
lemon (*Amazake*), 6 oz.	0	0
lemon (*Thank You*), ½ cup	2.0	0
rice (*Thank You*), ½ cup	3.0	2.0

tapioca:

(*Del Monte*), 4-oz. cup	4.0	1.0
(*Jell-O* Snacks), 4 oz.	4.0	1.5
(*Thank You*), ½ cup	4.0	2.0

vanilla:

(*Del Monte*), 4-oz. cup	4.0	1.0
(*Del Monte* Lite), 4-oz. cup	1.0	0
(*Jell-O* Snacks), 4 oz.	5.0	2.0
(*Rich's*), 3-oz. container	6.0	6.0
(*Thank You*), ½ cup	5.0	2.0
vanilla-chocolate swirl (*Jell-O* Snacks), 4 oz.	5.0	2.0

Pudding mix, ½ cup*, except as noted:

all varieties (*Jell-O* Fat /Sugar Free Instant)	0	0
banana cream (*Jell-O* Cook & Serve/Instant)	2.5	1.5
butter pecan (*Jell-O* Instant)	3.0	1.5
butterscotch (*Jell-O* Cook & Serve/Instant)	2.5	1.5

chocolate:

| (*D-Zerta*) | 0 | 0 |
| (*Jell-O* Cook & Serve/Instant) | 2.5 | 1.5 |

	total fat (grams)	saturated fat (grams)
milk (*Jell-O* Cook & Serve)	2.5	1.5
milk (*Jell-O* Instant)	3.0	2.0
chocolate fudge (*Jell-O* Cook & Serve)	2.5	1.5
chocolate fudge (*Jell-O* Instant)	3.0	1.5
chocolate or vanilla (*Jell-O* Sugar Free Cook & Serve)	2.5	1.5
coconut cream (*Jell-O* Cook & Serve)	5.0	4.0
coconut cream (*Jell-O* Instant)	4.5	3.5
creme caramel/flan (*Alsa*), ¼ pkg. mix	0	0
custard (*Jell-O* Americana)	2.5	1.5
flan (*Jell-O* Cook & Serve)	2.5	1.5
lemon:		
(*Durkee* Famous), 1 tbsp. mix	0	0
(*Jell-O* Cook & Serve)	2.0	.5
(*Jell-O* Instant)	2.5	1.5
mousse, dark or milk chocolate (*Alsa*), ¼ pkg. mix	4.0	4.0
mousse, white chocolate (*Alsa*), ¼ pkg. mix	3.5	3.0
pistachio (*Jell-O* Instant)	3.0	1.5
rice:		
(*Jell-O* Americana)	2.5	1.5
cinnamon raisin (*Lundberg Family Farms*)	0	0
coconut (*Lundberg Family Farms*)	2.0	1.5
honey almond (*Lundberg Family Farms*)	.5	0
tapioca (*Jell-O* Americana)	2.5	1.5
vanilla (*Jell-O* Cook & Serve)	2.5	1.5
vanilla or French vanilla (*Jell-O* Instant)	2.5	1.5
Puff pastry, see "Pastry shell"		
Pummelo:		
untrimmed, 1 lb.	.1	0
1 medium, about 2.5 lbs.	.2	<.1
Pumpkin:		
fresh:		
raw, untrimmed, 1 lb.	.3	.2
raw, 1" cubes, ½ cup	.1	<.1

	total fat (grams)	saturated fat (grams)

Pumpkin, fresh *(cont.)*

    boiled, drained, mashed, ½ cup .... .1 .... <.1

    canned:

      w/ or w/out winter squash, ½ cup 3 2

      (*Comstock*), ⅓ cup 0 0

      (*Libby's* Solid Pack), ½ cup 5 0

      (*Stokely*), ½ cup 0 0

      pie mix (*Libby's*), ½ cup 0 0

      pie mix (*Stokely*), ½ cup 0 0

Pumpkin butter (*Smucker's* Autumn Harvest),

    1 tbsp. 0 0

Pumpkin flower:

    raw, untrimmed, 1 lb. 7 4

    boiled, drained, ½ cup .... .1 .... <.1

Pumpkin leaf:

    raw, untrimmed, 1 lb. 7 4

    boiled, drained, ½ cup .... .1 .... <.1

Pumpkin pie, see "Pie"

Pumpkin pie filling, see "Pie filling" and

    "Pumpkin, canned"

Pumpkin pie spice, 1 tbsp. .... .7 .... n.a.

Pumpkin seed oil (*Hain*), 1 capsule 1.0 0

Pumpkin seeds, shelled, except as noted:

    roasted:

      in shell, 1 oz., about 85 seeds .... 5.5 .... 1.0

      in shell, 1 cup .... 12.4 .... 2.3

      1 oz. .... 12.0 .... 2.2

      1 cup .... 95.6 .... 18.1

      (*Eden*), 1 oz. .... 11.0 .... 2.5

    dried:

      in shell, 4 oz. .... 38.5 .... 7.3

      1 oz., about 142 kernels .... 13.0 .... 2.5

      1 cup .... 63.3 .... 12.0

Pumpkinseed fish, see "Sunfish"

	total fat (grams)	saturated fat (grams)
Purslane:		
raw, untrimmed, 1 lb.	.3	0
trimmed, 1 oz.	<.1	0
boiled, drained, ½ cup	.1	0

Q

	total fat (grams)	saturated fat (grams)
Quail, raw:		
meat w/skin, 1 bird, 3.8 oz. (4.3 oz. w/bone)	13.1	.... 3.7
meat only, 1 bird, 3.2 oz. (4.3 oz. w/bone and		
skin)	4.2	.... 1.2
meat only, 1 breast, about 2 oz.	1.8	5
Quiche, frozen, ⅙ carton:		
bacon and onion (*Stilwell Pour-A-Quiche*)	16.0	.... 12.0
broccoli and cheddar (*Stilwell Pour-A-Quiche*)	14.0	.... 8.0
cheese, three (*Stilwell Pour-A-Quiche*)	16.0	.... 12.0
ham (*Stilwell Pour-A-Quiche*)	15.0	.... 11.0
spinach and onion (*Stilwell Pour-A-Quiche*) :.....	13.0	.... 10.0
Quince:		
untrimmed, 1 lb.	.3	.... <.1
1 medium, about 5.3 oz.	.1	.... tr.
Quincy's, 1 serving:		
breakfast:		
apples, escalloped	2.0	 0
bacon	3.0	.... 1.0
beef hash, corned	15.0	.... 8.0
eggs, scrambled	7.0	.... 2.0
ham, country	6.0	.... 2.0

	total fat (grams)	saturated fat (grams)
oatmeal	2.0	0
pancakes, plain	3.0	1.0
pancakes, with syrup	3.0	1.0
sausage gravy	6.0	2.0
sausage links	22.0	8.0
sausage patties	23.0	9.0
steak fingers	25.0	11.0
entrees (entree only):		
chicken, grilled, 4.8 oz.	2.0	<1.0
chicken, grilled, 9.5 oz.	3.0	2.0
chicken, fillet, homestyle	24.0	6.0
chicken sandwich, grilled	5.0	2.0
hamburger, quarter-pound	20.0	9.0
prime rib, 8 oz.	46.0	18.0
prime rib, 16 oz.	93.0	36.0
steak:		
chopped	34.0	13.0
country style	29.0	15.0
sandwich, country style	29.0	15.0
fillet	12.0	5.0
ribeye, 7.3 oz.	60.0	24.0
ribeye, 9.5 oz.	78.0	31.0
sirloin, petite, 4 oz.	37.0	15.0
sirloin, regular, 5.8 oz.	54.0	21.0
sirloin, large, 7.8 oz.	70.0	27.0
sirloin tips	9.0	4.0
sizzlin' strip	37.0	15.0
t-bone	170.0	88.0
stir-fries:		
beef	77.0	14.0
chicken	66.0	11.0
rice pilaf	2.0	0
trout, grilled	12.0	3.0
side dishes:		
baked potato	0	0

	total fat (grams)	saturated fat (grams)

Quincy's, side dishes *(cont.)*

blackeyed peas	1.0	0
broccoli, plain	1.0	0
broccoli, w/ cheese sauce	13.0	5.0
broccoli and rice casserole	5.0	3.0
cabbage, steamed	5.0	1.0
candied yams	10.0	2.0
carrots, steamed	4.0	1.0
corn, on cob	1.0	0
corn, whole kernel	6.0	1.0
green beans	1.0	0
green peas	3.0	1.0
hash rounds	14.0	3.0
macaroni and cheese	9.0	2.0
mashed potatoes	1.0	0
mushrooms	12.0	2.0
new potatoes	11.0	2.0
pinto beans	0	0
refried beans	7.0	1.0
squash	10.0	2.0
turnip greens	6.0	1.0
vegetable medley	1.0	0

soups:

chili w/ beans	11.0	2.0
clam chowder	9.0	1.0
cream of broccoli	10.0	1.0
vegetable beef	2.0	1.0

desserts and breads:

banana nut bread	7.0	1.0
banana pudding	12.0	9.0
biscuit	15.0	4.0
brownie pudding cake	5.0	1.0
chocolate chip cookie	8.0	<1.0
cobbler, apple, cherry, or peach	8.0	2.0
cornbread	5.0	1.0

	total fat (grams)	saturated fat (grams)
frozen yogurt	2.0	1.0
hot toppings:		
caramel	1.0	<1.0
fudge	4.0	1.0
pineapple	0	0
sugar cookie	3.0	1.0
yeast roll	4.0	<1.0
Quinoa, dry:		
1 cup	9.9	1.0
(*Arrowhead Mills*), ¼ cup	2.0	0
(*Eden*), ¼ cup	2.5	0

R

	total fat (grams)	saturated fat (grams)
Rabbit, domesticated, meat only:		
roasted, 11 oz. (1 lb. raw boneless)	25.2	7.5
roasted, 4 oz.	9.1	2.7
stewed, 10.5 oz. (1 lb. boneless)	25.2	7.5
stewed, 4 oz.	9.5	2.8
stewed, diced, 1 cup	11.8	3.5
Rabbit, wild, meat only:		
stewed, 10.5 (1 lb. raw boneless)	10.5	3.1
stewed, 4 oz.	4.0	1.2
stewed, diced, 1 cup	4.9	1.5
Raccoon, meat only:		
roasted, 14 oz. (l lb. raw boneless)	57.9	n.a.
roasted, 4 oz.	16.4	n.a.
Radish:		
untrimmed, 1 lb.	2.2	.1
10 medium, 1.8 oz.	.2	<.1
sliced, ½ cup	.3	<.1
Radish, black, trimmed, 1 oz.	<.1	0
Radish, Oriental:		
raw, untrimmed, 1 lb.	.4	.1
raw, sliced, ½ cup	<.1	<.1

	total fat (grams)	saturated fat (grams)
boiled, drained, sliced, ½ cup	.2	.1
Radish, white icicle:		
untrimmed, 1 lb.	.3	.1
sliced, ½ cup	.1	<.1
Radish seeds, sprouted:		
½ cup	.5	.1
(*Jonathan's Sprouts*), 1 cup. 3 oz.	2.0	0
alfalfa sprouts with, see "Alfalfa sprouts"		
Rainbow baking morsels (*Nestlé*), 1 tbsp.	3.0	2.0
Raisin:		
w/seeds, seedless, or golden, 1 oz.	.1	<.1
w/seeds, seedless, or golden, ½ cup not packed	.3	.1
(*Dole*), ½ cup	0	0
(*Sun-Maid*), 2 oz.	.2	0
natural (*Del Monte*), 1.5 oz. box	.5	0
natural or golden (*Del Monte*), ¼ cup	0	0
Thompson/monukka (*Sonoma*), 1.4 oz., ¼ cup	0	0
Raisin, chocolate or yogurt coated, see "Candy"		
Raisin sauce (*Chelten House*), 2 tbsp.	0	0
Ranch dip:		
(*Heluva* Good Classic), 2 tbsp.	5.0	3.0
(*Kraft* Premium), 2 tbsp.	4.0	3.0
(*Nalley*), 2 tbsp.	11.0	2.0
creamy (*Keebler Chip Chasers*)	5.0	3.0
yogurt (*Crowley's* Cool), 2 tbsp.	2.0	1.5
Ranch dip mix, cracked pepper (*Knorr*), ¹⁄₂₀ pkg.	0	0
Ranchero beans, see "Mexican beans"		
Ranchero sandwich, frozen:		
(*Schwan's*), 5.5-oz. piece	18.0	8.0
Raspberry:		
fresh, untrimmed, 1 pint, 11.5 oz.	1.7	.1
fresh, trimmed, ½ cup	.3	<.1
canned, in syrup, ½ cup	.2	tr.
canned, in syrup (*Wilderness*), ½ cup	0	0
frozen, sweetened, 10-oz. pkg.	.5	<.1

	total fat (grams)	saturated fat (grams)
Raspberry *(cont.)*		
frozen, sweetened, ½ cup	.2	tr.
Raspberry pastry filling, red (*Solo*), 2 tbsp.	0	0
Raspberry juice or drink, all blends, all brands,		
8 fl. oz.	0	0
Raspberry nectar (*R. W. Knudsen*), 8 fl. oz.	0	0
Raspberry-peach juice (*R. W. Knudsen*), 8 fl. oz.	0	0
Raspberry-tamarind dipping sauce (*Helen's Tropical*		
Exotics), 2 tbsp.	1.0	0
Ravioli, canned or packaged:		
beef:		
(*Chef Boyardee* Suprema), 10.5-oz. bowl	5.0	2.0
(*Franco American Garfield*), 1 cup	10.0	4.0
(*Hormel Micro Cup*), 7.5 oz.	11.0	4.0
(*Libby's Diner*), 7.75 oz.	9.0	3.5
(*Nalley*), 7.5 oz. cup	9.0	4.0
(*Progresso*), 1 cup	5.0	2.0
cheese:		
(*Chef Boyardee* Suprema), 7.5-oz. cup	3.0	1.5
(*Nalley*), 7.5 oz. cup	10.0	5.0
(*Progresso*), 1 cup	2.0	1.0
mini (*Hormel Kid's Kitchen*), 7.5 oz.	6.0	3.0
Ravioli entree, frozen:		
(*Celentano*), 6.5 oz., 6 pieces	9.0	5.0
(*Celentano* Mini), 4 oz., 12 pieces	6.0	3.0
(*Celentano* Great Choice), 6.5 oz., 6 pieces	4.0	2.0
(*Celentano* Value Pack), 6.5 oz., 6 pieces	9.0	5.0
baked (*Healthy Choice*), 9 oz.	2.0	1.0
beef (*Stouffer's* Entree), 9.5 oz.	14.0	4.0
cheese:		
(*The Budget Gourmet*), 9.5 oz.	13.0	9.0
(*Lean Cuisine*), 8.5 oz.	7.0	3.0
(*Schwan's*), 5.5 oz., 5 pieces	13.0	7.0
(*Stouffer's Lunch Express*), 8.5 oz.	14.0	5.0
(*Swanson's Fun Feast*), 11 oz.	11.0	5.0

	total fat (grams)	saturated fat (grams)
mini (*Celentano* Round), 4 oz., 12 pieces	6.0	3.0
mini (*Kid Cuisine*), 9.52 oz.	4.0	1.0
w/tomato sauce (*Stouffer's* Entree), 9.5 oz.	14.0	5.0
chicken (*Schwan's*), 5.5 oz., 5 pieces	11.0	5.0
Florentine (*Weight Watchers Smart Ones*), 8.5 oz.	2.0	.5
Rax, 1 serving:		
sandwiches:		
barbecued beef	19.5	n.a.
barbecued beef, w/out mayo or oil	10.3	n.a.
BBC (beef, bacon, and cheddar)	50.9	n.a.
cheddar melt	22.6	n.a.
cheddar melt, w/out mayo or oil	15.6	n.a.
deluxe	34.6	n.a.
deluxe, w/out mayo or oil	13.2	n.a.
deluxe, Jr.	24.8	n.a.
deluxe Jr., w/out mayo or oil	8.1	n.a.
grilled chicken	33.4	n.a.
grilled chicken, w/out mayo or oil	6.8	n.a.
mushroom melt	37.4	n.a.
Philly melt	31.9	n.a.
regular *Rax*	21.9	n.a.
regular *Rax*, w/out mayo or oil	12.7	n.a.
turkey	31.7	n.a.
turkey, w/out mayo or oil	4.2	n.a.
turkey bacon club	46.5	n.a.
potatoes:		
plain	0	0
butter	11.3	n.a.
cheese	.2	n.a.
cheese/bacon	18.5	n.a.
cheese/broccoli	.2	n.a.
sour topping	4.0	n.a.
soups:		
chicken noodle	1.2	n.a.

	total fat (grams)	saturated fat (grams)

Rax, soups *(cont.)*

chili	9.4	n.a.
cream broccoli	3.8	n.a.

salad:

chicken Caesar, grilled	5.0	n.a.
gourmet garden	9.0	n.a.
side, Caesar	2.0	n.a.
side, regular	4.0	n.a.

salad dressings:

blue cheese	16.0	n.a.
buttermilk ranch	20.0	n.a.
Catalina, Italian or ranch, fat free	0	0
creamy Caesar	15.0	n.a.
honey French	5.0	n.a.
1000 Island	13.0	n.a.
vinaigrette	2.0	n.a.

shakes, chocolate, strawberry, or vanilla yogurt	.5	n.a.

Red beans (see also "Kidney beans" and "Mexican beans"), canned ½ cup:

(*Allens*)	.5	0
(*Green Giant/Joan of Arc*)	.5	0
Mexican style (*Stokely*)	.5	0

Red snapper, see "Snapper"

Redfish, see "Ocean perch"

Refried beans, canned, ½ cup, except as noted:

(*Allens*)	2.5	1.0
(*Chi-Chi's*)	6.0	1.0
(*Las Palmas*)	2.0	1.0
(*Las Palmas* No Fat)	0	0
(*Old El Paso*)	2.0	1.0
(*Old El Paso* Fat Free)	0	0
(*Taco Bell*), ⅓ cup	2.5	.5
black beans (*Las Palmas*)	2.0	0
black beans (*Old El Paso*)	2.0	0
and cheese (*Old El Paso*)	3.5	1.5

	total fat (grams)	saturated fat (grams)
w/green chilies (*Old El Paso*)	.5	0
w/sausage (*Old El Paso*), ¼ cup	13.0	5.0
spicy (*Old El Paso*)	3.0	1.5
vegetarian:		
(*Hain*)	1.0	n.a.
(*Hain* Fat Free)	0	0
(*Old El Paso*)	1.0	0
Refried beans, mix, instant (*Fantastic Foods International*), ⅓ cup	.5	0
Relish, pickle (see also specific listings):		
all varieties (*Del Monte*), 1 tbsp.	0	0
dill, chunky (*Nalley*), 1 tbsp.	0	0
hamburger and hotdog (*Nalley*), 1 tbsp.	0	0
piccalilli, sweet or corn (*Pickle Eater's*), 1 tbsp.	0	0
red hot (*Ron's*), 1 tbsp.	0	0
sweet:		
¼ cup	.4	0
1 tbsp.	.1	0
(*Hebrew National*), 1 tbsp.	0	0
(*Nalley*), 1 tbsp.	0	0
pickle (*Claussen*), 1 tbsp.	0	0
Rhubarb:		
fresh, untrimmed, 1 lb.	.7	n.a.
fresh, diced, ½ cup	.1	0
frozen (*Stilwell*), 1 cup	.5	0
Rice, plain, uncooked (see also "Rice glutinous," "Rice blends," and "Rice dishes, mix"), ¼ cup uncooked, except as noted:		
(*Minute* Original), ½ cup	0	0
arborio (*Fantastic Foods*)	0	0
basmati:		
(*Casbah*), 2 oz., 1 cup*	.1	0
(*Fantastic Foods*)	0	0
brown (*Fantastic Foods*)	2.0	0
brown (*Lundberg Family Farms* Organic)	1.5	0

	total fat (grams)	saturated fat (grams)

Rice, basmati *(cont.)*

brown (*Lundberg Family Farms* Premium)	2.0	0
brown, regular or Indian (*Arrowhead Mills*) ...	1.0	0
white (*Lundberg Family Farms* Organic)	.5	0
white (*Lundberg Family Farms* Premium)	.5	0
white, regular or Indian (*Arrowhead Mills*)	0	0

brown:

all grains and quick (*Arrowhead Mills*)	1.0	0
flour (*Lundberg Family Farms* Organic/ Premium)	1.5	0
long grain	1.4	.3
long grain (*Carolina*)	1.0	0
long grain (*Mahatma*)	1.0	0
medium grain	1.3	.3
instant or precooked (*Uncle Ben's*), ½ cup ...	1.5	0
parboiled (*Uncle Ben's*)	1.5	0
sweet (*Lundberg Family Farms*)	1.5	0
sweet (*Lundberg Family Farms* Organic)	1.0	0
quick (*Lundberg Family Farms*)	1.0	0
whole grain (*River*)	1.0	0
whole grain, instant (*Minute*), ½ cup	1.5	0
jasmine (*Fantastic Foods*)	0	0
jasmine, brown (*Fantastic Foods*)	2.0	0

white, long grain:

regular or parboiled	.3	.1
(*Carolina*)	1.0	0
(*Lundberg Family Farms* Organic)	2.0	0
(*Mahatma*)	0	0
(*Minute* Premium), ½ cup	0	0
instant (*Minute* Boil-in-Bag), ½ bag	0	0
instant (*Uncle Ben's*), ½ cup	.5	0
organic (*Lundberg Family Farms*)	1.5	0
parboiled (*Uncle Ben's Converted*)	0	0
precooked	<.1	tr.

	total fat (grams)	saturated fat (grams)
precooked (*Uncle Ben's Converted* Boil-in-Bag), ⅓ cup	.5	0
precooked (*Uncle Ben's Converted* Fast Cook), ½ cup	.5	0
w/wild rice (*Minute*), ⅓ box	.5	0
white, medium or short grain	.3	<.1
white, short-grain, (*Lundberg Family Farms* Organic)	1.5	0
white, sushi (*Lundberg Family Farms* Organic)	0	0
white, whole grain (*River*)	0	0
Rice, freeze-dried*, brown (*AlpineAire*), ½ cup	.4	0
Rice, glutinous:		
raw, ¼ cup	.3	.1
cooked, plain, 1 cup	.5	.1
Rice, wild, see "Wild rice"		
Rice beverage ("milk"), 8 fl. oz.:		
all varieties, except apricot, mocha Java, or original (*Amazake*)	4.0	.5
(*Amazake* Original)	0	0
(*EdenRice*)	3.0	.5
(*Rice Dream/Rice Dream Lite*)	2.0	n.a.
apricot (*Amazake*)	0	0
carob (*Rice Dream*)	3.0	n.a.
chocolate (*Rice Dream*)	3.0	n.a.
chocolate, enriched (*Rice Dream*)	2.5	0
mocha Java (*Amazake*)	2.0	0
rice and soy (*EdenRice*)	3.0	.5
vanilla lite or vanilla enriched (*Rice Dream*)	2.0	0
Rice blends, uncooked, ¼ cup:		
(*Lundberg Family Farms* Countrywild)	1.5	0
(*Lundberg Family Farms* Jubilee)	1.5	0
(*Lundberg Family Farms* Richvale Red)	1.5	0
black japonica (*Lundberg Family Farms*)	2.0	0
multigrain (*Uncle Ben's* Specialty Blends)	1.0	0
organic (*Lundberg Family Farms* Golden Rose)	1.0	0

	total fat (grams)	saturated fat (grams)
Rice blends *(cont.)*		
pilaf (*Uncle Ben's* Specialty Blends)	.5	0
rice trio (*Uncle Ben's* Specialty Blends)	1.0	0
Wehani (*Lundberg Family Farms*)	1.5	0
wild (*Uncle Ben's* Specialty Blends)	.5	0
wild (*Lundberg Family Farms*)	1.5	0
Rice bran, crude, ¼ cup	4.3	.9
Rice bran oil, 1 tbsp.	13.6	2.7
Rice cake, 1 cake, except as noted:		
all varieties:		
(*Lundberg Family Farms* Regular)	0	0
(*Mother's*)	0	0
(*Pritikin*)	0	0
(*Quaker*)	0	0
except butter flavor or cheese (*Hain*)	0	0
except sesame-garlic (*Mochi*)	1.0	0
butter flavor (*Hain*)	1.0	0
caramel (*Hain*)	0	0
cheese, nacho (*Hain*)	1.0	<1.0
cheese, white cheddar (*Hain*)	1.0	0
mini cakes:		
apple cinnamon, plain or teriyaki (*Hain*), .5 oz.	<1.0	0
barbecue or ranch (*Hain*), .5 oz.	3.0	n.a.
brown (*Lundberg Family Farms*), .6 oz.	0	0
cheese or nacho cheese (*Hain*), .5 oz.	2.0	0
creamy dill (*Lundberg Family Farms*), .6 oz.	1.0	0
honey nut or plain popcorn (*Hain*), .5 oz.	1.0	0
nacho (*Lundberg Family Farms*), .6 oz.	.5	0
popcorn, cheddar or butter flavor (*Hain*), .5 oz.	2.0	0
white cheddar (*Lundberg Family Farms*), .6 oz.	1.0	0
sesame-garlic (*Mochi*)	1.5	0

	total fat (grams)	saturated fat (grams)

Rice dishes, canned:

Mexican (*Old El Paso*), ½ cup	2.0	.5
Spanish (*Old El Paso*), 1 cup	1.0	n.a.
Spanish (*Van Camp's*), 1 cup	3.0	.5

Rice dishes, frozen:

and broccoli (*Green Giant*), 10-oz. pkg.	12.0	3.5
and chicken, stir-fry (*Lean Cuisine Lunch Express*), 9 oz.	9.0	1.0
fried, w/chicken (*Chun King*), 8 oz.	6.0	1.5
fried, w/pork (*Chun King*), 8 oz.	6.0	2.0
medley (*Green Giant*), 10-oz. pkg.	3.0	1.5
Mexican, w/chicken (*Lean Cuisine Lunch Express*), 9 oz.	8.0	1.5
Oriental (*Green Giant*), 8 oz.	.5	0
Oriental, w/vegetables (*The Budget Gourmet Side Dish*), 5.75 oz.	12.0	5.0
pilaf (*Green Giant*), 10-oz. pkg.	3.0	1.5
pilaf, w/green beans (*The Budget Gourmet Side Dish*), 5.62 oz.	12.0	3.0
teriyaki, stir fry (*Lean Cuisine Lunch Express*), 9 oz.	5.0	1.0
white and wild (*Green Giant*), 10-oz. pkg.	5.0	.5

Rice dishes, mix (see also "Rice blends"), dry form, except as noted:

Alfredo broccoli (*Lipton* Rice & Sauce), ½ cup	4.5	2.0
almond, toasted, pilaf (*Near East*), 1 cup*	6.0	1.0
basmati and lentils (*Lundberg Family Farms*), 1 cup*	1.0	0
basmati pilaf, tomato and herbs (*Knorr*), ¼ pkg.	.5	0
beef:		
(*Rice-A-Roni*), 1 cup*	10.0	2.0
(*Rice-A-Roni* ⅓ Less Salt), 1 cup*	5.0	1.0
broccoli (*Lipton* Rice & Sauce), ½ cup	1.0	0
and mushroom (*Rice-A-Roni*), 1 cup*	7.0	1.5

	total fat (grams)	saturated fat (grams)

Rice dishes, mix, beef *(cont.)*

Oriental (*Success*), ½ cup, 3.75 oz.	.5	0
pilaf (*Near East*), 1 cup*	4.5	1.0
beef flavor (*Lipton* Rice & Sauce), ½ cup	1.0	0

and beans (see also specific rice mix listings):

black beans (*Mahatma*), 2 oz.	1.5	0
black beans (*Near East* Mediterranean), 1 cup*	5.0	1.0
black beans, spicy (*Spice Islands*), 1 pkg.	0	0
Bombay curry (*Fantastic Foods*), 2.3 oz.	3.0	1.5
Cajun (*Fantastic Foods*), 2.3 oz.	2.0	0
Caribbean (*Fantastic Foods*), 2.1 oz.	1.5	0
Northern Italian (*Fantastic Foods*), 2.2 oz.	1.5	0
red beans (*Mahatma*), 2 oz.	1.0	0
red beans (*Near East*), 1 cup*	3.5	1.0
red beans (*Rice-A-Roni*), 1 cup*	7.0	1.5
red beans, spicy (*Spice Islands*), 1 pkg.	.5	0
Szechuan (*Fantastic Foods*), 1.9 oz.	2.0	0
Tex-Mex (*Fantastic Foods*), 2.4 oz.	2.0	0

broccoli:

au gratin (*Rice-A-Roni*), 1 cup*	17.0	4.5
au gratin (*Rice-A-Roni* ⅓ Less Salt), 1 cup* ..	11.0	3.0
au gratin (*Savory Classics*), 1 cup*	19.0	5.0
au gratin (*Uncle Ben's Country Inn Recipes*), 2.5 oz.	4.0	2.0
and cheese (*Mahatma*), 2 oz.	1.5	.5
and cheese (*Success*), ½ cup, 4.6 oz.	2.0	1.0
cheese flavor (*Rice-A-Roni* Fast Cook), 1 cup*	12.0	3.0
and white cheddar (*Uncle Ben's Country Inn Recipes*), 2.5 oz.	5.0	3.0

brown rice:

all varieties (*Arrowhead Mills* Quick), ¼ pkg. ..	1.0	0
and basmati, w/lentils (*Lundberg Family Farms*), 1 cup*	1.0	0
and lentils (*Lundberg Family Farms*), 1 cup* ..	1.0	0

	total fat (grams)	saturated fat (grams)
pilaf (*Near East*), 1 cup*	5.0	1.0
quick (*Lundberg Family Farms*), ¼ cup	1.5	0
and wild (*Success*), ½ cup, 4.5 oz.	1.0	0
and wild, mushroom (*Uncle Ben's*), 1.5 oz.	1.0	0
Cajun:		
(*Lipton* Rice & Sauce), ½ cup	1.0	0
and beans (*Lipton* Rice & Sauce), ½ cup	1.0	0
w/beans (*Rice-A-Roni*), 1 cup*	5.0	1.0
cheddar, white w/herbs (*Rice-A-Roni*), 1 cup*	14.0	4.0
cheddar broccoli (*Lipton* Rice & Sauce), ½ cup	3.0	1.0
chicken:		
(*Rice-A-Roni*), 1 cup*	10.0	2.0
(*Rice-A-Roni* Flex-Serve), 1 cup*	9.0	2.0
(*Rice-A-Roni* ⅓ Less Salt), 1 cup*	5.0	1.0
(*Savory Classics*), 1 cup*	8.0	1.5
(*Spice Islands*), 1 pkg.	1.5	0
(*Success* Classic), ½ cup, 4 oz.	1.0	0
almond, w/wild rice (*Savory Classics*), 1 cup*	9.0	1.5
creamy (*Lipton* Rice & Sauce), ½ cup	5.0	1.0
broccoli (*Lipton Golden Saute*), ½ cup	5.0	2.0
and broccoli (*Rice-A-Roni*), 1 cup*	7.0	1.5
and broccoli (*Uncle Ben's Country Inn Recipes*), 2.5 oz.	7.0	3.5
pilaf (*Near East*), 1 cup*	4.5	1.0
pilaf, w/brown rice (*Lundberg Family Farms*), 1 cup*	3.0	.5
pilaf, w/wild rice (*Near East* Mediterranean), 1 cup*	4.0	1.0
and vegetables (*Rice-A-Roni*), 1 cup*	7.0	1.5
and vegetable (*Uncle Ben's Country Inn Recipes* Homestyle), 2.5 oz.	6.0	3.0
w/mushrooms (*Rice-A-Roni*), 1 cup*	14.0	3.0
w/wild rice (*Uncle Ben's Country Inn Recipes*), 2 oz.	1.0	0

	total fat (grams)	saturated fat (grams)

Rice dishes, mix, chicken *(cont.)*

chicken flavor (*Lipton* Rice & Sauce), ½ cup	2.0	1.0
chicken flavor (*Rice-A-Roni* Fast Cook), 1 cup*	7.0	1.5
curry (*Near East*), 1 cup*	4.0	1.0
curry (*Spice Islands*), 1 pkg.	2.5	0
fried:		
(*Lipton Golden Saute*), ½ cup	1.0	0
(*Rice-A-Roni*), 1 cup*	11.0	2.0
beef flavor (*Lipton Golden Saute*), ½ cup	4.0	0
Oriental (*Lipton Golden Saute*), ½ cup	4.5	1.5
herb, savory (*Lipton Golden Saute*), ½ cup	4.0	1.0
herb and butter (*Lipton* Rice & Sauce), ½ cup	4.0	2.0
herb and butter (*Rice-A-Roni*), 1 cup*	9.0	2.0
herbed, au gratin (*Uncle Ben's Country Inn Recipes*), 2.5 oz.	3.5	1.5
jambalaya (*Mahatma*), 2 oz.	1.0	0
jasmine pilaf, lemon and herbs (*Knorr*), ¼ pkg.	1.0	0
long grain (*Lipton* Rice & Sauce), ½ cup	1.0	0
long grain and wild:		
(*Mahatma*), 2 oz.	.5	0
(*Near East*), 1 cup*	4.5	1.0
(*Rice-A-Roni*), 1 cup*	6.0	1.0
(*Success*), ½ cup, 4 oz.	0	0
(*Uncle Ben's* Original Natural), 2 oz.	.5	0
(*Uncle Ben's* Fast Cook), 2 oz.	1.0	0
chicken and almonds (*Rice-A-Roni*), 1 cup*	9.0	1.5
chicken and herb (*Uncle Ben's*), 2 oz.	1.5	0
garden vegetable (*Uncle Ben's*), 2 oz.	1.5	0
mushroom and herb (*Lipton*), ½ cup	1.0	.5
pilaf (*Rice-A-Roni*), 1 cup*	6.0	1.5
medley (*Lipton* Rice & Sauce), ½ cup	2.0	.5
Mexican (*Old El Paso*), ½ cup*	2.0	n.a.
Mexican (*Pritikin*), ⅓ cup	2.0	0
Mexican fiesta (*Savory Classics*), 1 cup*	7.0	1.5
mushroom (*Lipton* Rice & Sauce), ½ cup	1.0	1.0

	total fat (grams)	saturated fat (grams)
mushroom, creamy, and wild rice (*Uncle Ben's Country Inn Recipes*), 2.5 oz.	2.5	1.5
mushroom, savory (*Lundberg Family Farms*), 1 cup*	2.5	0
nutted pilaf (*Casbah*), 1 oz. dry, ½ cup*	2.0	0
onion mushroom (*Lipton Golden Saute* Rice & Sauce), ½ cup	4.0	1.5
Oriental:		
(*Pritikin*), ⅓ cup	1.5	0
(*Rice-A-Roni*), 1 cup*	6.0	1.0
(*Rice-A-Roni* Fast Cook), 1 cup*	11.0	2.0
(*Savory Classics*), 1 cup*	12.0	2.5
and vegetables (*Spice Islands*), 1 pkg.	2.5	0
pilaf (see also specific varieties):		
(*Casbah*), 1 oz. dry, ½ cup*	0	0
(*Lipton* Rice & Sauce), ½ cup	1.0	0
(*Mahatma*), 2 oz.	0	0
(*Near East*), 1 cup*	4.5	1.0
(*Rice-A-Roni*), 1 cup*	9.0	2.0
(*Savory Classics*), 1 cup*	6.0	1.5
(*Success*), ½ cup, 4.5 oz.	0	0
brown rice, w/miso (*Fantastic Foods* Quick Pilaf), about ½ cup	3.0	0
garlic herb (*Lundberg Family Farms*), 1 cup* ..	2.5	.5
harvest (*Knorr*), ¼ pkg.	.5	0
risotto, all varieties (*Knorr*), ¼ pkg.	.5	0
risotto (*Rice-A-Roni*), 1 cup*	9.0	2.0
sesame chicken (*Mahatma*), 2 oz.	1.5	0
Spanish:		
(*Lipton* Rice & Salad), ½ cup	1.0	0
(*Lundberg Family Farms* Fiesta), 1 cup*	2.0	0
(*Mahatma*), 2 oz.	.5	0
(*Rice-A-Roni*), 1 cup*	8.0	1.5
(*Success*), ½ cup, 4.3 oz.	.5	0
and beans (*Fantastic Only A Pinch*), 2.2 oz. ...	1.5	0

	total fat (grams)	saturated fat (grams)

Rice dishes, mix, Spanish *(cont.)*
    brown rice, pilaf *(Fantastic Foods* Quick Pilaf),
        about ½ cup . . . . 2.0 .. 0
    pilaf *(Casbah)*, 1 oz. dry, ½ cup* 0 0
    pilaf *(Near East)*, 1 cup* . . . . 6.0 . . . . 1.0
    Stroganoff *(Rice-A-Roni)*, 1 cup* . . . . 14.0 . . . . 3.5
    tomato and herb *(Uncle Ben's Country Inn*
        Recipes), 2.5 oz. 1.0 0
    tomato herb bean *(Near East)*, 1 cup* . . . . 5.0 . . . . 1.0
    vegetable bean, garden *(Near East)*, 1 cup* . . . . . 5.0 . . . . 1.0
    vegetable pilaf *(Uncle Ben's Country Inn Recipes)*,
        2 oz. 1.0 0
    and vegetables, country *(Spice Islands)*, 1 pkg. 5 0
    yellow *(Mahatma)*, 2 oz. 0 0
Rice flour:
    (Arrowhead Mills), ¼ cup 5 0
    brown, 1 cup 4.4 9
    white, 1 cup 2.2 6
Rice mix, see "Rice dishes, mix"
Rice seasoning mix:
    fried rice *(Durkee)*, ¼ pkg. 0 0
    fried rice *(Kikkoman)*, 1 oz. 2 0
Rice syrup, all varieties *(Lundberg Family*
    Farms Sweet Dreams), ¼ cup 0 0
Rigatoni entree, frozen:
    (Lean Cuisine), 9 oz. . . . . 4.0 . . . . 1.5
    in cream sauce, w/broccoli and chicken *(The*
        Budget Gourmet Light & Healthy), 10.8 oz. .. 6.0 . . . . 2.5
    w/chicken, vegetables *(Healthy Choice Generous*
        Serving), 12.5 oz. . . . . 4.0 . . . . 2.0
    in meat sauce *(Healthy Choice)*, 9.5 oz. . . . . 6.0 . . . . 2.0
Rigatoni entree, mix, w/cheddar and broccoli *(Golden*
    Grain Noodle Roni), 1 cup* . . . . 19.0 . . . . 5.0
Risotto, see "Rice dishes, mix"
Roast, vegetarian, see "Vegetarian dishes, frozen"

	total fat (grams)	saturated fat (grams)
Rockfish, Pacific, meat only:		
raw, 4 oz.	1.8	.4
baked, broiled, or microwaved, 4 oz.	2.3	.5
Roe (see also "Caviar"):		
carp (*Krinos*), 1 tbsp.	.5	.5
mixed species:		
raw, 4 oz.	7.3	1.7
raw, 1 tbsp.	1.0	.2
baked, broiled, or microwaved, 4 oz.	9.3	2.1
Roll (see also "Biscuit"), 1 piece, except as noted:		
(*Arnold Bran'nola* Buns)	2.0	0
(*Francisco*)	1.0	0
(*Roman Meal* Original Bun)	2.5	0
assorted (*Brownberry* Hearth)	1.5	0
brown and serve (*Pepperidge Farm* Hearth), 3 pieces	2.0	0
brown and serve (*Roman Meal* Original), 2 pieces	2.2	.3
butter, brown and serve (*Pepperidge Farm*)	5.0	3.0
club, brown and serve (*Pepperidge Farm*)	1.5	0
croissant, see "Croissant"		
dinner:		
(*Arnold Bran'nola*)	1.0	0
(*Francisco*)	1.0	0
(*Pepperidge Farm* Country Style Classic), 3 pieces	3.0	1.0
(*Roman Meal* Original), 2 pieces	2.7	.4
all varieties (*Awrey's*)	1.0	0
parker house (*Pepperidge Farm*), 3 pieces	4.5	1.5
plain or sesame (*Arnold*), 2 pieces	2.5	.5
poppy seed finger (*Pepperidge Farm*), 3 pieces	4.5	1.5
potato (*Arnold*), 2 pieces	1.5	0
sesame seed finger (*Pepperidge Farm*), 3 pieces	4.5	1.5

	total fat (grams)	saturated fat (grams)
Roll, dinner *(cont.)*		
wheat (*August Bros.*)	2.0	0
white (*August Bros.*)	1.0	0
egg, Dutch (*Arnold*)	3.0	<1.0
French style:		
(*Brownberry/Francisco* International, 6")	1.0	0
(*Francisco* 6")	2.5	0
(*Pepperidge Farm*), ⅛ loaf	1.5	1.0
(*Pepperidge Farm* 9 Pack)	1.0	0
(*Pepperidge Farm* Sliced), ⅛ loaf	1.5	.5
(*Pepperidge Farm* Twin), ⅛ of 2 loaves	1.5	.5
brown and serve (*Pepperidge Farm* 3 Pack)	2.5	.5
brown and serve (*Pepperidge Farm*), ½ piece	2.0	.5
mini (*Francisco*)	1.0	0
7-grain (*Pepperidge Farm*)	2.0	0
sourdough (*Pepperidge Farm*)	1.0	0
hamburger:		
(*Arnold*)	2.0	0
(*August Bros.*)	2.5	.5
(*Pepperidge Farm*)	2.5	1.0
(*Roman Meal* Original)	2.2	.3
wheat (*August Bros.*)	2.0	0
hoagie, multigrain (*Pepperidge Farm*)	4.5	2.5
hoagie, soft (*Pepperidge Farm* Deli)	4.5	2.5
hot dog (frankfurter):		
(*Arnold/Arnold* Sliced)	2.0	0
(*Arnold* Bran'nola)	1.5	0
(*Arnold* New England Style)	2.0	0
(*Pepperidge Farm*)	2.5	1.0
(*Roman Meal* Original)	2.1	.3
Dijon (*Pepperidge Farm*)	3.0	1.5
potato (*Arnold*)	2.0	0
wheat (*Brownberry*)	2.0	0
Italian (*Pepperidge Farm*), ⅛ loaf	2.0	1.0

	total fat (grams)	saturated fat (grams)
Italian (*Savoni* 8")	3.5	.5
kaiser:		
(*August Bros.*)	2.0	0
(*Brownberry* Hearth)	2.5	0
(*Brownberry Francisco*)	1.0	0
(*Francisco*)	2.0	0
(*Levy* Old Country)	2.0	0
w/sesame (*Arnold*)	4.0	.5
onion (*Arnold* Deli)	2.0	0
onion (*Levy* Old Country)	3.0	.5
potato:		
(*Arnold*)	2.0	0
(*Pepperidge Farm* Hearty)	2.5	.5
sesame (*Arnold*)	3.0	.5
sandwich:		
(*Pepperidge Farm* Hearty)	5.0	2.5
(*Roman Meal* Original)	3.0	.4
multi grain (*Pepperidge Farm*)	3.0	.5
onion (*Pepperidge Farm*)	3.0	1.5
potato (*Brownberry*)	2.5	0
potato (*Pepperidge Farm*)	4.0	.5
sesame (*Pepperidge Farm*)	3.0	1.5
soft, plain or sesame (*Arnold*)	3.0	.5
sourdough (*Pepperidge Farm*)	3.5	1.5
wheat (*Brownberry* Buns)	2.0	0
white, seeded (*Brownberry* Buns)	3.0	.5
white, unseeded (*Brownberry* Buns)	2.5	.5
sourdough:		
(*Francisco*)	1.0	0
(*Pepperidge Farm* Twin), 1/9 of 2 loaves	1.5	.5
brown and serve (*Francisco*)	1.0	0
steak (*August Bros./Arnold* Premium)	2.5	0
sub (*August Bros.*)	2.5	0
sub (*Levy* Old Country)	1.5	0

	total fat (grams)	saturated fat (grams)

Roll *(cont.)*
| twist, golden (*Pepperidge Farm* Heat & Serve) | 4.0 | 1.5 |

Roll, frozen or refrigerated:
(*Rich's* Homestyle), 2 pieces	3.0	1.0
butterflake dinner (*Pillsbury*), 1 piece	5.0	1.0
cheese crescent (*Pillsbury*), 2 pieces	12.0	3.0
crescent (*Pillsbury*), 2 pieces	11.0	2.5
garlic and cheese (*Pepperidge Farm*), 1 piece	5.0	1.5

Roll, mix, dry:
hot roll (*Dromedary*), 1/16 pkg.	.5	0
hot roll (*Pillsbury*), 1/4 cup mix	1.0	0
date nut (*Dromedary*), 1/3 pkg.	7.0	2.5

Roll, sweet (see also "Bun, honey"):
apple twist (*Hostess*), 2.5-oz. piece	4.0	1.5
caramel nut (*Aunt Fanny's*), 2-oz. piece	6.0	2.0
caramel pecan swirl (*Hostess*), 2-oz. piece	15.0	6.0
cinnamon:		
(*Aunt Fanny's*), 2-oz. piece	5.0	2.0
(*Hostess*), 2.3-oz. piece	6.0	2.5
(*Hostess* Home Baked), 1.6-oz. piece	5.0	1.0
(*Pepperidge Farm*), 2.3-oz. piece	12.0	2.5
mini (*Hostess Cinnaminis*), 2.4 oz., 5 pieces	17.0	4.0
or pecan cinnamon (*Aunt Fanny's* 8-Pack), 1.4-oz. piece	3.0	1.0
fruit, Dixie, or apple cinnamon (*Aunt Fanny's*), 2-oz. piece	4.0	2.0
pecan (*Hostess Spinners*), 1-oz. piece	5.0	1.0
strawberry (*Aunt Fanny's* 8-Pack), 1.4-oz. piece	3.0	1.0

Rolls, sweet, refrigerated or frozen, 1 piece:
| apple cinnamon, w/icing (*Pillsbury*) | 5.0 | 1.5 |
| caramel (*Pillsbury*) | 7.0 | 1.5 |

	total fat (grams)	saturated fat (grams)
cinnamon:		
glazed (*Weight Watchers*), 2.1 oz.	5.0	1.5
w/icing (*Pillsbury*)	5.0	1.5
w/icing (*Schwan's*), 1 piece, 2.7 oz.	4.5	1.0
raisin, w/icing (*Pillsbury*)	7.0	1.5
orange, w/icing (*Pillsbury*)	7.0	1.5
Root beer shake (*Nestlé Killer Shakes*), 1 carton	15.0	9.0
Rose apple, untrimmed, 1 lb.	.9	n.a.
Roselle:		
untrimmed, 1 lb.	1.8	n.a.
trimmed, ½ cup or 1 oz.	.2	0
Rosemary, dried:		
1 tbsp.	.5	0
1 tsp.	.2	0
Rotini, see "Pasta"		
Rotini dishes, mix:		
and cheese, broccoli (*Kraft Velveeta*), 4.5 oz.,		
about 1 cup*	16.0	10.0
primavera (*Lipton* Pasta & Sauce), ½ cup	5.0	2.0
Rotini entree, frozen:		
(*Green Giant Garden Gourmet Right for Lunch*),		
9.5 oz.	10.0	5.0
Roughy, orange, meat only:		
raw, 4 oz.	.8	<.1
baked, broiled, or microwaved, 4 oz.	1.0	<.1
Roughy, frozen, orange, fillets (*Schwan's*), 4 oz.	1.5	0
Roy Rogers, 1 serving:		
breakfast:		
bagel, plain	2.0	<1.0
bagel, cinnamon raisin	1.0	<1.0
Big Country Breakfast Platter, w/bacon	43.0	13.0
Big Country Breakfast Platter, w/ham	39.0	11.0
Big Country Breakfast Platter, w/sausage	61.0	19.0
biscuit	21.0	6.0

	total fat (grams)	saturated fat (grams)

Roy Rogers, breakfast *(cont.)*

biscuit, bacon	23.0	7.0
biscuit, bacon and egg	26.0	8.0
biscuit, *Cinnamon 'N' Raisin*	18.0	5.0
biscuit, ham and egg	23.0	7.0
biscuit, ham and cheese	24.0	8.0
biscuit, ham, egg, and cheese	27.0	10.0
biscuit, sausage	31.0	10.0
biscuit, sausage and egg	35.0	11.0
hash rounds	14.0	3.0
pancakes, 3 pieces	2.0	1.0
pancakes, 3 pieces, w/2 bacon strips	9.0	3.0
pancakes, 3 pieces, w/1 sausage patty	16.0	6.0
sourdough, ham, egg, and cheese	24.0	9.0

sandwiches and burgers:

bacon cheeseburger	28.0	13.0
bacon cheeseburger, sourdough	46.0	18.0
cheeseburger	13.0	7.0
cheeseburger, ¼ lb. (average precooked weight)	22.0	10.0
chicken fillet	24.0	5.0
chicken, grilled	11.0	2.0
chicken, grilled, sourdough	21.0	6.0
Fisherman's Fillet (seasonal)	21.0	5.0
hamburger	9.0	4.0
hamburger, ¼ lb. (average precooked weight)	18.0	8.0
roast beef	4.0	1.0

chicken:

fried breast	15.4	4.0
fried leg	7.0	2.0
fried thigh	15.0	4.0
fried wing	8.0	2.0
nuggets, 6 pieces	18.0	4.0
nuggets, 9 pieces	29.0	6.0

	total fat (grams)	saturated fat (grams)
¼ *Roy's Roaster*, white meat	29.0	9.0
¼ *Roy's Roaster*, white meat, skin off	6.0	2.0
¼ *Roy's Roaster*, dark meat	34.0	10.0
¼ *Roy's Roaster*, dark meat, skin off	10.0	3.0
salads:		
grilled chicken	4.0	1.0
garden	14.0	9.0
side	<1.0	<1.0
side dishes and potatoes:		
baked beans, 5 oz.	2.0	1.0
baked potato	1.0	0
baked potato, w/margarine	13.0	2.0
baked potato, w/margarine and sour cream	19.0	6.0
coleslaw, 5 oz.	25.0	4.0
cornbread	17.0	3.0
fries, regular	15.0	4.0
fries, large	18.0	5.0
gravy, 1.5 oz.	<1.0	<1.0
mashed potatoes, 5 oz.	<1.0	<1.0
desserts:		
frozen yogurt cone, vanilla	4.0	3.0
hot fudge sundae	10.0	5.0
strawberry shortcake	21.0	5.0
strawberry sundae	6.0	3.0
Rum liquor, all varieties and proofs, 3 fl. oz.	0	0
Rum runner mixer, frozen* (*Bacardi*), 8 fl. oz.	0	0
Rutabaga:		
fresh:		
raw, untrimmed, 1 lb.	.8	.1
raw, cubed, ½ cup	.1	<.1
boiled, drained, cubed, ½ cup	.1	<.1
canned, diced (*Allens/Sunshine*), ½ cup	0	0
Rye, whole grain:		
1 cup	4.2	.5
(*Arrowhead Mills*), ¼ cup	1.0	0

	total fat (grams)		saturated fat (grams)
Rye flour:			
(*Arrowhead Mills*), ¼ cup	1.0	....	0
dark, 1 cup	3.4	....	.4
light, 1 cup	1.4	....	.1
medium, 1 cup	1.8	....	.2
medium (*Pillsbury's Best*), 1 cup	2.0	....	0
and wheat (*Pillsbury's Best* Bohemian Style), 1 cup	1.0	....	0
Rye liquor, all varieties and proofs, 3 fl. oz.	0	....	0

S

	total fat (grams)	saturated fat (grams)
Saag sauce, see "Cooking sauce"		
Sablefish, meat only:		
raw, 4 oz.	17.4	3.6
smoked, 4 oz.	22.8	4.8
Safflower oil, 1 tbsp.:		
(*Hain*)	14.0	1.0
(*Hollywood*)	14.0	1.0
linoleic	13.6	1.2
oleic	13.6	.8
Safflower seed kernel, dried, 1 oz.	10.9	1.0
Safflower seed meal, partially defatted, 1 oz.	.7	.1
Saffron:		
1 tbsp.	1.4	.1
1 tsp.	.5	<.1
Sage, dried, ground:		
1 tbsp.	.3	.1
1 tsp.	.1	<.1
Salad dressing, 2 tbsp., except as noted:		
all varieties:		
(*Healthy Sensations!*)	0	0
(*Kraft Free*)	0	0

	total fat (grams)	saturated fat (grams)
Salad dressing, all varieties *(cont.)*		
(*Medford Farms* Fat Free)	0	0
(*Nalley's* Fat Free)	0	0
(*Paula's* No-Fat)	0	0
(*Pritikin*)	0	0
(*Seven Seas Free*)	0	0
(*Weight Watchers Salad Celebrations* Fat Free)	0	0
bacon and tomato (*Kraft*)	14.0	2.5
bacon and tomato (*Kraft Deliciously Right* Lowfat)	5.0	1.0
blue cheese:		
(*Bernstein's*)	20.0	2.5
(*Bernstein's* Lite)	8.0	1.5
(*Kraft Roka*)	7.0	4.0
chunky (*Marie's*)	19.0	3.5
chunky (*Marie's* Reduced Calorie)	7.0	1.0
chunky (*Seven Seas*)	7.0	4.0
chunky (*Wish-Bone*)	16.0	3.0
chunky (*Wish-Bone* Lite)	8.0	2.0
creamy (*Bernstein's* Restaurant)	13.0	1.5
buttermilk, old fashioned (*Hain*)	14.0	2.0
Caesar:		
(*Bernstein's*)	10.0	1.0
(*Bernstein's* Extra Rich)	11.0	1.0
(*Kraft*)	13.0	2.5
(*Kraft Deliciously Right* Lowfat)	5.0	1.0
(*Pfeiffer*)	16.0	2.5
(*Seven Seas Viva*)	12.0	2.0
cheese, three (*Weight Watcher Salad Celebrations*)	2.0	0
creamy (*Marie's*)	18.0	3.0
creamy (*Seven Seas*)	15.0	2.5
w/olive oil (*Wish-Bone*)	10.0	1.5
w/olive oil (*Wish-Bone* Lite)	5.0	1.0

	total fat (grams)	saturated fat (grams)
ranch (*Kraft*)	15.0	2.5
cheese (*Bernstein's* Fantastico!)	11.0	1.0
coleslaw (*Hellman's*)	16.0	2.5
coleslaw (*Kraft*)	12.0	2.0
Dijon vinaigrette (*Hain*)	13.0	2.0
Dijon vinaigrette (*Wish-Bone* Lite)	5.0	1.0
dill, creamy (*Bernstein's Light Fantastic*)	2.0	0
French:		
(*Bernstein's* Creamy Herbal)	11.0	1.0
(*Kraft*)	12.0	2.0
(*Kraft Deliciously Right* Lowfat)	3.0	.5
(*Marie's* Tangy)	11.0	1.5
(*Nalley's* Creamy)	9.0	.5
(*Seven Seas* Creamy)	12.0	2.0
(*Wish-Bone* Deluxe)	11.0	1.5
(*Wish-Bone* Lite)	2.0	.5
(*Wish-Bone* Sweet 'n Spicy)	12.0	2.0
Catalina (*Kraft*)	11.0	2.0
Catalina (*Kraft Deliciously Right* Lowfat)	4.0	.5
Catalina w/honey (*Kraft*)	12.0	2.0
garlic, creamy (*Kraft*)	11.0	2.0
green goddess (*Seven Seas*)	13.0	2.0
herbs and spices (*Seven Seas*)	12.0	2.0
honey Dijon (*Kraft*)	15.0	2.0
honey Dijon (*Wish-Bone*)	10.0	1.5
honey mustard (*Bernstein's*)	12.0	1.0
honey mustard (*Marie's*)	15.0	2.0
honey mustard (*Nalley's* Restaurant Style)	12.0	1.0
Italian:		
(*Bernstein's*)	16.0	1.0
(*Bernstein's* Restaurant Recipe)	4.0	.5
(*Bernstein's* Wine Country)	11.0	1.0
(*Kraft*)	12.0	2.0
(*Kraft Deliciously Right*)	7.0	1.0
(*Kraft* Presto)	15.0	2.5

	total fat (grams)	saturated fat (grams)
Salad dressing, Italian *(cont.)*		
(*Pfeiffer*)	13.0	2.0
(*Seven Seas Viva*)	11.0	1.5
(*Seven Seas Viva* Reduced Calorie)	4.0	1.0
(*Wish-Bone*)	9.0	1.5
(*Wish-Bone* Lite)	.5	0
(*Wish-Bone* Robusto, 8 oz.)	10.0	1.5
(*Wish-Bone* Robusto, 16 oz.)	9.0	1.5
(*Wish-Bone* Romano)	14.0	2.0
w/cheese (*Bernstein's* Reduced Calorie)	2.0	.5
w/cheese and garlic (*Bernstein's*)	11.0	1.0
creamy (*Hain*)	16.0	2.5
creamy (*Kraft*)	11.0	4.0
creamy (*Kraft Deliciously Right* Lowfat)	5.0	1.0
creamy (*Seven Seas* Reduced Calorie)	5.0	1.0
creamy (*Wish-Bone*)	12.0	2.0
creamy (*Wish-Bone* Lite)	3.5	1.0
garlic (*Marie's*)	19.0	3.0
garlic (*Marie's* Low Calorie)	7.0	.5
w/herbs and garlic (*Bernstein's*)	13.0	1.0
house, w/olive oil (*Kraft*)	2.0	2.0
olive oil (*Wish-Bone* Classic)	6.0	1.0
two cheese (*Seven Seas*)	7.0	1.0
wine and cheese (*Maple Grove Farms of Vermont*)	4.6	1.0
zesty (*Kraft*)	11.0	1.5
lemon pepper vinaigrette (*Chelten House*)	6.0	.5
mayonnaise type:		
(*Miracle Whip*), 1 tbsp.	7.0	1.0
(*Miracle Whip Free*)	0	0
(*Mrs. Filberts* Reduced Calorie), 1 tbsp.	3.0	0
(*Nalley* Whip), 1 tbsp.	5.0	.5
olive oil vinaigrette (*Wish-Bone*)	5.0	.5
Parmesan (*Bernstein's Light Fantastic*)	1.0	.5
Parmesan, creamy (*Wish-Bone*)	18.0	3.0

	total fat (grams)	saturated fat (grams)
pepper Parmesan (*Morgan's*), 1 tbsp.	7.0	2.0
peppercorn ranch (*Kraft*)	18.0	3.0
poppyseed (*Marie's*)	12.0	1.5
poppyseed ranch (*Hain*)	14.0	2.0
ranch:		
(*Bernstein's* Homestyle Recipe)	12.0	1.0
(*Bernstein's* Lite)	6.0	.5
(*Cains* Country)	15.0	2.0
(*Kraft*)	18.0	3.0
(*Kraft Deliciously Right* Lowfat)	11.0	2.0
(*Morgan's*), 1 tbsp.	5.5	<1.0
(*Nalley* Homestyle)	8.0	.5
(*Seven Seas*)	16.0	2.5
(*Seven Seas* Reduced Calorie)	9.0	1.5
(*Wish-Bone*)	17.0	2.5
(*Wish-Bone* Lite, 8 oz.)	8.0	1.5
(*Wish-Bone* Lite, 16 oz.)	9.0	2.0
buttermilk (*Kraft*)	16.0	3.0
creamy (*Marie's*)	20.0	3.0
cucumber (*Kraft*)	15.0	2.5
cucumber (*Kraft Deliciously Right* Lowfat)	5.0	1.0
Parmesan garlic (*Bernstein's*)	11.0	1.0
Salsa (*Kraft*)	13.0	2.0
sour cream and onion (*Kraft*)	18.0	3.0
raspberry vinaigrette (*Chelten House*)	6.0	.5
red wine vinegar and oil (*Seven Seas*)	11.0	2.0
red wine vinegar and oil (*Seven Seas* Reduced Calorie)	5.0	1.0
Roquefort (*Bernstein's*)	15.0	2.0
Russian:		
(*Kraft*)	10.0	1.5
(*Seven Seas Viva*)	16.0	2.5
(*Weight Watchers Salad Celebrations*)	1.5	0
(*Wish-Bone*)	6.0	1.0
salsa and sour cream (*Bernstein's*)	9.0	1.0

	total fat (grams)	saturated fat (grams)

Salad dressing *(cont.)*

Salsa, zesty garden (*Kraft*)	6.0	1.0
Sante Fe (*Wish-Bone*)	15.0	2.5
sesame vinaigrette (*Wish-Bone*)	5.0	.5
Sierra (*Wish-Bone*)	16.0	2.5
slaw (*Marzetti*), 2 tbsp.	16.0	2.5
sun-dried tomato vinaigrette (*Chelten House*)	6.0	.5
Thousand Island:		
(*Bernstein's*)	11.0	1.0
(*Hain*)	9.0	1.5
(*Kraft*)	10.0	1.5
(*Kraft Deliciously Right* Lowfat)	4.0	1.0
(*Nalley's*)	11.0	1.0
(*Weight Watchers Salad Celebrations*)	1.5	0
(*Wish-Bone*)	12.0	2.0
(*Wish-Bone* Lite)	5.0	1.0
w/bacon (*Kraft*)	12.0	2.0
vinaigrette, see specific varieties		

Salad dressing mix, 2 tbsp.*, except as noted:

all varieties (*Good Seasons* Fat Free)	0	0
all varieties (*Weight Watchers*), 1/6 pkg.	0	0
buttermilk, farm style (*Good Seasons*)	12.0	2.0
Caesar, gourmet (*Good Seasons*)	16.0	2.5
cheese garlic (*Good Seasons*)	16.0	2.5
garlic w/herbs (*Good Seasons*)	15.0	2.0
honey mustard (*Good Seasons*)	15.0	2.0
Italian:		
(*Good Seasons*)	15.0	2.0
(*Good Seasons* Reduced Calorie)	5.0	1.0
mild (*Good Seasons*)	15.0	2.5
zesty (*Good Seasons*)	15.0	2.0
zesty (*Good Seasons* Reduced Calorie)	5.0	1.0
Mexican spice (*Good Seasons*)	15.0	2.5
Oriental sesame (*Good Seasons*)	16.0	2.5
ranch (*Good Seasons*)	12.0	2.0

	total fat (grams)	saturated fat (grams)
ranch (*Good Seasons* Reduced Calorie)	4.5	1.0
Salad topper, 1 tbsp.:		
(*McCormick Salad Toppins*)	1.5	0
all varieties, except garlic Italian (*Pepperidge*		
Farm)	2.0	0
garlic Italian (*Pepperidge Farm*)	1.5	0
Salami:		
beef:		
(*Boar's Head* Chub), 2 oz.	9.0	3.0
(*Hebrew National*), 2 oz.	14.0	6.0
(*Hebrew National* Lean), 2 oz.	6.0	2.0
(*Hebrew National* Reduced Fat), 2 oz.	8.0	4.0
(*Oscar Mayer* Machiach), 2 slices, 1.6 oz.	10.0	5.0
cooked, 1 oz.	5.7	2.4
beef and pork, cooked, 1 oz.	5.7	2.3
beef (*Oscar Mayer* Salami for Beer), 1.6 oz.,		
2 slices	9.0	3.0
cooked (*Boar's Head*), 2 oz.	11.0	5.0
cooked (*Thorn Apple Valley*), 1-oz. slice	7.0	n.a.
cotto (*Oscar Mayer*), 1.6 oz., 2 slices	9.0	4.0
cotto, beef (*Oscar Mayer*), 2 slices, 1.6 oz. ...	7.0	3.0
dry or hard:		
(*Boar's Head*), 1 oz.	9.0	3.5
(*Hillshire Farms*), 1 oz.	9.0	n.a.
(*Hormel Homeland*), 1 oz.	10.0	4.0
(*Oscar Mayer*), 3 slices, 1 oz.	9.0	3.0
(*Oscar Mayer Deli-Thin*), 1.2 oz., 4 slices	11.0	4.0
(*Patrick Cudahy* Heritage), 1 oz.	11.0	4.0
pork, 1 oz.	9.6	3.3
pork and beef, 1 oz.	9.7	3.5
Genoa:		
(*Boar's Head* Natural Casing), 2 oz.	14.0	5.0
(*Hormel Di Lusso*), 1 oz.	7.0	3.0
(*Oscar Mayer*), 3 slices, 1 oz.	9.0	3.0
(*Patrick Cudahy* LaFortuna), 2 oz.	20.0	9.0

	total fat (grams)	saturated fat (grams)

Salami, Genoa *(cont.)*
    Italian (*Hillshire Farms*), 1 oz. .... 7.0 .... n.a.
    turkey, see "Turkey salami"
"Salami," vegetarian, frozen (*Worthington*),
    2 oz., 3 slices .... 8.0 .... 1.0
Salisbury steak, see "Beef dinner" and "Beef entree"
Salmon, meat only, 4 oz.:
    Atlantic, raw .... 7.2 .... 1.2
    chinook, raw .... 11.9 .... 2.9
    chinook, smoked or lox .... 4.9 .... 1.1
    chum, raw .... 4.3 .... 1.0
    coho, raw .... 6.8 .... 1.3
    coho, boiled, poached, or steamed .... 8.6 .... 1.6
    pink, raw 3.9 6
    red or sockeye, raw .... 9.7 .... 1.7
    red or sockeye, baked, broiled, or microwaved ... 12.4 .... 2.2
Salmon, canned:
    chum (*Peter Pan*), ¼ cup .... 4.0 .... 1.0
    coho (*Peter Pan*), ¼ cup .... 5.0 .... 1.0
    keta or pink (*Bumble Bee*), 3.5 oz. .... 8.0 .... 2.0
    king (*Peter Pan*), ¼ cup .... 10.0 .... 3.0
    pink:
        (*Libby's*), ¼ cup .... 5.0 .... 1.0
        (*Peter Pan*), ¼ cup .... 5.0 .... 1.0
        skinless, boneless (*Bumble Bee*), 3.25 oz. .... 5.0 .... 1.0
        skinless, boneless (*Libby's*), ⅓ cup 2.0 0
    red:
        (*Bumble Bee*), 3.5 oz. .... 10.0 .... 2.0
        (*Libby's*), ¼ cup .... 7.0 .... 1.5
        (*Peter Pan*), ¼ cup .... 7.0 .... 1.5
        skinless and boneless (*Bumble Bee*), 3.25 oz. ... 6.0 .... 1.0
Salmon, frozen:
    chum fillets (*Peter Pan*), 4 oz., about 1 fillet ..... 4.0 .... 1.0
    chum steaks (*Peter Pan*), 4 oz., about 1 steak .... 4.0 .... 1.0

	total fat (grams)	saturated fat (grams)
coho fillets (*Peter Pan*), 4 oz., about 1 fillet	7.0	1.0
Salmon, smoked (see also "Salmon"):		
lox (*Vita*), 3-oz. pkg.	1.5	0
lox, sliced (*Vita*), 2 oz.	1.0	0
nova (*Vita*), 3-oz. pkg.	1.5	0
nova, sliced (*Vita*), 2 oz.	1.0	0
Salmon, smoked, spread (see also "Cheese, cream"):		
(*Vita*), ¼ cup	5.0	1.0
cream cheese and (*Vita*), ¼ cup, 2 oz.	17.0	11.0
Salmon oil, 1 tbsp.	13.6	2.7
Salsa (see also specific listings), 2 tbsp.,		
except as noted:		
(*Garden of Eatin' Cha Cha Corn*)	0	0
(*Gracias*)	0	0
(*Nalley* Superba)	0	0
(*Pace*)	0	0
all varieties:		
(*Chi-Chi's*)	0	0
(*Del Monte*)	0	0
(*Hain* Thick & Chunky)	0	0
(*Keebler Chip Chasers*)	0	0
(*La Victoria*)	0	0
(*Las Palmas* Mexicana)	0	0
(*Old El Paso*)	0	0
(*Pace*)	0	0
(*Taco Bell*)	0	0
(*Tom's*), 1.1 oz.	0	0
dip (see also "Salsa dip"):		
mild or medium (*Doritos*)	0	0
mild or medium (*Eagle*)	0	0
mild or medium (*Old El Paso*)	0	0
mild, medium, or hot (*Tostitos*)	0	0
garlic (*Garden of Eatin' Great Garlic*)	0	0
hot (*Garden of Eatin' Hot Habanero*)	0	0

	total fat (grams)		saturated fat (grams)

Salsa *(cont.)*

Italian, all varieties (*Progresso*) 0 0

picante, see "Picante sauce"

Salsa dip, 2 tbsp.:

cheese, see "Cheese dip"

yogurt (*Crowley's*) .... 2.0 .... 1.5

Salsa seasoning mix (*Lawry's* Spices & Seasonings),

½ tsp. 0 0

Salsify:

raw, untrimmed, 1 lb. .... .8 .... <.1

sliced, ½ cup .... .1 .... tr.

boiled, drained, sliced ½ cup .... .1 .... tr.

Salt, all varieties, 1 tbsp. 0 0

Salt, seasoned, all varieties (*Lawry's*), ¼ tsp. 0 0

Salt pork, raw, 1 oz. .... 22.8 .... 8.3

Salt substitute, seasoned (*Lawry's*), ¼ tsp. 0 0

Sandwich, see specific listings

Sandwich sauce, see "Sloppy Joe sauce"

Sandwich and salad sauce (*Durkee* Famous),

1 tbsp. 6.0 5

Sandwich spread:

(*Kraft* Sandwich and Burger Sauce), 1 tbsp. 5.0 5

meat:

(*Oscar Mayer*), 2 oz. .... 10.0 .... 4.0

(*Spam*), 4 tbsp. .... 11.0 .... 4.0

pork and beef, 1 oz. .... 4.9 .... 1.7

pork and beef, 1 tbsp. 2.6 9

meatless:

mayonnaise-type, 1 oz. .... 9.6 .... 1.4

mayonnaise-type, 1 tbsp. .... 5.2 .... 5.8

relish (*Hellman's*), 1 tbsp. .... 5.0 .... 1.0

vegetarian, canned (*Loma Linda*), ¼ cup 4.5 9

Sapodilla:

untrimmed, 1 lb. .... 4.0 .... n.a.

	total fat (grams)	saturated fat (grams)
1 medium, about 2.3 oz.	1.9	n.a.
Sapote:		
untrimmed, 1 lb.	1.9	n.a.
1 medium, about 11.2 oz.	1.4	n.a.
Sardine, fresh, see		
Sardine, canned:		
Atlantic, in soybean oil, drained:		
3.2 oz. (3.75-oz. can)	10.5	1.4
2 oz.	6.5	.9
2 medium, 3" × 1" × ½"	2.8	.4
Pacific, in tomato sauce, drained, 2 oz.	6.8	1.8
Pacific, in tomato sauce, 1 medium, 4¾" long	4.6	1.2
in mustard sauce (*Underwood*), 1 can	12.0	3.0
in olive oil, skinless, boneless (*Granadaisa*),		
¼ cup, about 2 oz.	7.0	1.5
in soya oil (*Underwood*), 3-oz. can	16.0	3.5
in tomato sauce (*Del Monte*), 2 oz., ½ fish		
w/sauce	4.0	1.5
in tomato sauce (*Underwood*), 1 can	11.0	3.0
Sardine oil, 1 tbsp.	13.6	4.1
Sauce, see specific listings		
Sauerbraten seasoning mix (*Knorr* Recipe Mix),		
⅙ pkg.	1.0	.5
Sauerkraut, ½ cup, except as noted:		
(*Boar's Head*), 2 tbsp.	0	0
(*Claussen*)	0	0
(*Del Monte*)	0	0
(*Eden*)	0	0
(*Frank's* Quality Kraut), 2 tbsp.	0	0
(*Hebrew National*), 2 tbsp.	0	0
(*Hebrew National/Shorr's* New Kraut)	1.0	0
(*Pickle Eater's Kozmic Kraut*), ¼ cup	0	0
(*Pickle Eater's* Natural), 2 tbsp.	0	0
(*Rosoff* Home Style)	1.0	0
(*Seneca*), 2 tbsp.	0	0

	total fat (grams)	saturated fat (grams)

Sauerkraut *(cont.)*
all varieties (*Stokely*)	0	0
w/liquid, 4 oz. or ½ cup	.2	<.1
Sauerkraut juice, canned, 6 fl. oz.	.1	0

Sausage (see also "Frankfurter" and specific
sausage listings):
(*Hillshire Farm* Country Recipe), 2 oz.	16.0	n.a.
(*Schwan's*), 3 oz., 3 links	32.0	11.0
beef (see also "smoked," below):		
(*Hillshire Farm*), 2 oz.	16.0	n.a.
raw, cooked (*Jones Dairy Farm* Roll), 2 oz.	13.0	6.0
cooked (*Jones Dairy Farm* Golden Brown),		
1.6 oz., 2 links	15.0	6.0
smoked (*Thorn Apple Valley*), 2 oz.	16.0	n.a.
smoked, cooked (*Jones Dairy Farm*		
Brown & Serve), 1.6 oz., 2 links	17.0	7.0
beef and cheddar (*Hillshire Farm*), 2 oz.	15.0	n.a.
liver, see "Liverwurst"		
Mexican or Spanish, see "Chorizo"		
pork, raw, cooked:		
(*Hormel Little Sizzlers*), 3 links	20.0	7.0
(*Hormel Little Sizzlers*), 2 patties	23.0	8.0
(*Jones Dairy Farm* Dinner), 1.4 oz., 1 link	14.0	5.0
(*Jones Dairy Farm* Little Link), 1.9 oz.,		
3 links	17.0	7.0
(*Jones Dairy Farm* Light Links), 2 oz.,		
2 links	11.0	4.0
hot or roll (*Jones Dairy Farm*), 2 oz.	21.0	8.0
patty (*Jones Dairy Farm*), 1.1 oz., 1 patty	12.0	4.0
pork, cooked:		
(*Hormel Little Sizzlers*), 3 links	22.0	8.0
(*Hormel Little Sizzlers*), 2 patties	18.0	6.0
(*Jones Dairy Farm* Brown & Serve), 1.6 oz.,		
2 links	18.0	7.0

	total fat (grams)	saturated fat (grams)
(*Jones Dairy Farm* Brown & Serve/Golden Brown Light), 1.6 oz., 2 links	9.0	3.0
(*Jones Dairy Farm* Brown & Serve Microwave), 1.6 oz., 2 links	15.0	n.a.
(*Oscar Mayer*), 1.7 oz., 2 links	15.0	5.0
mild or spicy (*Jones Dairy Farm* Golden Brown), 1.6 oz., 2 links	18.0	6.0
patty (*Jones Dairy Farm* Golden Brown), 1 patty	14.0	5.0
pork patty (*Schwan's*), 2-oz. patty	22.0	8.0
pork patty, regular or extra mild (*Jimmy Dean*), 1 oz.	11.0	n.a.
pork and bacon, cooked (*Jones Dairy Farm* Brown & Serve), 1.6 oz., 2 links	17.0	7.0
smoked:		
(*Boar's Head*), 4.5 oz.	36.0	14.0
(*Healthy Choice* Low Fat), 2 oz.	2.0	<1.0
(*Hillshire Farm* Bun Size), 2 oz.	16.0	n.a.
(*Hillshire Farm* Flavorseal), 2 oz.	17.0	n.a.
(*Hillshire Farm* Lite), 2 oz.	11.0	n.a.
(*Hillshire Farm* Lit'l Smokies), 2 oz.	11.0	n.a.
(*Oscar Mayer* Little Smokies), 2 oz., 6 links	16.0	6.0
(*Oscar Mayer* Smokie Links), 1.5-oz. link	12.0	4.0
(*Thorn Apple Valley* Smoky Link), 1 link	7.0	n.a.
beef (*Hillshire Farm* Bun Size or Flavorseal), 2 oz.	16.0	n.a.
beef (*Oscar Mayer* Smokies), 1.5-oz. link	12.0	4.0
cheese (*Hillshire Farm* Lit'l Cheddar Smokies), 2 oz.	16.0	n.a.
cheese (*Oscar Mayer* Smokies), 1.5-oz. link	12.0	4.0
cheese, cheddar (*Thorn Apple Valley*), 2 oz.	16.0	n.a.
hot (*Boar's Head*), 3.2 oz.	25.0	10.0
hot (*Hillshire Farm* Flavorseal), 2 oz.	16.0	n.a.

	total fat (grams)	saturated fat (grams)

Sausage, canned (see also "Vienna sausage"), pickled, hot or smoked (*Hormel*), 6 links, 2 oz. .... 11.0 .... 5.0

"Sausage," vegetarian:

1 oz. 5.1 8

.9-oz. link 4.5 7

1.3-oz. patty .... 6.9 .... 1.1

"Sausage," vegetarian, canned (see also " 'Frankfurter,' vegetarian, canned"), (*Worthington Saucettes*), 1.3-oz. link .... 6.0 .... 1.0

"Sausage," vegetarian, frozen (see also " 'Frankfurter,' vegetarian, frozen"):

(*Green Giant* Breakfast Patties), 2 oz., 2 patties ... 6.0 5

(*Morningstar Farms* Breakfast Links), 1.6 oz., 2 links .... 5.0 .... 1.0

(*Morningstar Farm* Breakfast Patties), 1.3-oz. patty .... 5.0 .... 1.5

(*Morningstar Farms* Garden Vege), 2.4-oz. patty .. 4.0 5

(*Worthington Prosage* Links), 1.6 oz., 2 links .... 9.0 .... 1.5

(*Worthington Prosage* Patties), 1.3-oz. patty ..... 7.0 .... 2.0

ground (*Worthington*), 1.9 oz., ½ cup .... 6.0 .... 1.5

links (*Green Giant* Breakfast Links), 2.4 oz., 3 links 8.0 5

roll (*Worthington Prosage*), 1.9 oz., ⅝" slice ..... 10.5 .... 2.0

Sausage breakfast sandwich, see "Sausage sandwich"

Sausage gravy mix (*Durkee/French's*), ⅛ pkg. .... 2.0 .... 1.0

Sausage sandwich, frozen:

biscuit:

(*Hormel Quick Meal*), 1 piece .... 22.0 .... 6.0

(*Schwan's*), 3.2 oz. .... 23.0 .... 8.0

(*Weight Watchers*), 3 oz. .... 11.0 .... 3.5

and cheese (*Hormel Quick Meal*), 1 piece .... 26.0 .... 10.0

and gravy (*Schwan's*), 1 piece .... 15.0 .... 5.0

and egg (*Hormel Quick Meal*), 1 piece .... 24.0 .... 8.0

egg and cheese (*Great Starts*), 5.5 oz. .... 30.0 .... 12.0

	total fat (grams)	saturated fat (grams)
muffin, egg and cheese (*Hormel Quick Meal*), 1 piece	23.0	10.0
Savory, ground:		
1 tbsp.	.3	0
1 tsp.	.1	0
Scallion, see "Onion, green"		
Scallop, mixed species, meat only:		
raw, 4 oz.	.9	.1
raw, 2 large or 5 small, about 1.1 oz.	.2	<.1
breaded, fried, 2 large, about 1.1 oz.	3.4	.8
"Scallop," vegetarian, canned (*Worthington Skallops*), 3 oz., ½ cup	1.5	.5
Scallop squash:		
raw, untrimmed, 1 lb.	.9	.2
raw, sliced, ½ cup	.1	<.1
boiled, drained, sliced, or mashed, ½ cup	.2	<.1
Scrapple (*Jones Dairy Farm*), 2 oz.	8.0	3.0
Scrod, fresh, see "Cod, Atlantic"		
Scrod entree, frozen, New England style (*Schwan's*), 5-oz. piece	13.0	2.5
Scup, meat only, raw, 4 oz.	3.1	n.a.
Sea bass, mixed species, meat only:		
raw, 4 oz.	2.3	.6
baked, broiled, or microwaved, 4 oz.	2.9	.7
Sea trout, mixed species, meat only, raw, 4 oz.	4.1	1.2
Seafood, see specific listings		
Seafood entree, frozen, and okra gumbo (*Bodin's*), 7 oz.	1.0	0
Seafood cocktail sauce, see "Cocktail sauce"		
Seasoning (see also specific listings):		
all-purpose (*Perc*), 1 tsp.	.3	0
all-purpose and herb (*Perc*), 1 tsp.	<.1	0
country, zesty (*Perc*), 1 tsp.	0	0
garden (*Perc*), 1 tsp.	0	0

	total fat (grams)	saturated fat (grams)
Seasoning *(cont.)*		
garden, extra spicy (*Perc*), 1 tsp.	.1	0
hot and spicy (*Perc*), 1 tsp.	.1	0
salt-free (*Lawry's* 17), ¼ tsp.	0	0
spice and herb medley (*Perc*), 1 tsp.	.1	0
Seasoning and coating mix (see also specific listings):		
country mild (*Shake'N Bake*), ⅛ pkg.	2.0	1.0
honey mustard (*Shake'N Bake*), ⅛ pkg.	1.0	0
Italian herb (*Shake'N Bake*), ⅛ pkg.	.5	0
tangy honey (*Shake'N Bake*), ⅛ pkg.	1.0	0
Seaweed:		
agar:		
raw, 1 oz.	tr.	tr.
dried, 1 oz.	.1	<.1
bars (*Eden* Gelatin), 1 tbsp.	0	0
flakes (*Eden*), 1 tbsp.	0	0
arame, wakame, or hiziki (*Eden*), ½ cup	0	0
Irish moss, raw, 1 oz.	<.1	tr.
kelp, raw, 1 oz.	.2	.1
kombu, pressed (*Eden*), ½ of 7" sheet	0	0
laver, raw, 1 oz.	.1	<.1
nori, pressed (*Eden*), 1 sheet	0	0
wakame, raw, 1 oz.	.1	<.1
Semolina, whole grain, 1 cup	1.8	.3
Sesame butter (see also "Tahini"):		
(*Roaster Fresh*), 1 oz.	15.0	2.2
paste from whole seeds, 1 oz.	14.5	2.0
paste from whole seeds, 1 tbsp.	8.1	1.1
Sesame flour:		
high fat, 1 oz.	10.5	1.5
partially defatted, 1 oz.	3.4	.5
low-fat, 1 oz.	.5	.1
Sesame meal, partially defatted, 1 oz.	13.6	1.9
Sesame oil:		
1 tbsp.	13.6	1.9

	total fat (grams)	saturated fat (grams)
(*Eden*), regular/hot pepper, 1 tbsp.	14.0	2.0
(*Hain*), 1 tbsp.	14.0	2.0
Sesame paste, see "Sesame butter" and "Tahini"		
Sesame seasoning, regular, w/garlic		
or w/seaweed (*Eden* Organic), ½ tsp.	.5	0
Sesame seeds:		
whole:		
dried, 1 oz.	14.1	2.0
dried, ¼ cup	17.9	2.5
dried, 1 tbsp.	4.5	.6
roasted and toasted, 1 oz.	13.6	1.9
hulled kernels:		
dried, 1 oz.	15.5	2.2
dried, ¼ cup	20.6	2.9
dried, 1 tbsp.	4.4	.6
toasted, 1 oz.	13.6	1.9
hulled or unhulled (*Arrowhead Mills*), ¼ cup	20.0	2.5
Sesame sticks (*Barbara's*), 1.1 oz., 30 pieces	2.5	0
Sesbania flower:		
raw, untrimmed, 1 lb.	.2	0
raw or steamed, 1 cup	<.1	0
Shad, American, meat only, raw, 4 oz.	3.9	n.a.
Shallot:		
fresh, untrimmed, 1 lb.	.4	.1
fresh, chopped, 1 tbsp.	<.1	0
freeze-dried, ¼ cup	<.1	0
Shark, mixed species, meat only, raw, 4 oz.	5.1	1.1
Sheanut oil, 1 tbsp.	13.6	6.3
Sheepshead, meat only:		
raw, 4 oz.	2.7	.7
baked, broiled, or microwaved, 4 oz.	1.8	.4
Shellie beans, canned:		
(*Stokely*), ½ cup	0	0
w/liquid, ½ cup or 4 oz.	.2	<.1

	total fat (grams)	saturated fat (grams)

Shells, pasta, entree, see "Pasta shells entree"
Shepherd's pie, see "Beef entree, frozen"
Sherbet:

all flavors (*Blue Bell*), ½ cup	1.0	1.0
all flavors (*Schwan's*), ½ cup	1.0	.5
all flavors (*Weeks*), ½ cup	1.0	.5
lime or orange (*Blue Bell* Snack Cups), 3-fl.-oz. cup	1.0	0
(*Nestlé Flintstones* Push-Up Treats), 2.75 oz.	2.0	1.0
orange, ½ cup	1.9	1.1

Sherbet and cream, orange (*Borden/Meadow Gold Low Fat*), ½ cup ... 2.0 .... 1.0

Shortening, 1 tbsp.:

(*Crisco/Crisco* Butter Flavor)	12.0	3.0
lard or vegetable oil	12.8	5.2
hydrogenated soy and cottonseed oil	12.8	3.2
hydrogenated soy and palm oil	12.8	3.9

Shrimp, mixed species, meat only:

raw, 4 oz., about 16 large	2.0	.4
boiled, poached, or steamed, 4 oz.	1.2	.3
boiled, poached, or steamed, .8 oz., about 4 large	.2	.1
breaded, fried, 4 large, about 1.1 oz.	3.7	.6

Shrimp, canned, drained:

4 oz.	2.2	.4
1 cup, about 4.5 oz.	2.5	.5

"Shrimp," imitation, made from surimi, 4 oz. ... 1.7 .... n.a.
Shrimp cocktail (*Vita*), 4-oz. jar ... 0 0
Shrimp dinner, frozen:

Creole (*Armour Classics* Lite), 10 oz.	.5	0
marinara (*Healthy Choice*), 10.5 oz.	1.0	<1.0
mariner (*The Budget Gourmet* Light & Healthy), 11 oz.	6.0	2.0

Shrimp entree, freeze-dried*:

Alfredo (*AlpineAire*), 1½ cups	3.0	n.a.

	total fat (grams)	saturated fat (grams)
Newburg (*AlpineAire*), 1½ cups	6.0	n.a.
Shrimp entree, frozen:		
battered, beer (*Gorton's* Premium), 6 pieces	15.0	2.5
battered, fantail (*SeaPak* Shrimp 'n Batter), 6 pieces	9.0	2.0
breaded:		
(*Gorton's* Original Premium), 6 pieces	13.0	2.5
whole (*Gorton's* Microwavable), 4-oz. pkg.	16.0	2.5
whole (*Mrs. Paul's* Special Recipe), 5.5 oz., 8 pieces	10.0	2.0
whole (*Schwan's*), 7 pieces	9.0	1.5
whole (*Van de Kamp's*), 7 pieces	10.0	1.5
butterfly (*Van de Kamp's*), 7 pieces	14.0	2.5
butterfly, raw (*SeaPak*), 4 oz., about 8 pieces	1.0	0
butterfly (*SeaPak* Oven Crunchy), 3 oz., about 4 pieces	9.0	1.0
fantail (*Schwan's*), 4 pieces	1.5	0
marinara (*Weight Watchers Smart Ones*), 9 oz.	2.0	.5
popcorn:		
(*Gorton's*), 1 cup	16.0	3.0
(*SeaPak* Oven Crunchy), 3 oz., 15 pieces	12.0	2.0
breaded (*Van de Kamp's*), 20 pieces	13.0	2.0
garlic and herb (*Gorton's*), 1¼ cup	13.0	3.0
microwave (*SeaPak*), 3 oz., about 14 pieces	9.0	1.0
poppers (*SeaPak* Oven Crunchy), 3 oz., 20 pieces	12.0	2.0
scampi (*Gorton's*), 6 pieces	16.0	3.0
stir-fry, see "Stir-fry entree"		
Shrimp hors d'oeuvre, frozen, Newberg, (*Pepperidge Farm* Kit), 1 filled shell	20.0	7.0
Sisymbrium seeds, whole, dried, 1 oz.	1.3	.3

	total fat (grams)	saturated fat (grams)

Sloppy Joe sauce:
  canned:

(*Green Giant*), ¼ cup	0	0
(*Hormel Not-So-Sloppy Joe Sauce*), ¼ cup	0	0
all varieties (*Del Monte*), ¼ cup	0	0
regular or barbecue (*Libby's*), ⅓ cup	0	0
frozen (*Banquet Hot Sandwich Toppers*), 4 oz.	7.0	3.0

Sloppy Joe seasoning mix:

(*Durkee/French's*), ⅙ pkg.	0	0
(*Lawry's* Spices & Seasonings), 1 tsp.	0	0
(*McCormick*), ⅛ pkg.	0	0

Smelt, rainbow, meat only:

raw, 4 oz.	2.8	.5
baked, broiled, or microwaved, 4 oz.	3.5	.7

Snack chips, hot and spicy (*Eden* Wasabi Chips),
  1.1 oz., 50 chips ... 4.0 .... 1.5

Snack mix (see also "Trail mix" and specific
  snack listings), ½ cup, except as noted:

(*Chex Mix* Traditional), ⅔ cup	3.5	1.0
(*Chex Mix* Bold n' Zesty)	7.0	1.5
(*Eagle*)	7.0	1.0
(*Pepperidge Farm Goldfish* Original)	8.0	1.5
honey mustard and onion (*Pepperidge Farm*)	10.0	1.5

  cheddar:

(*Chex Mix*), ⅔ cup	4.5	1.0
smokey (*Pepperidge Farm*)	10.0	1.5
zesty (*Pepperidge Farm Goldfish*)	10.0	1.5
w/*Goldfish* (*Pepperidge Farm*)	8.0	1.0
nutty, extra (*Pepperidge Farm*)	9.0	1.5
pepperoni cheese pizza-flavored (*Combos*), 1.7-oz. bag	11.0	2.0
pepperoni cheese pizza-flavored (*Combos*), 1 oz.	7.0	1.0
savory, seasoned, or spicy (*Pepperidge Farm*)	8.0	1.0

Snail, sea, see "Whelk"

Snap beans, see "Green

	total fat (grams)	saturated fat (grams)
beans"		
Snapper, mixed species, meat only:		
raw, 4 oz.	1.5	.3
baked, broiled, or microwaved, 4 oz.	2.0	.1
Snow peas, see "Peas, edible-podded"		
Soba noodles, see "Noodle, Japanese"		
Soft drinks, carbonated, all flavors and brands,		
8 fl. oz.	0	0
Sole:		
fresh, see "Flatfish"		
frozen (*Van de Kamp's* Natural), 4 oz.	1.5	1.0
Sole entree, frozen, fillets, lightly breaded		
(*Van de Kamp's*), 1 piece	11.0	2.0
Sopressata sausage:		
(*Ideal*), 2 oz.	19.0	5.0
mini (*Cinghiale*), 1 oz.	8.0	3.0
Sorbet (see also "Ice" and "Sherbet"), ½ cup:		
all fruit varieties (*Garden of Eatin'* Fruit Glace)	0	0
orange and cream (*Häagen-Dazs*)	8.0	4.0
raspberry and cream (*Häagen-Dazs*)	7.0	4.0
Sorghum, whole grain, 1 cup	6.3	.9
Sorghum syrup:		
½ cup	0	0
(*Arrowhead Mills*), 1 tbsp.	0	0
Sorrel, see "Dock"		
Soup, canned, ready-to-serve, 1 cup, except as noted:		
all varieties (*Health Valley* Fat Free)	0	0
bean:		
black (*Progresso* Hearty)	1.5	0
black, w/bacon (*Old El Paso*)	1.5	.5
and ham (*Campbell's Chunky*)	2.0	.5
and ham (*Campbell's Chunky*), 10.5-oz. can	3.0	1.0
and ham (*Healthy Choice*), 7.5 oz.	2.0	1.0
and ham (*Hormel*), 7.5 oz.	4.0	1.5
and ham (*Progresso*)	2.0	.5

	total fat (grams)	saturated fat (grams)
Soup, canned, bean *(cont.)*		
w/ham, chunky	8.5	3.3
beef:		
(*Healthy Choice* Hearty), 7.5 oz.	1.0	<1.0
(*Old El Paso* Hearty)	2.5	1.5
barley (*Progresso*)	4.0	1.5
barley (*Progresso* Healthy Classics)	2.0	1.0
chowder, chunky (*Nalley*), 7.5 oz.	3.0	1.5
chunky	5.1	2.6
minestrone (*Progresso*)	4.0	1.5
noodle (*Progresso*)	3.0	1.5
and pasta (*Campbell's Chunky*)	3.0	1.0
and potato (*Healthy Choice*), 7.5 oz.	1.0	<1.0
w/vegetables (*Campbell's Chunky*)	4.0	1.0
vegetable (*Hormel*), 7.5 oz.	1.0	0
vegetable (*Progresso* Healthy Classics)	1.5	.5
vegetable, country (*Campbell's Chunky*)	5.0	1.5
vegetable and rotini (*Progresso* Pasta Soups)	3.5	1.5
beef broth (*Weight Watchers*)	0	0
beef broth or bouillon	.5	.3
black bean, see "bean," above		
borscht (*Gold's*)	0	0
broccoli:		
cheese w/ham (*Hormel*), 1 cup	13.0	5.0
cream of (*Progresso*)	3.0	.5
and shells (*Progresso* Pasta Soups)	1.0	0
chickarina (*Progresso*)	5.0	2.0
chicken:		
(*Healthy Choice* Hearty), 7.5 oz.	2.0	<1.0
(*Progresso* Hearty), 10.5-oz. can	2.5	.5
barley (*Progresso*)	2.5	.5
broccoli cheese w/potato (*Campbell's Chunky*)	12.0	5.0
chowder, chunky (*Nalley*), 7.5 oz.	3.5	1.5
chowder w/mushrooms (*Campbell's Chunky*)	12.0	4.0

	total fat (grams)	saturated fat (grams)
chunky	6.6	2.0
corn chowder (*Campbell's Chunky*)	15.0	7.0
cream of (*Progresso*)	10.0	3.5
minestrone (*Progresso*)	3.5	1.0
noodle (*Campbell's* Low Sodium), 10.75-oz. can	5.0	1.5
noodle (*Campbell's* Microwave), 10.5-oz. cup	4.0	1.0
noodle (*Campbell's Chunky* Classic)	4.0	1.0
noodle (*Campbell's Healthy Request*)	3.0	1.0
noodle (*Campbell's Home Cookin'*)	3.5	1.0
noodle (*Healthy Choice* Old Fashioned), 7.5 oz.	2.0	<1.0
noodle (*Hormel*), 7.5 oz.	3.0	1.0
noodle (*Old El Paso* Hearty)	3.0	1.0
noodle (*Progresso*), 10.5-oz can	2.5	.5
noodle (*Progresso*), 19 oz.	2.0	.5
noodle (*Progresso* Healthy Classics)	2.0	.5
noodle (*Weight Watchers*), 10.5-oz. can	2.0	.5
noodle, w/meatballs	3.6	1.1
noodle, w/mushroom (*Campbell's Chunky*)	5.0	1.5
noodle, w/mushroom (*Campbell's Chunky*), 10.5-oz. can	6.0	2.0
w/pasta (*Healthy Choice*), 7.5 oz.	2.0	1.0
w/pasta (*Pritikin*)	1.0	0
w/rice (*Campbell's* Microwave), 10.5-oz. cup	2.5	1.0
w/rice (*Campbell's Healthy Request*)	3.0	1.0
w/rice (*Campbell's Home Cookin'*)	3.0	1.0
w/rice (*Healthy Choice*), 7.5 oz.	1.0	<1.0
w/rice (*Hormel*), 7.5 oz.	3.0	1.0
w/rice (*Old El Paso*)	2.5	.5
w/rice (*Pritikin*)	1.0	0
w/rice (*Weight Watchers*), 10.5 oz.	1.5	0
rice, chunky	3.2	1.0
rice, w/vegetable (*Progresso*), 10.5-oz. can	4.0	1.0

	total fat (grams)	saturated fat (grams)

Soup, canned, chicken *(cont.)*

rice, w/vegetable (*Progresso* 19 oz.)	3.0	1.0
rice, w/vegetable (*Progresso* Healthy Classics)	1.5	0
and rotini (*Progresso* Hearty Pasta Soups)	2.0	.5
spicy, and penne (*Progresso* Hearty Pasta Soups)	4.0	1.0
vegetable, chunky	4.8	1.4
vegetable (*Campbell's Healthy Request*)	2.0	1.0
vegetable (*Old El Paso*)	2.5	.5
vegetable (*Progresso* Homestyle)	2.5	.5
vegetable and penne (*Progresso* Pasta Soups)	2.5	.5
and wild rice (*Progresso*)	2.0	.5
chicken broth:		
(*Campbell's Healthy Request*)	0	0
(*College Inn*)	4.0	1.0
(*Pritikin*)	0	0
(*Progresso*)	.5	0
(*Weight Watchers*), .16 oz.	0	0
chili bean (*Pritikin*)	.5	0
chili beef (*Healthy Choice*), 7.5 oz.	1.0	<1.0
clam chowder, Manhattan (*Progresso*)	2.0	0
clam chowder, Manhattan, chunky	3.4	2.1
clam chowder, New England:		
(*Campbell's Chunky*)	15.0	6.0
(*Campbell's Chunky*), 10.5-oz. can	18.0	7.0
(*Campbell's Healthy Request*)	3.0	1.0
(*Campbell's Home Cookin'*), 10.75-oz. can	19.0	6.0
(*Campbell's Home Cookin'*)	14.0	5.0
(*Hormel*), 7.5 oz.	5.0	2.5
(*Nalley* Puget Sound), 7.5 oz.	6.0	4.0
(*Progresso*), 10.5-oz. can	12.0	3.5
(*Progresso*), 18.5 oz.	10.0	3.0
(*Progresso* Healthy Classics)	2.0	.5

	total fat (grams)	saturated fat (grams)
clam and rotini chowder (*Progresso* Pasta Soups)	9.0	2.0
corn chowder (*Progresso*)	10.0	4.0
crab	1.5	.4
escarole	1.8	.5
escarole in chicken broth (*Progresso*)	1.0	0
garlic and pasta (*Progresso* Healthy Classics)	1.5	0
gazpacho	2.2	.3
lentil:		
(*Healthy Choice*), 7.5 oz.	1.0	<1.0
(*Pritikin*)	.5	0
(*Progresso*), 10.5-oz. can	2.5	0
(*Progresso*), 19 oz.	2.0	0
(*Progresso* Healthy Classics)	1.5	0
w/ham	2.8	1.1
w/sausage (*Progresso*)	7.0	2.0
and shells (*Progresso* Pasta Soups)	1.5	0
vegetarian (*Hain* 99% Fat Free), 10.5-oz. can	2.0	0
vegetarian (*Hain* 99% Fat Free), ½ of 19-oz. can	1.0	0
macaroni and bean (*Progresso*)	4.0	1.0
meatballs and pasta pearls (*Progresso* Pasta Soups)	7.0	3.0
minestrone:		
(*Campbell's Healthy Request*)	2.0	.5
(*Campbell's Home Cookin'*)	2.0	1.0
(*Healthy Choice*), 7.5 oz.	1.0	<1.0
(*Pritikin*)	1.0	0
(*Progresso*), 10.5-oz. can	3.5	.5
(*Progresso*), 19 oz.	2.5	.5
(*Progresso* Healthy Classics)	2.5	0
(*Weight Watchers*), 10.5 oz.	2.0	.5
chunky	2.8	1.5
and shells (*Progresso* Hearty Pasta Soups)	1.5	0
Tuscany-style (*Campbell's Home Cookin'*)	7.0	1.5

	total fat (grams)	saturated fat (grams)

Soup, canned, minestrone *(cont.)*

zesty (*Progresso*)	6.0	2.5
mushroom, cream of:		
(*Campbell's* Low Sodium), 10.75-oz. can	14.0	4.0
(*Campbell's Healthy Request*)	3.0	1.0
(*Campbell's Home Cookin'*)	13.0	6.0
(*Progresso*)	8.0	3.5
pea, split:		
(*Campbell's* Low Sodium), 10.75-oz. can	4.0	3.0
(*Pritikin*)	.5	0
(*Progresso* Healthy Classics)	2.5	1.0
green (*Progresso*)	3.0	1.0
w/ham (*Campbell's Home Cookin'*)	1.5	.5
w/ham (*Healthy Choice*), 7.5 oz.	3.0	1.0
w/ham (*Progresso*)	4.0	1.5
penne, in broth (*Progresso* Hearty Pasta Soups)	1.0	0
pepper steak (*Campbell's Chunky*)	2.5	1.0
potato cheese w/ham (*Hormel*), 1 cup	13.0	5.0
potato ham chowder (*Campbell's Chunky*)	14.0	8.0
sirloin burger, w/vegetables (*Campbell's Chunky*)	9.0	3.5
sirloin burger, w/vegetables (*Campbell's Chunky*), 10.5-oz. can.	11.0	4.5
tomato:		
(*Campbell's Healthy Request*)	2.0	.5
(*Progresso*)	2.0	0
beef, w/rotini (*Progresso*)	4.5	1.5
garden (*Healthy Choice*), 7.5 oz.	3.0	1.0
and rotini (*Progresso* Hearty Pasta Soups)	1.0	0
w/tomato pieces (*Campbell's* Low Sodium), 10.75-oz. can	6.0	2.5
tortellini (*Progresso* Pasta Soups)	5.0	1.5
vegetable (*Progresso* Hearty Classics)	1.0	0
tortellini, w/chicken broth (*Progresso*)	2.0	.5
tortellini, creamy (*Progresso*)	15.0	8.0

	total fat (grams)	saturated fat (grams)
turkey rice, white and wild (*Healthy Choice*), 7.5 oz.	2.0	1.0
turkey vegetable (*Healthy Choice*), 7.5 oz.	3.0	1.0
vegetable:		
(*Campbell's Chunky*)	3.0	1.0
(*Campbell's Chunky*), 10.5-oz. can	4.0	1.0
(*Campbell's Home Cookin'* Fiesta)	2.5	.5
(*Pritikin* Hearty)	.5	0
(*Progresso*)	2.0	.5
(*Progresso* Healthy Classics)	1.5	0
(*Weight Watchers*), 10.5 oz.	1.0	0
beef (*Campbell's Chunky*)	5.0	1.5
beef (*Healthy Choice*), 7.5 oz.	1.0	<1.0
beef (*Campbell's Healthy Request*)	2.5	1.0
beef (*Campbell's Home Cookin'*), 10.75 oz. can	2.5	1.5
beef (*Campbell's Home Cookin'*)	2.0	1.0
beef, chunky (*Campbell's* Low Sodium), 10.75-oz. can	4.5	1.5
chunky	3.7	.6
country (*Campbell's Home Cookin'*), 10.75-oz. can	2.0	0
country (*Campbell's Home Cookin'*)	1.0	0
country (*Healthy Choice*), 7.5 oz.	1.0	<1.0
garden (*Healthy Choice*), 7.5 oz.	1.0	<1.0
garden (*Old El Paso*)	2.5	.5
hearty (*Campbell's Healthy Request*)	1.0	0
Italian (*Campbell's Home Cookin'*)	4.0	1.5
w/pasta (*Campbell's Chunky*)	3.0	.5
and rotini (*Progresso* Hearty Pasta Soups)	1.0	0
Southwestern, w/black beans & rice (*Campbell's Healthy Request*)	1.5	.5
vegetarian (*Pritikin*)	0	0
vegetable broth (*Pritikin*)	0	0

	total fat (grams)	saturated fat (grams)

Soup, canned, condensed, undiluted, ½ cup:

asparagus, cream of (*Campbell's*)	7.0	2.0
bean, w/bacon (*Campbell's*)	5.0	2.0
beef broth or bouillon (*Campbell's*)	0	0
beef noodle (*Campbell's*)	2.5	1.0
broccoli, cheese (*Campbell's*)	7.0	3.0
broccoli, creamy (*Campbell's Healthy Request*)	2.0	1.0
celery, cream of (*Campbell's*)	7.0	2.5
cheese, cheddar (*Campbell's*)	10.0	5.0
cheese, nacho, fiesta (*Campbell's*)	8.0	4.0
chicken:		
cream of (*Campbell's*)	8.0	3.0
cream of, and broccoli (*Campbell's*)	8.0	2.5
gumbo (*Campbell's*)	1.5	.5
mushroom, creamy (*Campbell's*)	9.0	2.5
noodle (*Campbell's*)	2.5	1.0
noodle (*Campbell's NoodleO's*)	3.0	1.0
noodle, creamy (*Campbell's*)	7.0	2.0
w/rice, hearty (*Campbell's*)	2.5	1.0
w/rice, white and wild (*Campbell's*)	2.0	.5
and stars (*Campbell's*)	2.0	.5
vegetable (*Campbell's*)	2.0	.5
chicken broth (*Campbell's*)	2.0	.5
clam chowder:		
Manhattan (*Bookbinder's*)	.5	0
Manhattan (*Campbell's*)	2.0	.5
New England (*Bookbinder's*)	3.0	.5
New England (*Campbell's*)	2.5	.5
New England (*Snow's*)	1.5	0
corn, golden (*Campbell's*)	3.5	1.0
crab bisque (*Bookbinder's*)	7.0	3.0
lobster bisque (*Bookbinder's*)	4.0	3.0
minestrone (*Campbell's*)	2.0	1.0
mushroom, cream of (*Campbell's*)	7.0	2.5
mushroom, golden (*Campbell's*)	3.0	1.0

	total fat (grams)		saturated fat (grams)
noodle, double, in chicken broth (*Campbell's*)	2.5	....	1.0
onion, French (*Campbell's*)	2.5	....	0
oyster stew (*Bookbinder's*)	5.0	....	1.5
pea, split, w/ham and bacon (*Campbell's*)	3.5	....	2.0
potato, cream of (*Campbell's*)	3.0	....	1.5
seafood bisque (*Bookbinder's*)	8.0	....	3.0
shrimp bisque (*Bookbinder's*)	7.0	....	3.0
snapper (*Bookbinder's*)	6.0	....	1.5
tomato:			
(*Campbell's*)	2.0	....	0
(*Campbell's* Healthy Request)	2.0	....	.5
bisque (*Campbell's*)	3.0	....	1.5
Italian, w/basil and oregano (*Campbell's*)	.5	....	0
rice (*Campbell's* Old Fashioned)	2.0	....	.5
vegetable, hearty, w/pasta (*Campbell's*)	1.0	....	0
vegetable beef (*Campbell's*)	2.0	....	1.0
Soup, freeze-dried, 1½ cup*:			
bean, multi (*AlpineAire*)	.5	....	0
broccoli, cream of (*AlpineAire*)	5.0	....	n.a.
minestrone (*AlpineAire* Alpine)	2.0	....	n.a.
potato cheddar, creamy (*AlpineAire*)	7.0	....	n.a.
Soup, frozen:			
barley mushroom (*Tabatchnick*), 7.5 oz.	0	....	0
bean (*Tabatchnick* Yankee), 7.5 oz.	1.5	....	0
beef, hearty (*Old El Paso*), 1 cup	2.5	....	1.5
black bean, w/bacon (*Old El Paso*), 1 cup	1.5	....	.5
Boston clam chowder (*Schwan's*), 1 cup	8.0	....	2.5
broccoli, cream of (*Schwan's*), 1 cup	10.0	....	6.0
broccoli, cream of (*Tabatchnick*), 7.5 oz.	4.0	....	2.0
cabbage (*Tabatchnick*), 7.5 oz.	0	....	0
cheddar vegetable (*Tabatchnick* Wisconsin), 7.5 oz.	9.0	....	3.0
chicken:			
(*Tabatchnick* New York), 7.5 oz.	0	....	0
w/dumplings (*Tabatchnick*), 7.5 oz.	2.0	....	0

	total fat (grams)	saturated fat (grams)

Soup, frozen, chicken *(cont.)*

noodle, hearty (*Old El Paso*), 1 cup	3.0	1.0
rice or vegetable (*Old El Paso*), 1 cup	2.5	.5
corn chowder (*Tabatchnick*), 7.5 oz.	6.0	2.0
minestrone (*Tabatchnick*), 7.5 oz.	1.0	0
pea (*Tabatchnick*), 7.5 oz.	1.5	0
potato (*Tabatchnick* New England), 7.5 oz.	6.0	2.5
potato (*Tabatchnick* Old Fashioned), 7.5 oz.	0	0
spinach, cream of (*Tabatchnick*), 7.5 oz.	4.0	2.0
vegetable (*Tabatchnick*), 7.5 oz.	1.0	0
vegetable, garden (*Old El Paso*), 1 cup	2.5	.5
Wisconsin cheese (*Schwan's*), 1 cup	10.0	5.0

Soup mix, dry:

all varieties (*Health Valley* Fat Free), ⅓ cup	0	0
almond chicken (*Casbah*), 1.5-oz. container	1.5	0
asparagus au gratin (*Casbah*), 1.5-oz. container	2.0	0
barley:		
(*Aunt Patsy's Pantry*), 1 cup	.5	0
(*Buckeye* Beefed Up), ⅛ pkg.	1.0	0
chowder (*Buckeye* Burgoo), ⅛ pkg.	1.0	0
bean:		
(*Buckeye* Northwest Bean Pot), ⅛ pkg.	1.0	0
black (*Aunt Patsy's Pantry/Buckeye*), ⅙ pkg.	1.0	0
black (*Fantastic Jumpin' Black Beans*), 2 oz.	1.0	0
black (*Knorr*), 1.9-oz. container	1.0	0
black, and rice (*Uncle Ben's*), 1.5 oz., about ¼ pkg.	1.5	0
five (*Fantastic Foods*), 2.2 oz.	1.0	0
many (*Aunt Patsy's Pantry*), 1 cup	.5	0
navy (*Aunt Patsy's Pantry*), 1 cup	0	0
navy (*Knorr*), 1.3-oz. container	0	0
7, and barley, all varieties (*Arrowhead Mills*), ¼ cup	0	0
(*Buckeye* Many Mac), ⅒ pkg.	1.0	0

	total fat (grams)	saturated fat (grams)
broccoli, cream of (*Knorr Chef's Collection*), ½ pkg.	3.0	1.0
broccoli and cheddar, creamy (*Fantastic Foods*), 1.5 oz.	2.0	1.0
broccoli and cheese (*Cup-a-Soup*), 1 pkt.	3.0	1.5
(*Casbah* La Fresta), 1.5-oz. container	1.0	0
cheddar, broccoli (*Casbah*), 1.3-oz. container	2.0	1.0
chicken:		
broth (*Cup-a-Soup*), 1 pkt.	1.0	0
cream of (*Cup-a-Soup*), 1 pkt.	2.5	.5
noodle (*Cup-a-Soup*), 1 pkt.	1.0	.5
noodle, hearty (*Cup-a-Soup*), 1 pkt.	1.0	.5
noodle, hearty (*Lipton*), ¼ cup	2.0	.5
supreme (*Cup-a-Soup*), 1 pkt.	4.0	2.0
thyme (*Aunt Patsy's Pantry*), 1 cup	.5	0
vegetable (*Cup-a-Soup*), 1 pkt.	1.0	.5
chicken flavor noodle (*Knorr*), ⅓ pkg.	1.0	.5
chicken flavor vegetable (*Knorr*), 1.1-oz. container	0	0
chili (*Fantastic Foods Cha-Cha Chili*), 2.3 oz.	1.5	0
corn and potato chowder, creamy (*Fantastic Foods*), 1.7 oz.	1.0	0
couscous, w/lentils (*Fantastic Foods*), 2.1 oz.	1.0	0
harvest, heart (*Casbah*), 1 container	1.0	0
herb:		
fine (*Knorr* Soup & Recipe), ⅓ pkg.	5.0	1.5
golden, w/lemon (*Lipton* Recipe Secrets), 2 tbsp.	.5	0
Italian (*Lipton* Recipe Secrets), 2 tbsp.	0	0
savory, w/garlic (*Lipton* Recipe Secrets), 2 tbsp.	.5	0
hot and sour (*Knorr*), ⅓ pkg.	1.5	.5
jambalaya (*Casbah*), 1.3-oz. container	0	0
leek (*Knorr* Soup & Recipe), ⅓ pkg.	3.0	1.0

	total fat (grams)	saturated fat (grams)

Soup mix *(cont.)*
  lentil:

(*Buckeye* Great Lean N'Lentils), ⅛ pkg.	1.0	0
(*Knorr* Hearty), 2-oz. container	0	0
country (*Fantastic Foods*), 2.2 oz.	1.0	0
minestrone (*Fantastic Foods*), 1.4 oz.	1.0	0
red (*Aunt Patsy's Pantry*), 1 cup	.5	0
Moroccan stew (*Casbah*), 2-oz. container	0	0

  mushroom:

beefy (*Lipton* Recipe Secrets), 1 tbsp.	0	0
creamy (*Cup-a-Soup*), 1 pkt.	2.5	.5
creamy (*Fantastic Foods*), 1.4 oz.	0	0
wild, cream of (*Knorr* Chef's Collection), ½ pkg.	3.0	.5

  noodle:

(*Lipton*), 3 tbsp.	1.0	0
w/chicken (*Lipton*), 3 tbsp.	2.5	1.0
w/real chicken broth (*Lipton*), 2 tbsp.	2.0	1.0
w/real chicken broth (*Lipton* Giggle Noodle), 2 tbsp.	2.0	1.0
w/real chicken broth (*Lipton* Ring-O-Noodle), 2 tbsp.	2.0	1.0
chicken free (*Fantastic Foods*), 1.5 oz. ..	.5	0
ring (*Cup-a-Soup*), 1 pkt.	1.0	0
w/vegetables (*Lipton*), 3 tbsp.	2.0	1.0
vegetable curry (*Fantastic Foods*), 1.5 oz.	1.0	0
vegetable miso (*Fantastic Foods*), 1.3 oz.	1.0	0
vegetable tomato (*Fantastic Foods*), 1.5 oz. ...	1.0	0

  onion:

(*Campbell's* Soup & Recipe Mix), 1 tbsp.	0	0
(*Lipton* Recipe Secrets), 1 tbsp.	0	0
beefy (*Lipton* Recipe Secrets), 1 tbsp.	.5	0
French (*Knorr* Soup & Recipe), ⅓ pkg.	1.0	.5
golden (*Lipton* Recipe Secrets), 2 tbsp.	1.5	0
mushroom (*Lipton* Recipe Secrets), 2 tbsp. ...	1.0	0

	total fat (grams)		saturated fat (grams)
orzo thyme (*Buckeye*), ¼ pkg.	1.0	....	0
oxtail (*Knorr* Soup & Recipe), ⅓ pkg.	2.5	....	1.0
pasta (*Buckeye* Starry Pasta), ¹⁄₁₀ pkg.	0	....	0
pasta (*Casbah* Pasta Fasul), 1.5-oz. container	0	....	0
pea:			
(*Aunt Patsy's Pantry* Plentiful), 1 cup	.5	....	0
(*Buckeye* Country Pea Patchwork), ⅛ pkg.	1.0	....	0
green (*Cup-a-Soup*), 1 pkt.	4.0	....	1.5
snow, cream of (*Knorr Chef's Collection*),			
½ pkg.	2.0	....	.5
split (*Fantastic Foods*), 1.8 oz.	.5	....	0
Virginia (*Cup-a-Soup*), 1 pkt.	5.0	....	2.0
potato leek (*Knorr*), 1.2-oz. container	0	....	0
spinach, cream of (*Knorr* Soup & Recipe),			
⅓ pkg.	2.5	....	1.0
tomato (*Cup-a-Soup*), 1 pkt.	2.0	....	1.0
tomato Parmesan (*Casbah*), 1.8-oz. container	1.5	....	0
tomato rice Parmesano (*Fantastic Foods*),			
1.9 oz.	2.0	....	.5
vegetable:			
(*Knorr* Soup & Recipe), ¼ pkg.	0	....	0
(*Lipton* Recipe Secrets), 3 tbsp.	0	....	0
barley (*Fantastic Foods*), 1.4 oz.	.5	....	0
creamy chicken flavor (*Cup-a-Soup*), 1 pkt.	4.0	....	1.0
hearty harvest (*Cup-a-Soup*), 1 pkt.	1.5	....	.5
spring (*Cup-a-Soup*), 1 pkt.	1.0	....	.5
spring (*Knorr* Soup & Recipe), ⅓ pkg.	0	....	0
Sour cream, see "Cream, sour"			
Sour cream dip mix (*Durkee*), ¼ pkg.	.5	....	0
Soursop:			
untrimmed, 1 lb.	.9	....	n.a.
1 medium, about 2 lbs.	1.9	....	n.a.
Soy bean, see "Soybean"			
Soy beverage ("milk"), 8 fl. oz.:			
(*EdenSoy* Original)	4.0	....	.5

	total fat (grams)	saturated fat (grams)

Soy beverage *(cont.)*
   (*EdenSoy* Extra Original) .... | 5.0 .... | .5
   (*Health Valley Soy Moo*) .... | 0 .... | 0
   carob (*EdenSoy*) .... | 4.0 .... | .5
   vanilla (*EdenSoy/EdenSoy* Extra) .... | 3.0 .... | 0

Item	total fat (grams)	saturated fat (grams)
Soy beverage *(cont.)*		
(*EdenSoy* Extra Original)	5.0	.5
(*Health Valley Soy Moo*)	0	0
carob (*EdenSoy*)	4.0	.5
vanilla (*EdenSoy/EdenSoy* Extra)	3.0	0
Soy beverage mix, dry, all varieties (*Loma Linda Soyagen*), ¼ cup	6.4	1.1
Soy flour:		
(*Arrowhead Mills* Soybean), ¼ cup	9.0	1.5
full-fat, raw, 1 cup stirred	17.6	2.5
full-fat, roasted, 1 cup stirred	18.6	2.7
defatted, 1 cup stirred	1.2	.1
low-fat, 1 cup stirred	2.4	.9
Soy meal, defatted, raw, 1 cup	2.9	.3
Soy milk, see "Soy beverage"		
Soy nuggets (see also "Burger, vegetarian"), dry (*Love* Organic), 2 oz.	3.0	n.a.
Soy protein:		
concentrate, 1 oz.	.1	.1
isolate, 1 oz.	1.0	.1
Soy sauce, 1 tbsp.:		
all varieties (*House of Tsang*)	0	0
hot or honey (*Chun King Oriental Traditions*)	0	0
(*Kikkoman/Kikkoman* Lite)	0	0
(*Trappey's* Chef Magic)	0	0
shoyu (*Eden/Eden* Reduced Sodium)	0	0
tamari (*Eden*)	0	0
Soybean:		
green:		
raw, in pods, 1 lb.	16.4	1.8
raw, shelled, ½ cup	8.7	1.0
boiled, drained, ½ cup	5.8	.7
dried:		
raw, ½ cup	18.5	2.7
raw (*Arrowhead Mills*), ¼ cup	8.0	1.0

	total fat (grams)	saturated fat (grams)
boiled, ½ cup	7.7	1.1
dry-roasted, ½ cup	18.6	2.7
roasted, ½ cup	21.8	3.2
Soybean, fermented or paste, see "Miso" and "Natto"		
Soybean, sprouted, mature seeds:		
raw, 1 lb.	30.4	4.2
raw, ½ cup	2.3	.3
steamed, ½ cup	2.1	.3
Soybean cake or curd, see "Tofu"		
Soybean dishes, see "Vegetarian dishes" and specific listings		
Soybean grits, see "Cereal, hot or cooking"		
Soybean oil:		
1 tbsp.	13.6	2.0
(*Hain*)	14.0	2.0
(*Hollywood*)	14.0	3.0
Soybean and cottonseed oil, hydrogenated, 1 tbsp.	13.6	2.4
Soybean lecithin oil, 1 tbsp.	13.6	2.1
Spaghetti, dry or plain, see "Pasta"		
Spaghetti dinner, frozen (*Morton*), 8.5 oz.	3.0	1.0
Spaghetti entree, canned or packaged:		
(*Franco American*), 1 cup	2.0	1.0
(*Franco American Spaghetti O's*), 1 cup	2.0	.5
(*Kraft* Mild American), 1 cup	4.5	1.0
and ground beef (*Chef Boyardee* Suprema), 10.5 oz. bowl	6.0	3.0
w/frankfurters:		
(*Franco American*), 1 cup	11.0	5.0
(*Van Camp's* Spaghetti Weenee), 1 can	8.0	2.0
meat sauce (*Hormel* Micro Cup), 7.5-oz. cup	5.0	2.0
meat sauce (*Hormel Top Shelf*), 10-oz. bowl	5.0	2.5
w/meat sauce (*Kraft*), 1 cup	11.0	4.0
w/meatballs:		
(*Chef Boyardee*), 7.5-oz. cup	10.0	4.0
(*Franco American*), 1 cup	10.0	5.0

	total fat (grams)	saturated fat (grams)
Spaghetti entree, canned or packaged, w/meatballs *(cont.)*		
(*Franco American Spaghetti O's*), 1 cup	9.0	4.0
(*Franco American Where's Waldo?*), 1 cup	11.0	5.0
(*Hormel*), 7.5-oz. can	7.0	4.0
(*Hormel Kid's Kitchen*), 7.5 oz.	7.0	3.0
(*Hormel Micro Cup*), 7.5 oz.	7.0	3.0
(*Libby's Diner*), 7.75 oz.	5.0	2.0
rings (*Hormel Kid's Kitchen*), 7.5 oz.	1.0	1.0
tangy (*Kraft*), 1 cup	4.5	1.0
Spaghetti entree, freeze-dried*:		
w/meat and sauce (*Mountain House*), 1 cup	5.0	3.0
in mushroom sauce (*AlpineAire*), 1½ cups	1.0	n.a.
Spaghetti entree, frozen:		
(*Healthy Choice Quick Meal*), 10 oz.	6.0	2.0
w/meat sauce:		
(*The Budget Gourmet* Light & Healthy), 10 oz.	7.0	2.5
(*Lean Cuisine*), 11.5 oz.	6.0	1.5
(*Stouffer's Lunch Express*), 9⅝ oz.	10.0	3.5
(*Weight Watchers*), 10 oz.	6.0	2.0
w/meatballs (*Stouffer's*), 12⅝ oz.	15.0	4.0
w/meatballs (*Swanson* Budget), 10 oz.	13.0	6.0
w/meatballs and sauce (*Lean Cuisine*), 9.5 oz.	7.0	2.0
Spaghetti sauce, see "Pasta sauce"		
Spaghetti sauce seasoning mix:		
all varieties (*Durkee*), ⅕ pkg.	0	0
American, Italian, or thick (*French's*), ⅕ pkg.	0	0
mushroom (*French's*), ⅕ pkg.	1.0	0
Spaghetti squash:		
raw, untrimmed, 1 lb.	1.8	.4
raw, cubed, ½ cup	.3	.1
baked or boiled, drained, ½ cup	.2	<.1
Sparerib seasoning mix:		
(*Durkee* Roasting Bag), 1/7 pkg.	0	0
Spareribs, see "Pork," "Pork, frozen or refrigerated," and "Pork dinner"		

	total fat (grams)	saturated fat (grams)
Spelt flour (*Arrowhead Mills*), ¼ cup	.5	0
Spinach:		
fresh:		
raw, untrimmed, 1 lb.	1.1	.2
raw, partially trimmed, 10-oz. pkg.	.7	.1
raw, trimmed, 1 oz. or ½ cup chopped	.1	<.1
boiled, drained, ½ cup	.2	<.1
canned, ½ cup:		
w/liquid	.4	.1
drained	.5	.1
(*Stokely*)	0	0
leaf or chopped (*Allens/Popeye*)	1.0	0
leaf or chopped (*Del Monte*)	0	0
frozen (see also specific listings):		
10-oz. pkg.	.9	.1
boiled, drained, ½ cup	.2	<.1
(*Green Giant/Green Giant Harvest Fresh*), ¾ cup	0	0
au gratin (*The Budget Gourmet* Side Dish), 5.5 oz.	11.0	7.0
in butter sauce (*Green Giant*), ½ cup	1.5	1.0
Spinach, creamed, frozen:		
(*Green Giant*), ½ cup	3.0	1.5
(*Stouffer's* Side Dish), ½ of 9-oz. pkg.	12.0	4.0
(*Tabatchnick*), 7.5 oz.	2.0	1.0
Spinach, New Zealand, see "New Zealand spinach"		
Spinach soufflé, frozen (*Stouffer's* Side Dish), ⅓ of 12-oz. pkg.	10.0	2.0
Spiny lobster, meat only, raw, 4 oz.	1.7	.3
Spleen, braised, 4 oz.:		
beef	4.8	n.a.
lamb	5.4	n.a.
pork	3.6	1.2
veal	3.3	n.a.
Split peas, see "Peas, split"		

	total fat (grams)	saturated fat (grams)
Sponge gourd, raw, trimmed, 1 oz.	.1	tr.
Spot, meat only, raw, 4 oz.	5.6	1.7
Spring onion, see "Onion, green"		
Sprouts, see specific listings		
Sprouts, blended (*Jonathan's Gourmet Sprouts*), 3 oz., 1 cup	0	0
Squab, raw:		
meat w/skin, 1 bird, 7 oz. (9.1 oz. w/bone)	47.4	16.8
meat only, 1 bird, 5.9 oz. (9.1 oz. w/bone and skin)	12.6	3.3
meat only, 1 breast, about 3.6 oz.	4.6	1.2
Squash (see also "Summer squash," "Winter squash," and specific squash listings):		
frozen, sliced (*Stilwell*), ⅔ cup	0	0
Squash seeds, see "Pumpkin seeds"		
Squid, mixed species, meat:		
raw, 4 oz.	1.6	.4
dried, 1 oz.	1.2	n.a.
dipped in flour and fried, 4 oz.	8.5	2.1
Squirrel, meat only:		
roasted, 4 oz.	5.3	.6
roasted, diced, 1 cup	6.5	.7
Star fruit, see "Carambola"		
Steak, see "Beef" and "Beef entree"		
"Steak," vegetarian, see " 'Beef,' vegetarian"		
Steak sandwich, frozen, 1 piece:		
biscuit (*Hormel Quick Meal*)	14.0	4.0
and mushroom (*Mrs. Paterson's Aussie Pie*)	26.0	10.0
Steak sauce, 1 tbsp.:		
(*A.1./A.1.* Bold)	0	0
(*Heinz 57*)	0	0
(*Kikkoman*)	0	0
(*Maull's*)	0	0
(*Tabasco/McIlhenny*)	1.0	0
Carribean style (*Tabasco*)	.2	.1

	total fat (grams)	saturated fat (grams)
Steak spice (*Durkee*), ½ tsp.	0	0
Stew, vegetarian, see "Vegetarian dishes, canned"		
Stir-fry entree, frozen (see also specific listings):		
broccoli (*Green Giant Create-A-Meal*), 2⅓ cups ...	3.5	.5
fajita (*SeaPak* Meal Kit), ½ pkg., 3 fajitas	7.0	0
lo mein (*Green Giant Create-A-Meal*), 2⅓ cups ...	.5	0
Oriental (*SeaPak* Meal Kit), ½ pkg.	2.5	0
primavera (*SeaPak* Meal Kit), ½ pkg.	8.0	.5
scampi primavera (*Gorton's*), 10 oz., ½ pkg.	14.0	8.0
sweet and sour (*Gorton's*), 10 oz., ½ pkg.	1.5	0
sweet and sour (*Green Giant Create-A-Meal*), 1¾ cups	0	0
Szechuan (*Green Giant Create-A-Meal*), 1¾ cups	5.0	.5
teriyaki (*Gorton's*), 10 oz., ½ pkg.	1.5	0
teriyaki (*Green Giant Create-A-Meal*), 1¾ cups ...	0	0
vegetable almond (*Green Giant Create-A-Meal*), 1¾ cups	4.5	0
Stir-fry sauce:		
(*Kikkoman*), 1 tbsp.	0	0
(*House of Tsang Saigon Sizzle*), 1 tbsp.	1.0	0
(*House of Tsang Szechuan Spicy*), 1 tbsp.	.5	0
sweet and sour (*House of Tsang*), 1 tbsp.	0	0
Thai peanut (*San-J* Stir-fry and Dipping Sauce), 2 tbsp.	3.0	.5
Stir-fry sauce mix (Kikkoman), 1 oz.	.3	n.a.
Stomach, pork, raw, 1 oz.	2.7	n.a.
Strawberry:		
fresh:		
untrimmed, 1 lb.	1.6	.1
untrimmed, 1 pint, about 12 oz.	1.2	.1
trimmed, ½ cup	.3	<.1
canned, in syrup, ½ cup	.3	<.1
canned, in syrup (*Wilderness*), ½ cup	0	0
freeze-dried (*AlpineAire*), 1 oz.	.6	0

	total fat (grams)	saturated fat (grams)

Strawberry *(cont.)*
  frozen, sweetened:
    10-oz. pkg. .... .4 .... <.1
    whole or sliced, ½ cup .... .2 .... tr.
    (*Schwan's*), 1¼ cup 0 0
    (*Stilwell*), ⅔ cup 1.0 0
Strawberry float (*R.W. Knudsen*), 8 fl. oz. 0 0
Strawberry juice or drink, all blends, all brands,
    8 fl. oz. 0 0
Strawberry milk, 8 fl. oz.:
    whole (*Nestlé Quik*) .... 9.0 .... 5.0
    lowfat (*Nestlé Quik*) .... 5.0 .... 3.0
Strawberry milk drink, canned:
    (*Sego* Very Strawberry), 1 can .... 5.0 .... 1.0
    (*Sego* Lite Very Strawberry), 1 can .... 4.0 .... n.a.
    creme (*Carnation* Instant Breakfast), 10 fl. oz. 3.0 5
Strawberry milk drink mix:
    (*Nestlé Quik*), 2 tbsp. 0 0
    (*Pillsbury* Instant Breakfast), 1 pkt. 0 0
    creme (*Carnation* Instant Breakfast), 1 pkt. 0 0
Strawberry pastry filling (*Solo*), 2 tbsp. 0 0
Strawberry pie glaze (*Smucker's*), 2 oz. 0 0
Strawberry shake (*Nestlé Killer Shakes*), 1 carton .... 14.0 .... 8.0
Strawberry syrup (*Hershey's*), 2 tbsp. 0 0
Strawberry topping, 2 tbsp.:
    (*Kraft*) 0 0
    (*Mrs. Richardson's*) 0 0
    (*Smucker's*) 0 0
Strawberry-banana drink (*R. W. Knudsen*),
    8 fl. oz. 0 0
Strawberry-banana milk, low fat (*Nestlé Quik*),
    1 carton .... 5.0 .... 3.0
Strawberry-banana shake (*Nestlé Quik*), 1 carton ... 5.0 5
Strawberry-guava juice (*R. W. Knudsen*
    Tropical Blend), 8 fl. oz. 0 0

	total fat (grams)	saturated fat (grams)

String bean, see "Green bean"

Stroganoff entree, see "Beef entree"

Stroganoff seasoning mix:

(*Durkee*), ⅛ pkg.	0	0
(*French's*), ¼ pkg.	2.0	1.0
beef (*Lawry's* Spices & Seasonings), 1 tbsp.	0	0

Stroganoff sauce, see "Cooking sauce"

Stroganoff sauce mix:

½ cup*	5.4	3.4
(*Natural Touch*), 4 tbsp.	3.5	2.0

Strudel, see "Cake"

Stuffing, bread (see also "Bread cubes" and "Stuffing, mix"):

(*Croutettes* Mix), 1 cup	0	0
apple and raisin (*Pepperidge Farm* Distinctive), ½ cup	1.5	0
chicken, classic (*Pepperidge Farm* Distinctive), ½ cup	1.5	0

corn bread:

(*Arnold*), 2.4 oz., 2 cups	4.0	1.0
(*Brownberrry*), 2.4 oz., 2 cups	3.5	.5
(*Pepperidge Farm*), ¾ cup	2.0	0
honey pecan (*Pepperidge Farm* Distinctive), ½ cup	5.0	.5
country style or cube (*Pepperidge Farm*), ¾ cup	1.5	0
herb, country garden (*Pepperidge Farm* Distinctive), ½ cup	5.0	1.0

herb, seasoned:

(*Arnold*), 2.4 oz., 2 cups	3.0	.5
(*Brownberry*), 2 oz., 1 cup	2.5	.5
(*Pepperidge Farm*), ¾ cup	1.5	0

sage and onion:

(*Arnold/Brownberry*), 2.4 oz., 2 cups	3.0	.5
(*Pepperidge Farm* For Turkey), ½ cup	1.5	0

	total fat (grams)	saturated fat (grams)
Stuffing *(cont.)*		
seasoned or unspiced (*Arnold*), 2.4 oz., 2 cups ..	3.0	.5
vegetable harvest and almond (*Pepperidge Farm*		
Distinctive), ½ cup	3.0	.5
wild rice and mushroom (*Pepperidge Farm*		
Distinctive), ½ cup	6.0	1.5
Stuffing, mix:		
beef (*Stove Top*), ⅙ box dry	1.0	0
beef (*Stove Top*), ½ cup*	9.0	1.5
chicken:		
(*Stove Top/Stove Top* Lower Sodium),		
1 oz. dry	1.0	0
(*Stove Top/Stove Top* Lower Sodium),		
½ cup*	9.0	1.5
(*Stove Top* Flexible Serving), 1 oz. dry	3.0	0
(*Stove Top* Flexible Serving), ½ cup*	8.0	1.5
(*Stove Top* Microwave), ⅙ box dry	3.5	.5
(*Stove Top* Microwave), ½ cup*	7.0	1.5
w/rice (*Rice-A-Roni*), 1 cup*	9.0	2.0
cornbread:		
(*Stove Top*), ⅙ box dry	1.0	0
(*Stove Top*), ½ cup*	8.0	1.5
(*Stove Top* Flexible Serving), 1 oz. dry	2.5	0
(*Stove Top* Flexible Serving), ½ cup*	8.0	1.5
homestyle (*Stove Top* Microwave), ⅙ box		
dry	3.5	.5
homestyle (*Stove Top* Microwave), ½ cup* ...	7.0	1.5
w/rice (*Rice-A-Roni*), 1 cup*	8.0	1.5
herb:		
homestyle (*Stove Top* Flexible Serving), 1 oz.		
dry	3.0-	0
homestyle (*Stove Top* Flexible Serving),		
½ cup*	8.0	1.5
savory (*Stove Top*), ⅙ box dry	1.0	0
savory (*Stove Top*), ½ cup*	9.0	1.5

	total fat (grams)	saturated fat (grams)
herb and butter (*Rice-A-Roni*), 1 cup*	9.0	2.0
mushroom and onion (*Stove Top*), ⅙ box dry	1.5	0
mushroom and onion (*Stove Top*), ½ cup*	9.0	1.5
pork (*Stove Top*), ⅙ box dry	1.0	0
pork (*Stove Top*), ½ cup*	9.0	1.5
rice, long grain and wild (*Stove Top*), ⅙ box dry	1.0	0
rice, long grain and wild (*Stove Top*), ½ cup*	9.0	1.5
San Francisco style (*Stove Top*), ⅙ box dry	1.0	0
San Francisco style (*Stove Top*), ½ cup*	9.0	1.5
turkey (*Stove Top*), ⅙ box dry	1.0	0
turkey (*Stove Top*), ½ cup*	9.0	1.5
wild rice (*Rice-A-Roni*), 1 cup*	9.0	2.0
Sturgeon, mixed species, meat only:		
raw, 4 oz.	4.6	1.1
baked, broiled, or microwaved, 4 oz.	5.9	1.3
smoked, 4 oz.	5.0	1.2
Sturgeon roe, see "Caviar"		
Succotash:		
canned, ½ cup:		
(*Seneca*)	0	0
(*Stokely*)	1.0	n.a.
w/whole kernel corn, w/liquid	.6	.1
w/cream style corn	.7	.1
frozen, 10-oz. pkg.	2.5	.5
frozen, boiled, drained, ½ cup	.8	.1
Sugar, all varieties, 1 lb.	0	0
Sugar, substitute, all varieties, 1 tbsp.	0	0
Sugar apple:		
untrimmed, 1 lb.	.7	tr.
1 medium, about 9.9 oz.	.5	tr.
Sugar cane juice, 1 oz.	tr.	0
Sugar cane sticks (*Frieda's*), 3.5 oz.	.4	n.a.
Sugar snap peas, see "Peas, edible-podded"		

	total fat (grams)	saturated fat (grams)
Sukiyaki sauce (*Kikkoman*), 1 tbsp.	0	0
Summer sausage (see also "Thuringer cervelat"):		
(*Hillshire Farm*), 2 oz.	16.0	n.a.
(*Hillshire Farm* Light), 2 oz.	12.0	n.a.
(*Schwan's*), 2 oz.	13.0	5.0
beef (*Hillshire Farm*), 2 oz.	17.0	n.a.
beef (*Usinger's* Lite), 2 oz.	10.2	4.1
w/cheese (*Hillshire Farm*), 2 oz.	18.0	n.a.
Summer squash (see also specific squash listings):		
all varieties:		
raw, untrimmed, 1 lb.	.9	.2
raw, sliced, ½ cup	.1	<.1
boiled, drained, sliced, ½ cup	.3	.1
Sunfish, pumpkinseed, meat only, raw, 4 oz.	.8	.2
Sunflower seed butter:		
1 oz.	13.6	1.4
1 tbsp.	7.6	.8
(*Roaster Fresh*), 1 oz.	13.6	1.6
Sunflower seed flour:		
partially defatted, 1 cup	1.3	.1
partially defatted, 1 tbsp.	.1	tr.
Sunflower seed oil:		
(*Hain*), 1 tbsp.	14.0	2.0
hydrogenated, 1 tbsp.	13.6	1.8
linoleic, 1 tbsp.	13.6	1.4
Sunflower seeds:		
(*Arrowhead Mills*), ¼ cup	15.0	1.5
(*Frito-Lay*), ⅓ cup	8.0	1.0
dried, in shell, 4 oz.	30.5	3.2
dried, kernels, ½ cup	35.7	3.8
dry-roasted:		
in shell (*Planters/Planters* Bull Pen Chew),		
1 oz.	15.0	1.5
kernels, 1 oz.	14.1	1.5

	total fat (grams)	saturated fat (grams)
kernels, ¼ cup	15.9	1.7
kernels (*Planters*), ¼ cup	17.0	1.5
oil-roasted, kernels:		
1 oz.	16.3	1.7
¼ cup	19.4	2.0
(*Planters*), 1 oz.	14.5	1.5
barbecue (*Planters*), .9 oz.	13.0	1.5
tamari-roasted (*Eden*), 1 oz.	11.0	1.5
toasted, 1 oz.	16.1	1.7
toasted, ¼ cup	19.0	2.0
Surimi, processed from walleye pollock, 4 oz.	1.0	n.a.
Surinam cherry, see "Pitanga"		
Swamp cabbage:		
raw, untrimmed, 1 lb.	.7	tr.
raw, trimmed, 1 oz. or ½ cup chopped	.1	tr.
boiled, drained, chopped, ½ cup	.1	tr.
Swedish meatballs, see "Meatball entree"		
Sweet potato:		
fresh:		
raw, untrimmed, 1 lb.	1.0	.2
1 medium, 5" x 2", about 6.3 oz.	.4	.1
baked in skin, pulp only, 1 medium	.1	<.1
boiled, w/out skin, mashed, ½ cup	.3	.1
canned:		
in syrup, w/liquid, 4 oz. or ½ cup	.2	<.1
vacuum pack, pieces, 4 oz. or ½ cup	.2	<.1
whole (*Royal Prince/Trappey's*), 4 pieces	.5	0
cut or mashed (*Allens/Princella/Sugary Sam*), ⅔ cup	.5	0
candied, regular or w/pineapple (*Royal Prince*), ½ cup	.5	0
frozen:		
10-oz. pkg.	.5	.1
baked, cubed, 4 oz. or ½ cup	.1	<.1

	total fat (grams)	saturated fat (grams)

Sweet potato, frozen *(cont.)*
    candied (*Mrs. Paul's*), 5 oz. w/¼ cup sauce
       mix 1.0 5
Sweet potato chips, see "Potato chips and crisps"
Sweet potato leaf:
    raw, untrimmed, 1 lb. 1.3 3
    steamed, ½ cup .... .1 .... <.1
Sweet and sour drink mixer:
    (*Holland-House*), 4 fl. oz. 0 0
    (*Mr. & Mrs. "T"*), 4 fl. oz. 0 0
    (*Rose's*), 4 fl. oz. 0 0
Sweet and sour sauce (see also "Cooking sauce"),
    2 tbsp., except as noted:
    (*Contadina*) 1.0 0
    (*House of Tsang*), 1 tsp. 0 0
    (*Kraft*) 5 0
    (*Kraft Sauceworks*) 0 0
    (*Kikkoman*), 1 tbsp. 0 0
    duck sauce (*Chelten House*) 0 0
    duck sauce (*Dai-Day*) 0 0
    duck sauce, all varieties (*Gold*) 0 0
    Hawaiian style (*World Harbors Maui Mountain*) ... 1.0 0
Sweet and sour sauce mix (*Kikkoman*),
    2⅛-oz. pkg. .... .5 .... n.a.
Sweetbreads, see "Pancreas" and "Thymus"
Swiss chard:
    raw, untrimmed, 1 lb. .... .8 .... <.1
    raw, chopped, ½ cup .... <.1 .... tr.
    boiled, drained, chopped, ½ cup .... .1 .... <.1
Swiss steak seasoning/gravy mix:
    (*Durkee*), ½ pkg. 0 0
    (*French's*), ⅛ pkg. 0 0
    (*McCormick Bag'n Season*), ⅙ pkg. 0 0

	total fat (grams)	saturated fat (grams)
Swordfish, meat only:		
raw, 4 oz.	4.6	1.3
baked, broiled, or microwaved, 4 oz.	5.8	1.6
Swordfish, frozen, steaks (*Peter Pan*), 4 oz.,		
about 1 steak	5.0	1.5
Syrup, see specific listings		

T

	total fat (grams)	saturated fat (grams)
Tabbouleh mix:		
(*Casbah*), 1 oz. dry or ⅔ cup*	<1.0	0
(*Fantastic Foods* Salad), ¼ dry, about ½ cup*	.5	0
(*Near East* Salad), ⅔ cup*	3.0	.5
Taco (see also "Taco dinner mix"), frozen, 4.9 oz., 5 pieces:		
beef, mini (*Schwan's* Taquito)	15.0	2.5
chicken, mini (*Schwan's* Taquito)	16.0	2.5
Taco Bell, 1 serving:		
burritos:		
bean burrito	12.0	4.0
beef burrito	19.0	8.0
big beef *Burrito Supreme*	25.0	11.0
Burrito Supreme	19.0	9.0
chicken burrito	13.0	5.0
chicken *Burrito Supreme*	23.0	9.0
chili cheese burrito	18.0	9.0
combo burrito	16.0	6.0
7 layer burrito	21.0	8.0
steak *Burrito Supreme*	23.0	11.0

	total fat (grams)	saturated fat (grams)
tacos and tostadas:		
soft taco	11.0	5.0
soft taco, chicken	10.0	4.0
soft taco, steak	9.0	4.0
soft *Taco Supreme*	15.0	8.0
taco	11.0	5.0
Taco Supreme	15.0	7.0
tostada	11.0	4.0
specialty items:		
beef *MexiMelt*	14.0	7.0
cinnamon twists	6.0	0
Mexican pizza	38.0	12.0
nachos	18.0	6.0
nachos *BellGrande*	34.0	12.0
nachos supreme	18.0	5.0
pintos 'n cheese	9.0	4.0
taco salad	55.0	16.0
side orders and condiments:		
green sauce	0	0
guacamole	3.0	1.0
nacho cheese sauce	4.0	2.0
picante sauce or pico de gallo	0	0
ranch dressing	14.0	3.0
red sauce	0	0
salsa	0	0
seasoned rice	3.0	1.0
sour cream	4.0	3.0
taco sauce, hot or mild	0	0
Taco dinner mix:		
(*Lawry's*), 2 shells, 1 tbsp. seasoning, 1½ tsp. sauce	7.0	1.5
(*Old El Paso*), 2 shells, seasoning and sauce	7.0	1.0
(*Old El Paso*), 2 pieces*	13.0	5.0
(*Pancho Villa*), 2 shells, seasoning and sauce	8.0	1.5
(*Pancho Villa*), 2 pieces*	13.0	5.0

	total fat (grams)	saturated fat (grams)
Taco dinner mix *(cont.)*		
soft (*Old El Paso*), 2 tortillas, seasoning and sauce	3.5	1.0
soft (*Old El Paso*), 2 pieces*	10.0	4.0
Taco John's, 1 serving:		
burritos:		
bean	11.1	3.0
beef	18.9	6.4
combination	13.4	5.6
smothered burrito platter	37.5	14.6
super	18.8	6.7
chimichanga platter	35.2	13.5
enchilada platter, double	36.5	13.0
fajitas:		
chicken fajita burrito	11.9	5.0
chicken fajita salad, w/out dressing	34.6	9.6
chicken fajita, softshell	8.3	3.1
Mexi Rolls:		
w/guacamole	45.6	11.8
w/nacho cheese	43.0	10.5
w/salsa	37.1	10.5
w/sour cream	47.0	10.5
Mexican pizza	35.9	13.5
nachos, super	49.9	15.4
Sampler platter	51.0	18.5
Sierra Chicken Fillet Sandwich	21.0	5.7
tacos:		
crispy	10.3	3.7
kid's meal, w/crispy taco	33.3	9.5
kid's meal, w/soft shell taco	32.7	9.7
kid's meal w/taco burger	34.1	10.1
salad	30.5	8.5
soft shell	11.3	4.2
Taco Bravo	13.6	4.4

	total fat (grams)	saturated fat (grams)
taco burger	11.2	4.3
side dishes and condiments:		
beans, refried	7.8	1.5
chili, Texas-style, w/2 crackers	14.3	6.5
Mexican rice	17.7	4.7
nachos	16.8	3.8
nacho cheese	6.0	2.0
Potato Oles	27.5	6.6
Potato Oles, w/nacho cheese	33.7	8.6
salad dressing, house	11.4	1.7
sour cream	5.0	n.a.
desserts:		
choco taco	17.0	11.0
churro	7.8	1.8
flauta, apple	1.1	.2
flauta, cherry	3.6	.7
flauta, cream cheese	7.9	3.1
Taco sauce (see also "Salsa"):		
(*Chi-Chi's* Thick & Chunky), 1 tbsp.	0	0
(*Old El Paso*), 1 tbsp.	0	0
(*Pancho Villa*), 2 tbsp.	0	0
all varieties (*Lawry's*), 2 tbsp.	0	0
all varieties (*Old El Paso*), 1 tbsp.	0	0
green or red (*La Victoria*), 1 tbsp.	0	0
hot (*Chi-Chi's*), 1 oz.	<2.0	<2.0
Taco seasoning mix:		
(*McCormick*), ⅙ pkg.	0	0
(*Old El Paso*), 2 tsp.	0	0
(*Taco Bell*), 2 tbsp.	0	0
all varieties (*Durkee/French's*), ⅛ pkg.	0	0
regular or chicken (*Lawry's* Spices & Seasonings), 1 tbsp.	0	0
salad (*Lawry's* Spices & Seasonings), 1 tsp.	0	0
vegetarian (*Natural Touch*), 3 tbsp.	1.0	0

	total fat (grams)	saturated fat (grams)

Taco shell (see also "Tostaco shell" and "Tostada shell"):

(*Lawry's* 12/18 Pack), 2 pieces	6.0	1.5
(*Old El Paso*), 3 pieces	10.0	1.5
(*Pancho Villa*), 3 pieces	11.0	2.5
(*Taco Bell*), 2 pieces	4.0	.5
mini (*Old El Paso*), 7 pieces	10.0	1.5
super (*Lawry's* 10-Pack), 2 pieces	10.0	2.0
super (*Old El Paso*), 2 pieces	12.0	2.0
tortilla, soft taco (*Old El Paso*), 2 pieces	3.5	.5
white corn (*Chi-Chi's*), 2 pieces	6.0	1.0
white corn (*Old El Paso*), 3 pieces	10.0	1.5

Tahini (see also "Sesame butter"):

(*Krinos*), 2 tbsp.	23.0	3.5
from raw kernels, 1 oz.	13.6	1.9
from raw kernels, 1 tbsp.	7.2	1.0
from unroasted kernels, 1 oz.	16.0	2.2
from unroasted kernels, 1 tbsp.	7.9	1.1
from roasted, toasted kernels, 1 oz.	15.3	2.1
from roasted, toasted kernels, 1 tbsp.	8.1	1.1

Tahini sauce mix (*Casbah*), 1 oz. dry or ¼ cup* 13.0 0

Tamale, canned:

(*Old El Paso*), 3 pieces	19.0	7.0
(*Van Camp's*), 2 pieces	13.0	5.0

beef:

(*Hormel*), 7.5-oz. can	21.0	8.0
(*Nalley*), 7.5 oz.	17.0	7.0
regular or hot-spicy (*Hormel*), 3 pieces	21.0	8.0
jumbo (*Hormel*), 2 pieces	20.0	8.0
chicken (*Hormel*), 3 pieces	10.0	4.0

Tamale, frozen (*Schwan's*), 4 pieces .... 15.0 .... 6.0

Tamari, see "Soy sauce"

Tamarind:

untrimmed, 1 lb.	.9	.4

	total fat (grams)	saturated fat (grams)
trimmed, ½ cup	.4	.2
Tandoori paste, mild (*Patak's* Original), 2 tbsp.	1.0	0
Tangerine:		
fresh:		
untrimmed, 1 lb.	.6	.1
1 medium, 2⅜" diameter, 4.1 oz.	.2	<.1
sections, ½ cup	.2	<.1
canned:		
in juice, ½ cup	.1	tr.
in syrup, ½ cup	.1	<.1
segments (*Dole* Mandarin), ½ cup	<1.0	0
Tangerine drink, all blends and brands, 8 fl. oz.	0	0
Tangerine juice:		
fresh, 6 fl. oz.	.4	<.1
frozen, undiluted, 6 fl. oz.	.8	.1
Tapioca, pearl, dry, 1 oz.	tr.	0
Tarama, see "Caviar"		
Taramosalata (*Krinos*), 1 tbsp.	10.0	2.0
Taro:		
raw, untrimmed, 1 lb.	.8	.2
raw or cooked, sliced, ½ cup	.1	<.1
Taro, Tahitian:		
raw, trimmed, 1 oz.	.3	.1
raw, trimmed, sliced, ½ cup	.6	.1
cooked, sliced, ½ cup	.5	.1
Taro chips:		
1 oz.	7.1	1.8
10 chips, about .8 oz.	5.7	1.5
(*Ray's*), 1 oz., 1 cup	6.0	1.0
Taro leaf:		
raw, untrimmed, lb.	2.0	.4
raw, ½ cup	.1	<.1
steamed, ½ cup	.3	.1
Taro shoots:		
raw, untrimmed, 1 lb.	.4	.1

	total fat (grams)	saturated fat (grams)

Taro shoots *(cont.)*

    raw, sliced, ½ cup .... <.1 .... tr.

    cooked, sliced, ½ cup .... .1 .... <.1

Tarpon, Atlantic, meat only, raw, 4 oz. .... .5 .... n.a.

Tarragon, ground:

    1 tbsp. .... .4 .... <.1

    1 tsp. .... .1 .... tr.

Tart crust or shell, see "Pastry shell"

Tartar sauce, 2 tbsp., except as noted:

    (*Bookbinder's*) .... 11.0 .... 1.5

    (*Hellmann's*) .... 16.0 .... 2.5

    (*Kraft Sauceworks*) .... 10.0 .... 4.0

    (*Kraft* Nonfat) 0 0

    (*Lyon* Fish Shop), 1 tbsp. .... 1.0 .... n.a.

    (*Nalley*) .... 20.0 .... 3.0

    lemon and herb flavor (*Kraft Sauceworks*) .... 16.0 .... 2.5

TCBY, ½ cup:

    all flavors, regular .... 3.0 .... 1.0

    all flavors, nonfat or sugar free .... <1.0 .... <1.0

Tea, brewed:

    hot, regular or herbal, 1 cup 0 0

    iced, plain or flavored, all varieties and brands,

        8 fl. oz. 0 0

Teaseed oil, 1 tbsp. .... 13.6 .... 2.9

Teff, whole grain (*Arrowhead Mills*), ¼ cup 1.0 0

Teff flour (*Arrowhead Mills*), ¼ cup 1.0 0

Tempeh:

    1 oz. 2.2 3

    ½ cup 6.4 9

Tempura sauce (*Kikkoman*), 1 tbsp. 0 0

Tendergreen, see "Mustard spinach"

Tequila, distilled liquor, 3 fl. oz. 0 0

Teriyaki sauce (see also "Barbecue sauce"), 1 tbsp.:

    (*Kikkoman/Kikkoman* Lite) 0 0

    and marinade (*World Harbors Maui Mountain*) ... 0 0

	total fat (grams)	saturated fat (grams)
baste and glaze or marinade (*Kikkoman*)	0	0
Teriyaki entree (see also "Stir-fry entree" and specific listings), frozen (*Lean Cuisine Lunch Express*), 9 oz.	5.0	1.0
Teriyaki seasoning mix, beef (*Durkee* "Easy" Pouch), ⅕ pkg.	1.0	0
Thirst quencher drink, all varieties, all brands, 8 fl. oz.	0	0
Thuringer cervelat (see also "Summer sausage"):		
(*Oscar Mayer*), 1.6 oz., 2 slices	13.0	5.0
beef (*Oscar Mayer*), 1.6 oz., 2 slices	12.0	5.0
beef and pork, 1 oz.	8.5	.3.4
Thyme, ground:		
1 tbsp.	.3	.1
1 tsp.	.1	<.1
Thymus, braised:		
beef, 13.4 oz. (1 lb. raw)	95.2	n.a.
beef, 4 oz.	28.3	n.a.
veal, 9.1 oz. (1 lb. raw)	11.1	n.a.
veal, 4 oz.	4.9	n.a.
Tilefish, meat only:		
raw, 4 oz.	2.6	.5
baked, broiled, or microwaved, 4 oz.	5.3	1.0
Toaster pastries and muffins, 1 piece, except as noted:		
all varieties (*Toastettes*)	5.0	1.5
apple (*Pillsbury Toaster Strudel*)	7.0	1.5
apple cinnamon (*Kellogg's Pop-Tarts*)	5.0	1.0
banana nut (*Thomas' Toast-r-Cakes*)	5.0	.5
blueberry:		
(*Kellogg's Pop-Tarts*)	7.0	1.0
(*Pillsbury Toaster Strudel*)	7.0	1.5
(*Thomas' Toast-r-Cakes*)	3.0	.5
frosted (*Kellogg's Pop-Tarts*)	5.0	1.0
brown sugar cinnamon (*Kellogg's Pop-Tarts*)	9.0	1.0

	total fat (grams)	saturated fat (grams)

Toaster pastries and muffins *(cont.)*

brown sugar cinnamon, frosted (*Kellogg's Pop-Tarts*)	7.0	1.0
cherry (*Kellogg's Pop-Tarts*)	5.0	1.0
cherry (*Pillsbury Toaster Strudel*)	7.0	1.5
cherry, frosted (*Kellogg's Pop-Tarts*)	5.0	1.0
chocolate, frosted (*Kellogg's Pop-Tarts Minis*), 1 pouch	4.0	1.0
chocolate fudge, frosted (*Kellogg's Pop-Tarts*)	5.0	1.0
chocolate graham (*Kellogg's Pop-Tarts*)	6.0	2.0
chocolate vanilla creme, frosted (*Kellogg's Pop-Tarts*)	5.0	1.0
cinnamon (*Pillsbury Toaster Strudel*)	8.0	1.5
cinnamon apple (*Thomas' Toast-r-Cakes*)	3.0	.5
corn (*Thomas' Toast-r-Cakes*)	4.0	.5
cream cheese (*Pillsbury Toaster Strudel*)	10.0	3.5
cream cheese, w/strawberry or blueberry (*Pillsbury Toaster Strudel*)	9.0	3.0
French toast style (*Pillsbury Toaster Strudel*)	7.0	1.5
grape, frosted (*Kellogg's Pop-Tarts*)	5.0	1.0
grape, frosted (*Kellogg's Pop-Tarts Minis*), 1 pouch	4.0	1.0
graham, milk chocolate (*Kellogg's Pop-Tarts*)	6.0	1.0
raspberry (*Pillsbury Toaster Strudel*)	7.0	1.5
raspberry, frosted (*Kellogg's Pop-Tarts*)	6.0	1.0
S'mores, frosted (*Kellogg's Pop-Tarts*)	5.0	.5
strawberry:		
(*Kellogg's Pop-Tarts*)	5.0	1.5
(*Pillsbury Toaster Strudel*)	7.0	1.5
frosted (*Kellogg's Pop-Tarts*)	5.0	1.5
frosted (*Kellogg's Pop-Tarts Minis*), 1 pouch	4.0	1.0

Tofu:

raw:		
1 oz.	1.4	.2
¼ block, 4.1 oz., 2¼" × 1¾" × 1½"	5.6	.8

	total fat (grams)	saturated fat (grams)
½ cup	5.9	.9
extra firm (*Frieda's* Mori-Nu), 5.25 oz.	3.0	n.a.
firm, 1 oz.	2.5	.4
firm, ½ cup	11.0	1.6
firm (*Frieda's* Mori-Nu), 5.25 oz.	4.0	n.a.
firm (*Frieda's* Kikkoman), 5.25 oz.	7.0	n.a.
firm and soft (*Frieda's*), 4.2 oz.	3.7	.8
soft (*Frieda's* Mori-Nu), 5.25 oz.	4.0	n.a.
soft (*Frieda's* Kikkoman), 5.25 oz.	6.0	n.a.
dried-frozen (koyadofu), 1 oz.	8.6	1.2
grilled (yakidofu), 1 oz.	1.7	n.a.
okara, 1 oz.	.5	.1
okara, ½ cup	1.1	.1
salted and fermented (fuyu), 1 oz.	2.3	.3
Tofu "cheese," see "Cheese, fat free and nondairy"		
Tofu dishes, see specific listings		
Tofu entree mix, 1 cup w/tofu*:		
chow mein, mandarin (*Fantastic Foods* Tofu Classics)	5.0	1.0
shells 'n curry (*Fantastic Foods* Tofu Classics)	6.0	1.0
Stroganoff, creamy (*Fantastic Foods* Tofu Classics)	12.0	6.0
Tofu patty, frozen, 2.3-oz. patty:		
(*Natural Touch* Okara)	12.0	2.0
garden grain (*Natural Touch*)	7.0	1.0
garden vegetable (*Natural Touch*)	4.0	1.0
Tom Collins mixer (*Holland House*), 3 fl. oz.	0	0
Tomatillo, in jars:		
(*La Victoria* Entero), 5 pieces	1.0	0
crushed (*La Victoria*), 4.5 oz.	.5	0
Tomato, red, ripe:		
raw, untrimmed, 1 lb.	1.4	.2
raw, 2⅜" diameter, about 4.75 oz.	.4	.1
raw, chopped, ½ cup	.3	<.1

	total fat (grams)	saturated fat (grams)
Tomato *(cont.)*		
boiled, 4 oz. or ½ cup	.5	.1
Tomato, canned (see also "Tomato sauce"):		
all varieties:		
(*Contadina*), ½ cup	0	0
(*Del Monte*), ½ cup	0	0
(*Progresso*), ½ cup	0	0
crushed (*Eden*), ¼ cup	0	0
diced, w/green chilies (*Chi-Chi's*), ¼ cup	0	0
and green chili or jalapeño (*Old El Paso*), ¼ cup	0	0
for pasta, see "Pasta sauce"		
paste or puree, see "Tomato paste" and "Tomato puree"		
stewed, 4 oz. or ½ cup	.2	<.1
stewed or Italian (*Del Monte*), ½ cup	0	0
stewed, all varieties (*Green Giant*), ½ cup	0	0
whole, 4 oz. or ½ cup	.3	<.1
wedges, in tomato juice, 4 oz. or ½ cup	.2	<.1
Tomato, dried (sun-dried):		
1 oz. or ½ cup	.8	0
1 piece (32 pieces per cup)	.1	0
(*Sonoma* Pasta Toss), ½ cup	0	0
halves (*Sonoma*), 2–3 pieces, .2 oz.	0	0
marinated (*Sonoma*), 2–3 pieces, .35 oz.	2.5	0
Tomato, green:		
raw, untrimmed, 1 lb.	.8	.1
1 medium, 2⅜" diameter, about 4.75 oz.	.3	<.1
Tomato, pickled:		
(*Claussen*), 1 oz.	0	0
(*Hebrew National/Rosoff/Shorr's*), 1 oz., ⅓ tomato	0	0
Tomato, sun-dried, see "Tomato, dried"		
Tomato chili cocktail (*Snap-E-Tom*), 8 fl. oz.	0	0

	total fat (grams)	saturated fat (grams)
Tomato juice:		
6 fl. oz.	.1	<.1
(*Campbell's/Campbell's* Low Sodium), 10.5 fl. oz.	0	0
(*R.W. Knudsen*), 8 fl. oz.	0	0
Tomato paste, canned:		
1 oz.	.3	<.1
½ cup	1.2	.2
(*Contadina*), 2 tbsp.	0	0
(*Del Monte*), 2 tbsp.	0	0
(*Progresso*), 2 tbsp.	0	0
Italian (*Contadina*), 2 tbsp.	1.0	0
Tomato pesto, see "Pesto"		
Tomato powder, 1 oz.	.1	<.1
Tomato puree, canned:		
4 oz. or ½ cup	.1	<.1
(*Contadina*), ½ cup	0	0
(*Progresso*), ¼ cup	0	0
Tomato sauce (see also "Pasta sauce" and "Pizza sauce"):		
4 oz. or ½ cup	.2	<.1
(*Contadina*), ¼ cup	0	0
(*Del Monte*), ¼ cup	0	0
(*Eden*), ¼ cup	0	0
(*Hunt's*), ¼ cup	0	0
(*Progresso*), ½ cup	0	0
w/herbs and cheese, 4 oz.	2.2	.7
w/herbs and cheese, ½ cup	2.4	.8
Italian or thick and zesty (*Contadina*), ¼ cup	0	0
w/mushrooms, 4 oz.	.1	<.1
w/mushrooms, ½ cup	.2	<.1
w/onions, 4 oz. or ½ cup	.2	<.1
w/onion, green pepper and celery, 4 oz.	.8	.2
Spanish style, 4 oz. or ½ cup	.3	<.1
w/tomato tidbits, 4 oz.	.4	.1
w/tomato tidbits, ½ cup	.5	.1

	total fat (grams)	saturated fat (grams)
Tomato seasoning, dried tomato (*Sonoma* Season It), 2–3 tsp.	0	0
Tomato tapenade, dried tomato (*Sonoma*), 1 tbsp.	6.0	1.0
Tomato-beef cocktail (*Mott's Beefamato*), 8 fl. oz.	0	0
Tomato-clam juice cocktail (*Mott's Clamato/Clamato Caesar*), 8 fl. oz.	0	0
Tomatoseed oil, 1 tbsp.	13.6	2.7
Tongue:		
beef:		
simmered, 9.1 oz. (1 lb. raw)	53.7	23.1
simmered, 4 oz.	23.5	10.1
pickled, corned (*Hebrew National*), 2 oz.	9.0	3.5
pickled, corned (*Hebrew National* Deli Xpress Sliced), 2 oz.	9.0	4.0
lamb, braised, 9 oz. (1 lb. raw)	51.8	20.0
lamb, braised, 4 oz.	23.0	8.9
pork, braised, 4 oz.	21.1	7.3
veal, braised, 4 oz.	11.5	n.a.
Tonic water, all brands, 8 fl. oz.	0	0
Tonkatsu sauce (*Kikkoman*), 1 tbsp.	0	0
Topping, dessert, see specific listings		
Tortellini entree, canned or packaged:		
cheese (*Chef Boyardee*), 7.5-oz. cup	1.0	0
cheese (*Schwan's*), 1 cup	6.0	2.5
chicken (*Schwan's*), 1 cup	5.0	1.5
w/ground beef (*Chef Boyardee*), 10.5-oz. bowl	4.0	1.5
and meat sauce (*Chef Boyardee*), 7.5-oz. cup	3.0	1.5
Tortellini entree, frozen:		
(*Green Giant Garden Gourmet Right for Lunch*), 9.5 oz.	6.0	2.0
cheese:		
(*The Budget Gourmet* Side Dish), 6.25 oz.	8.0	2.0
w/Alfredo sauce (*Stouffer's*), 8⅞ oz.	33.0	18.0

	total fat (grams)	saturated fat (grams)
w/tomato sauce (*Stouffer's*), 9¼ oz.	6.0	5.0
Tortilla (see also "Taco shells"):		
(*Buena Vida* Fat Free), 1 piece	0	0
corn, 2 pieces:		
(*Garden of Eatin'* Corntillas)	1.5	0
blue corn (*Garden of Eatin'*)	1.5	0
white or yellow (*Azteca*)	1.0	0
flour (wheat), 1 piece, except as noted:		
(*Azteca*), 2 pieces	3.0	.5
(*Azteca* Homestyle)	2.0	0
(*Azteca* Super Size)	2.5	.5
(*Old El Paso*)	3.0	.5
burrito size (*Azteca*)	3.0	.5
whole wheat (*Garden of Eatin'*)	3.0	0
whole wheat, apple cinnamon or red chile (*Garden of Eatin'*)	3.0	0
whole wheat, lowfat (*Garden of Eatin'*)	1.0	0
Tortilla chips, see "Corn chips, puffs and similar snacks"		
Tortilla crisps, 1.1 oz., 36 pieces:		
(*Pepperidge Farm* Original)	6.0	1.0
chili cheese or salsa (*Pepperidge Farm*)	7.0	1.0
Tostaco shell (*Old El Paso*), 1 piece	7.0	1.0
Tostada shell:		
(*Lawry's* 10-Pack), 2 pieces	6.0	1.5
(*Old El Paso*), 3 pieces	10.0	2.0
Towel gourd, see "Gourd, dishcloth"		
Trail mix:		
(*Del Monte* Sierra), 1-oz. bag	6.0	2.0
(*Del Monte* Sierra), ¼ cup	8.0	2.5
(*Eden*), 1 oz.	10.0	1.5
(*Eden* California Harvest Mix), 1 oz.	7.0	1.5
(*Sonoma*), 1.4 oz., ¼ cup	7.0	3.0
Tree fern, cooked, 4 oz. or ½ cup chopped	.1	0
Tripe (see also "Stomach"), beef, raw, 1 oz.	1.1	.6

	total fat (grams)	saturated fat (grams)
Triticale, whole grain, 1 cup	4.0	.7
Triticale flour, whole grain, 1 cup	2.4	.4
Trout, meat only, 4 oz.:		
mixed species, raw	7.5	1.3
rainbow, raw	3.8	.7
rainbow, baked, broiled, or microwaved	4.9	.9
Trout, sea, see "Sea trout"		
Tuna, meat only, 4 oz.:		
bluefin, raw	5.6	1.4
bluefin, baked, broiled, or microwaved	7.1	1.8
skipjack, raw	1.2	.8
yellowfin, raw	1.1	.3
Tuna, canned:		
in oil, 2 oz., w/liquid except as noted:		
chunk light (*Carnation*)	12.0	n.a.
chunk light, drained (*StarKist*)	6.0	1.0
chunk light, drained (*StarKist* 3 oz.), 2.7 oz.	8.0	1.5
chunk light or white (*Bumble Bee*)	12.0	3.0
solid (*Progresso*), ¼ cup	12.0	2.0
solid white (*Bumble Bee*)	8.0	2.0
solid white, drained (*StarKist*)	3.0	.5
solid white, drained (*StarKist* 3 oz.), 2.8 oz.	5.0	1.0
in water, 2 oz., except as noted:		
chunk light, drained (*Bumble Bee*)	.5	0
chunk light, drained (*Bumble Bee* 3 oz.), 2.6 oz.	1.0	0
chunk light, drained (*StarKist*)	.5	0
chunk light, drained (*StarKist* 3 oz.), 2.7 oz.	1.0	0
chunk white, drained (*Bumble Bee*)	1.0	0
chunk white, drained (*Bumble Bee* 3 oz.), 2.6 oz.	1.0	1.0
chunk white, drained (*Bumble Bee* Diet Low Salt)	1.0	0
chunk white, drained (*StarKist* Low Salt /Fat)	.5	0

	total fat (grams)	saturated fat (grams)
solid light (*StarKist* Prime Catch)	1.0	0
solid light (*StarKist* Prime Catch 3 oz.), 2.8 oz.	1.0	0
solid white, drained (*Bumble Bee*)	1.0	0
solid white, drained (*Bumble Bee* 3 oz.), 2.7 oz.	1.0	0
solid white, drained (*Empress*)	1.0	0
solid or chunk white, drained (*StarKist*)	1.0	0
solid or chunk white, drained (*StarKist* 3 oz.), 2.8 oz.	1.0	0
smoked, hickory, solid light or white, drained (*StarKist* Prime Catch)	1.0	0
Tuna, frozen, yellowfin, steak (*Peter Pan*), 4 oz., about 1 steak	.5	0
"Tuna," vegetarian, frozen (*Worthington Tuno*), 1.9 oz., ½ cup	6.0	1.0
Tuna noodle entree, freeze dried, w/cheese (*AlpineAire*), 1½ cups*	7.0	n.a.
Tuna noodle entree, frozen:		
casserole (*Stouffer's*), 10 oz.	14.0	2.0
casserole (*Weight Watchers*), 9.5 oz.	7.0	2.5
Tuna noodle entree, packaged, casserole (*Dinty Moore American Classics*), 10 oz.	7.0	4.0
Tuna salad (*Longacre*), 1 oz.	4.0	n.a.
Tuna salad seasoning mix, all varieties (*Bumble Bee Tuna Mix-Ins*), ⅓ pkt.	0	0
Tuna spread (*Libby Spreadables*), ⅓ cup	8.0	1.0
Turkey, fryer-roaster, fresh, roasted:		
dark and light meat:		
meat w/skin, ½ bird, 1.8 lbs. (2.4 lbs. w/bone)	46.2	13.3
meat w/skin, 4 oz.	6.5	1.9
meat only, 4 oz.	3.0	1.0
meat only, chopped or diced, 1 cup	3.7	1.2

	total fat (grams)	saturated fat (grams)
Turkey, dark and light meat *(cont.)*		
meat only, chopped or diced, 1 oz.	6.6	1.7
dark meat:		
w/skin, 4 oz.	8.0	2.4
meat only, 4 oz.	4.9	1.6
meat only, chopped or diced, 1 cup	6.0	2.0
light meat:		
w/skin, 4 oz.	5.2	1.4
meat only, 4 oz.	1.3	1.4
meat only, chopped or diced, 1 cup	1.7	.5
breast:		
meat w/skin, ½ breast, 12.1 oz. (1.7 lbs. w/bone)	11.0	3.0
meat w/skin, 4 oz.	3.6	1.0
meat only, ½ breast, 10.8 oz. (1.7 lbs. w/bone and skin)	2.3	.7
meat only, 4 oz.	.8	.3
leg:		
meat w/skin, 1 leg, 8.6 oz. (11.4 oz. w/bone)	13.3	4.1
meat w/skin, 4 oz.	6.1	1.9
meat only, 1 leg, 7.9 oz. (11.4 oz. w/bone and skin)	8.5	2.8
meat only, 4 oz.	4.3	1.4
wing:		
meat w/skin, 1 wing, 3.2 oz. (5.2 oz. w/bone)	8.9	2.4
meat w/skin, 4 oz.	11.2	3.1
meat only, 1 wing, 2.1 oz. (5.2 oz. w/bone and skin)	2.1	.7
meat only, 4 oz.	3.9	1.2
Turkey, canned:		
w/broth, 5-oz. can	9.7	2.8
chunk *(Hormel)*, 2 oz.	3.0	1.0
chunk, white *(Hormel)*, 2 oz.	1.0	.5

	total fat (grams)	saturated fat (grams)
Turkey, freeze-dried, diced (*AlpineAire*), 1 oz.	1.0	n.a.
Turkey, frozen or refrigerated (see also "Turkey"):		
baby (*Boar's Head Maple Glazed Honey Coat*),		
3 oz.	1.0	.5
barbecued (*Empire* Kosher), 5 oz. w/out bone	12.0	3.5
barbecued (*Hebrew National/Falls* BBQ), 3 oz.		
w/out bone	8.0	n.a.
barbecued, breast (*Louis Rich*), 2 oz.	.5	0
breast, chops (*Longacre*), 4 oz.	1.0	n.a.
breast, raw:		
(*Longacre* Chef's Select /Cook-in-Bag), 1 oz. ..	1.0	n.a.
boneless (*Perdue/Perdue Fit 'N Easy*), 4 oz. ...	1.0	0
cutlets (*Norbest Tasti-Lean*), 3.5 oz.	.9	.4
cutlets (*Perdue* Thin Sliced), 3.5 oz.	1.0	0
cutlets or tenders (*Norbest* Saddle Pack),		
3.5 oz.	1.5	.6
fillets (*Perdue/Perdue Fit 'N Easy*), 4 oz.	1.0	.5
roast (*Norbest* Sweetheart), 3.5 oz.	1.6	.6
skinless (*Longacre*), 1 oz.	<1.0	n.a.
steaks (*Norbest* Saddle Pack), 3.5 oz.	.7	.3
steaks, cubed (*Norbest /Norbest Tasti-Lean*),		
3.5 oz.	.7	.3
strips or tips (*Norbest Tasti-Lean*), 3.5 oz.	.9	.4
tenders (*Norbest Tasti-Lean*), 3.5 oz.	1.5	.6
breast, cooked:		
(*Hebrew National/Falls* Gourmet), 3 oz.	1.0	n.a.
(*Hebrew National/Falls* Premium), 3 oz.	2.0	n.a.
(*Perdue/Perdue Fit 'N Easy*), 3 oz.	1.0	.5
(*Perdue/Perdue Fit 'N Easy* Thin Sliced),		
2.5 oz.	1.0	0
boneless (*Perdue/Perdue Fit 'N Easy*), 3 oz. ...	1.0	0
half (*Perdue*), 3 oz.	7.0	2.5
hickory smoked (*Louis Rich*), 2 oz.	.5	0
hickory smoked, dinner slices (*Louis Rich*),		
2.8-oz. slice	1.0	0

	total fat (grams)	saturated fat (grams)
Turkey, frozen or refrigerated, breast, cooked *(cont.)*		
honey roasted (*Louis Rich*), 2 oz.	.5	0
honey roasted, dinner slices (*Louis Rich*),		
2.8-oz. slice	1.0	.5
oven roasted (*Louis Rich*), 2 oz.	.5	0
oven roasted, dinner slices (*Louis Rich*),		
2.8-oz. slice	1.0	0
roast, without gravy (*Norbest*), 3.5 oz.	2.0	.7
smoked, slices (*Louis Rich*), 2.8 oz.	1.0	0
whole (*Perdue*), 3 oz.	8.0	2.5
dark and light meat, roasted, 4 oz.	6.6	n.a.
drumstick, cooked (*Perdue*), 3 oz.	7.0	2.0
ground, see "Turkey, ground"		
roast, seasoned or unseasoned (*Longacre*),		
1 oz.	2.0	n.a.
tenderlings, all varieties (*Longacre*), 4 oz.	<1.0	n.a.
tenderloins, raw or cooked (*Perdue/Perdue Fit 'N*		
Easy), 3 oz.	1.0	.5
thigh, cooked (*Perdue*), 3 oz.	11.0	3.5
thigh, roast (*Longacre* Cook-in-the-Bag),		
1 oz.	2.0	n.a.
whole, brown and roasted or smoked (*Longacre*),		
1 oz.	3.0	n.a.
whole, white meat, cooked (*Perdue*), 3 oz.	9.0	3.0
whole, dark meat, cooked (*Perdue*), 3 oz.	14.0	5.0
wing, cooked:		
(*Perdue*), 5.5-oz. piece	18.0	5.0
drummettes (*Perdue*), 3.5-oz. piece	9.0	3.0
tom, (*Perdue*), 3 oz.	8.0	2.5
tom, portions (*Perdue*), 2.5 oz.	8.0	2.5
tom, portions (*Perdue*), 3.5 oz.	12.0	3.5
Turkey, ground (see also "Turkey burger" and "Turkey sausage"):		
(*Longacre* Chubs), 1 oz.	3.0	n.a.
(*Louis Rich*), 4 oz. raw, 3 oz. cooked	12.0	3.5

	total fat (grams)	saturated fat (grams)
(*Norbest*), 2 oz.	6.2	2.4
raw:		
1 oz.	2.1	.6
(*Longacre*), 1 oz.	4.0	n.a.
(*Perdue*), 4 oz.	8.0	2.5
breast (*Perdue*), 4 oz.	1.5	.5
cooked:		
11.6 oz. (1 lb. raw)	45.5	12.4
4 oz.	15.6	4.3
breast (*Perdue*), 4 oz.	1.0	.5
patty, 2.9 oz. (4 oz. raw patty)	11.4	3.1
(*Perdue*), 4 oz.	9.0	3.0
"Turkey," vegetarian, canned (*Worthington Turkee*),		
3 slices, 3.3 oz.	14.0	2.5
"Turkey," vegetarian, frozen, smoked (*Worthington*),		
3 slices, 2 oz.	10.0	2.0
Turkey bacon (*Louis Rich*), .5-oz. slice	2.5	.5
Turkey bologna:		
(*Empire* Kosher), 3 slices, 1.8 oz.	5.5	1.5
(*Longacre*), 1 oz.	5.0	n.a.
(*Longacre* Sliced), .5-oz. slice	3.0	n.a.
(*Louis Rich*), 2 oz.	10.0	3.0
(*Norbest*), 2 oz.	11.3	3.8
Turkey burger (see also "Turkey, ground" and "Turkey		
patty"), 4-oz. burger, except as noted:		
1 oz.	4.3	n.a.
(*Longacre*), 3-oz. burger	13.0	n.a.
(*Longacre*)	17.0	n.a.
(*Perdue*)	8.0	2.5
barbecue (*Longacre*)	17.0	n.a.
cooked (*Perdue*)	9.0	3.0
Turkey dinner, frozen:		
(*Banquet Extra Helping*), 18.8 oz.	20.0	5.0
(*Morton*), 9 oz.	8.0	3.0
(*Swanson*), 11.5 oz.	7.0	2.0

	total fat (grams)	saturated fat (grams)

Turkey dinner *(cont.)*

breast, stuffed (*The Budget Gourmet* Light &
    Healthy), 11 oz. .... | 6.0 .... | 2.0 |

breast, stuffed (*The Budget Gourmet* Light & Healthy), 11 oz.	6.0	2.0
breast of (*Healthy Choice*), 10.5 oz.	3.0	2.0
w/dressing and gravy (*Armour Classics*), 11.25 oz.	7.0	4.0
and gravy (*Banquet* Meals), 9.25 oz.	10.0	3.0
tetrazzini (*Healthy Choice*), 12.25 oz.	4.0	1.0
white meat, mostly (*Swanson Hungry-Man*), 16.5 oz.	13.0	6.0
Turkey entree, canned or packaged:		
dressing, gravy and (*Libby's Diner*), 7 oz.	7.0	1.5
dressing, gravy (*Dinty Moore American Classics*), 10 oz.	7.0	2.0
w/mashed potatoes (*Dinty Moore American Classics*), 10 oz.	7.0	3.0
Turkey entree, freeze dried*:		
(*AlpineAire* Wild Thyme), 1¼ cups	6.0	n.a.
teriyaki (*AlpineAire*), 1⅓ cups	2.0	n.a.
tetrazzini (*Mountain House*), 1 cup	8.0	2.0
Turkey entree, frozen:		
(*Lean Cuisine* Homestyle), 9⅜ oz.	6.0	1.5
breast:		
boneless, w/gravy (*Schwan's*), 5 oz.	0	0
filet, unbreaded (*Schwan's*), 3-oz. piece	0	0
roasted, and stuffing, cinnamon apples (*Lean Cuisine*), 9¾ oz.	4.0	1.0
stuffed (*Weight Watchers*), 8.75 oz.	8.0	3.0
glazed (*The Budget Gourmet* Light & Healthy), 9 oz.	4.0	2.0
gravy and (*Banquet* Family), 4.8 oz.	5.0	1.5
gravy and (*Banquet Hot Sandwich Toppers*), 5 oz.	4.0	1.5
medallions, w/vegetables (*Healthy Choice Generous Serving*), 12.5 oz.	6.0	3.0

	total fat (grams)	saturated fat (grams)
open face, and gravy, w/mashed potatoes		
(*The Budget Gourmet*), 9 oz.	15.0	4.0
pie:		
(*Banquet*), 7 oz.	20.0	8.0
(*Banquet* Supreme), 7 oz.	13.0	5.0
(*Empire* Kosher), 8.2 oz.	23.0	5.0
(*Lean Cuisine*), 9.5 oz.	9.0	2.0
(*Morton*), 7 oz.	18.0	9.0
(*Stouffer's*), 10 oz.	33.0	9.0
(*Stouffer's*), ½ of 16-oz. pkg.	31.0	8.0
(*Swanson*), 7 oz.	21.0	9.0
roast:		
and homestyle stuffing (*Stouffer's*), 7⅞ oz.	11.0	2.5
medallions (*Weight Watchers Smart Ones*),		
8.5 oz.	2.0	.5
mushrooms, gravy (*Healthy Choice*), 8.5 oz.	3.0	1.0
sliced, gravy, dressing (*Healthy Choice* Homestyle),		
10 oz.	4.0	2.0
tetrazzini (*Stouffer's*), 10 oz.	19.0	3.0
w/vegetables (*Healthy Choice* Homestyle), 9.5 oz.	3.0	1.0
Turkey entree, refrigerated:		
breast nuggets (*Perdue Done It!*), 3 oz.	9.0	2.0
chili (*Longacre*), 4 oz.	3.0	n.a.
hickory barbecue (*Turkey By George*), 5 oz.	5.0	n.a.
lemon pepper (*Turkey By George*), 5 oz.	4.0	1.0
meat loaf, original, Italian, or Mexican (*Longacre*),		
4 oz.	5.0	n.a.
mustard tarragon (*Turkey By George*), 5 oz.	6.0	n.a.
Parmesan, Italian (*Turkey By George*), 5 oz.	5.0	n.a.
shaped (*Perdue Done It!* Fun Shapes), 3 oz.	9.0	2.0
teriyaki (*Longacre*), 4 oz.	<1.0	n.a.
Turkey frankfurter:		
(*Empire* Kosher), 2-oz. link	6.0	1.5
(*Longacre*), 2-oz. link	11.0	n.a.

	total fat (grams)	saturated fat (grams)

Turkey frankfurter *(cont.)*

(*Longacre*), 1.6-oz. link	9.0	n.a.
(*Longacre*), 1.2-oz. link	7.0	n.a.
and beef (*Oscar Mayer Healthy Favorites*), 2-oz. link	1.5	.5

and chicken:

(*Louis Rich,* 16 oz.), 1.6-oz. link	7.0	2.0
(*Louis Rich,* 12 oz.), 1.5-oz. link	6.0	2.0
(*Louis Rich Bun Length*), 2-oz. link	8.0	2.5
cheese (*Louis Rich*), 1.6-oz. link	7.0	2.5

Turkey giblets:

| raw, 1 oz. | 1.2 | .4 |
| simmered, chopped or diced, 1 cup | 7.4 | 2.2 |

Turkey gizzard, simmered, chopped or diced,

| 1 cup | 5.6 | 1.6 |

Turkey gravy:

| canned, ¼ cup | 1.3 | .4 |
| canned (*Swanson*), ¼ cup | 1.0 | 0 |

Turkey gravy mix:

¼ cup*	.5	.1
(*Durkee/French's*), ¼ pkg.	0	0
(*McCormick*), ¼ pkg.	0	0
roasted turkey (*Knorr Gravy Classics*), ⅕ pkg.	.5	0

Turkey ham:

1 oz.	1.4	.5
(*Healthy Choice*), 2 oz.	2.0	1.0
(*Hansel'n Gretel Healthy Deli*), 2 oz.	2.5	.5
(*Hillshire Farm* Deli Select), 1 slice	<1.0	n.a.
(*Longacre* Baked 12% Water), 1 oz.	3.0	n.a.
(*Longacre* Baked 20% Water), 1 oz.	2.0	n.a.
(*Longacre* Roll), 1 oz.	2.0	n.a.
(*Louis Rich*), 2 oz.	2.0	1.0
(*Louis Rich* 15% Water Added), 2 oz.	3.0	1.0
(*Louis Rich* Round), 1-oz. slice	1.0	0
(*Louis Rich* Square), 2.2 oz., 3 slices	2.5	.5

	total fat (grams)	saturated fat (grams)
(*Louis Rich Deli-Thin*), 1.8 oz., 4 slices	1.5	.5
(*Norbest/Norbest* Sliced), 2 oz.	2.8	1.0
(*Norbest* Tavern Ham), 2 oz.	2.9	1.0
Canadian style (*Norbest*), 2 oz.	2.8	1.0
canned, chunk (*Hormel*) 2 oz.	4.0	1.5
chopped (*Louis Rich*), 1-oz. slice	2.5	1.0
cured (*Norbest* Gourmet), 2 oz.	4.4	1.4
honey cured (*Louis Rich*), 2.2 oz.	2.0	.5
Turkey ham salad (*Longacre*), 1 oz.	4.0	0
Turkey liver, see "Liver"		
Turkey luncheon meat (see also "Turkey, frozen and refrigerated"), 2 oz., except as noted:		
all varieties (*Louis Rich* Fat Free), 1-oz. slice	0	0
bologna, see "Turkey bologna"		
breast:		
(*Boar's Head* Premium Lower Sodium Skin-on)	2.0	.5
(*Boar's Head* Premium Lower Sodium, Skinless)	.5	0
(*Hormel* Premium)	1.0	.5
(*Hormel Light & Lean* Deli)	.5	0
(*Hormel Light & Lean* Boneless), 3 oz.	1.0	.5
(*Hormel Sandwich Maker*)	.5	0
(*Jones Dairy Farm* Lean Choice), 3 oz.	1.5	n.a.
cuts, regular or smoked (*Hormel Light & Lean*), 16 pieces	.5	0
skinless and no-salt (*Hormel*)	.5	0
breast, Black Forest (*Hansel'n Gretel Healthy Deli*)	.5	0
breast, honey cured (*Hillshire Farm*), 1 oz.	1.0	n.a.
breast, honey roasted:		
(*Hansel'n Gretel Healthy Deli*)	.5	0
(*Hillshire Farm* Deli Select/Flavor Pack), 1 slice	<1.0	0
(*Hormel Light & Lean*)	.5	0

	total fat (grams)		saturated fat (grams)

Turkey luncheon meat, breast, honey roasted *(cont.)*

(*Louis Rich*), 1-oz. slice	1.0	....	0
breast, maple honey (*Boar's Head*)	.5	....	0
breast, oven roasted:			
(*Boar's Head* Golden Skin-on)	2.0	....	.5
(*Boar's Head* Golden Skinless)	.5	....	0
(*Boar's Head Ovengold* Skinless)	1.0	....	0
(*Empire* Kosher), 1.8 oz., 3 slices	.5	....	0
(*Hansel'n Gretel Healthy Deli*)	.5	....	0
(*Hebrew National* Thin), 1.8 oz., 5 slices	.5	....	0
(*Hillshire Farm* Deli Select), 1-oz. slice	<1.0	....	0
(*Hillshire Farm* Flavor Pack), .75-oz. slice	<1.0	....	0
(*Louis Rich*), 1-oz. slice.	.5	....	0
(*Louis Rich Carving Board* Thin), 2.1 oz., 6 slices	.5	....	0
(*Louis Rich Carving Board* Traditional), 1.5 oz., 2 slices	.5	....	0
(*Louis Rich Deli-Thin*), 1.8 oz., 4 slices	1.0	....	0
(*Louis Rich Deli-Thin* Fat Free), 1.8 oz., 4 slices	0	....	0
(*Oscar Mayer*), 1-oz. slice	.5	....	0
(*Oscar Mayer Healthy Favorites* Fat Free), 1.8 oz., 4 slices	0	....	0
breast, smoked:			
(*Empire* Kosher), 1.8 oz., 3 slices	0	....	0
(*Healthy Choice*)	2.0	....	<1.0
(*Hebrew National* Thin), 1.8 oz., 5 slices	.5	....	0
(*Hillshire Farm*), 1 oz.	1.0	....	n.a.
(*Hillshire Farm* Deli Select/Flavor Pack), 1 slice	<1.0	....	0
(*Longacre* Sliced), .75-oz. slice	<1.0	....	n.a.
(*Louis Rich*), 1-oz. slice	.5	....	0
(*Louis Rich Carving Board*), 1.5 oz., 2 slices	.5	....	0
(*Louis Rich Deli-Thin*), 1.8 oz., 4 slices	1.0	....	0
(*Oscar Mayer Deli-Thin*), 1.8 oz., 4 slices	1.0	....	0

	total fat (grams)	saturated fat (grams)
(*Oscar Mayer Healthy Favorites* Fat Free), 1.8 oz., 4 slices	0	0
hickory (*Boar's Head* Lower Sodium)	2.0	.5
hickory (*Hebrew National*)	.5	0
honey roasted (*Healthy Choice*)	2.0	<1.0
mesquite (*Hansel'n Gretel Healthy Deli*)	.5	0
pepper (*Boar's Head Cracked Pepper Mill*)	.5	0
lemon garlic (*Hebrew National* Thin), 1.8 oz., 5 slices	.5	0
ham, see "Turkey ham"		
pastrami, see "Turkey pastrami"		
roast, regular or smoked (*Oscar Mayer Deli-Thin*), 1.8 oz., 4 slices	1.0	0
roll, white or combo (*Longacre*), 1 oz.	3.0	n.a.
salami, see "Turkey salami"		
sausage, see "Turkey sausage"		
smoked, cured (*Longacre* Sliced), .5-oz. slice	1.0	n.a.
smoked, cured, dark (*Longacre*), 1 oz.	3.0	n.a.
smoked, white (*Louis Rich*), 1-oz. slice	1.0	0
Turkey nuggets, breaded		
(*Louis Rich*), 3.3 oz., 4 pieces	16.0	3.0
Turkey pastrami:		
2 oz.	3.5	1.0
(*Empire* Kosher), 1.8 oz., 3 slices	2.0	.5
(*Hansel'n Gretel Healthy Deli*), 2 oz.	2.5	.5
(*Hebrew National*), 2 oz.	2.5	.5
(*Longacre*), 1 oz.	2.0	n.a.
(*Louis Rich*), 2 oz.	2.0	1.0
(*Louis Rich* Square), 1.6 oz., 2 slices	1.5	0
(*Norbest*), 2 oz.	2.4	.8
breast, pastrami seasoned (*Boar's Head*), 2 oz.	.5	0
Turkey patty (see also "Turkey, ground" and "Turkey burger"):		
(*Empire* Kosher), 3.1-oz. patty	10.0	2.0
breaded (*Louis Rich*), 3-oz. patty	13.0	2.5

	total fat (grams)	saturated fat (grams)

Turkey patty *(cont.)*
| breaded or battered, fried, 1 oz. | 5.1 | n.a. |

Turkey pie, see "Turkey entree, frozen"

| **Turkey salad** (*Longacre*), 1 oz. | 4.0 | n.a. |

Turkey salami:
(*Empire* Kosher), 3 slices, 1.8 oz.	3.5	1.0
(*Longacre*), 1 oz.	3.0	n.a.
(*Longacre* Sliced), .8-oz. slice	3.0	n.a.
(*Longacre* Sliced), .5-oz. slice	1.0	n.a.
(*Louis Rich*), 2 oz.	9.0	2.5
(*Norbest*), 2 oz.	5.4	1.7
cotto (*Louis Rich*), 1-oz. slice	2.5	1.0

Turkey sandwich, frozen:
| hand-held, w/broccoli (*Mrs. Patterson's Aussie Pie*), 1 piece | 26.0 | 10.0 |
| honey Dijon (*Weight Watchers*), 4 oz. | 4.0 | 1.5 |

Turkey sausage:
(*Longacre* Links), 1 oz. raw	4.0	n.a.
(*Longacre* Patties), 2 oz. raw	8.0	n.a.
(*Louis Rich* Original/Hot), 2.5 oz.	6.0	2.5
(Louis Rich Links), 2 oz., 2 links	6.0	1.5
(*Norbest* Chub), 2 oz.	4.6	1.6
(*Norbest* Links), 2 oz.	5.3	1.9
breakfast, cooked (*Longacre*), 2.8-oz. link	12.0	n.a.
breakfast, cooked or raw (*Perdue*), 2 oz.	7.0	2.0
Italian, cooked (*Longacre*), 2.8-oz. link	12.0	n.a.
Italian, sweet or hot, raw or cooked (*Perdue*), 2-oz. link	4.0	1.0
Polish (*Hillshire Farm* Flavorseal Polska), 2 oz.	5.0	n.a.
Polish (*Louis Rich* Polska Kielbasa), 2 oz.	4.5	1.5
smoked:		
(*Hillshire Farm* Flavorseal), 2 oz.	5.0	n.a.
(*Louis Rich*), 2 oz.	5.0	1.5
and cheddar (*Louis Rich*), 2 oz.	5.0	2.0
and pork, cooked (*Jimmy Dean* Light), 1 oz.	7.0	n.a.

	total fat (grams)	saturated fat (grams)

and pork, hot or w/sage (*Jimmy Dean* Light),

   1 oz. .... 6.0 .... n.a.

Turkey spread:

   (*Libby Spreadables*), ⅓ cup .... 10.0 .... 1.5

   chunky (*Underwood* Light), 2⅛ oz. .... 2.0 .... <1.0

Turkey sticks:

   breaded (*Louis Rich*), 3 sticks, 3 oz. .... 15.0 .... 3.0

   breaded or battered, fried, 1 oz. .... 4.8 .... n.a.

Turmeric, ground:

   1 tbsp. .... .7 .... n.a.

   1 tsp. .... .2 .... n.a.

Turnip:

  fresh:

    raw, untrimmed, 1 lb. .... .4 .... <.1

    raw, cubed, ½ cup .... .1 .... <.1

    boiled, drained, cubed or mashed, ½ cup .... .1 .... tr.

  frozen:

    10-oz. pkg. .... .5 .... <.1

    boiled, drained, chopped, ½ cup .... .2 .... <.1

    (*McKenzie's*), 1 cup 0 0

Turnip greens:

  fresh:

    raw, untrimmed, 1 lb. 1.0 2

    raw, chopped, ½ cup .... .1 .... <.1

    boiled, drained, chopped, ½ cup .... .2 .... <.1

   canned, w/liquid, ½ cup 4 1

   canned, w/ or w/out turnips (*Allens/Sunshine*),

    ½ cup 5 0

  frozen, w/diced turnips:

    10-oz. pkg. 5 1

    boiled, drained, 4 oz. .... .2 .... <.1

    (*Stilwell*), 1 cup 0 0

Turnover, frozen or refrigerated:

  apple:

   (*Pepperidge Farm*), 3.2-oz. piece .... 14.0 .... 3.0

	total fat (grams)	saturated fat (grams)

Turnover, apple *(cont.)*

(*Pillsbury*), 4 oz., 2 pieces	17.0	3.5
iced (*Pepperidge Farm*), 3.4-oz. piece	14.0	3.0
mini (*Pepperidge Farm*), 1.4-oz. piece	8.0	2.0
blueberry (*Pepperidge Farm*), 3.2-oz. piece	16.0	3.0
cherry:		
(*Pepperidge Farm*), 3.2-oz. piece	13.0	3.0
(*Pillsbury*), 4 oz., 2 pieces	17.0	3.5
iced (*Pepperidge Farm*), 3.4-oz. piece	13.0	3.0
mini (*Pepperidge Farm*), 1.4-oz. piece	8.0	2.0
peach (*Pepperidge Farm*), 3.2-oz. piece	15.0	3.0
peach cobbler, mini (*Pepperidge Farm*), 1.6-oz. piece	8.0	2.0
raspberry (*Pepperidge Farm*), 3.2-oz. piece	14.0	3.0
raspberry, iced (*Pepperidge Farm*), 3.4-oz. piece	14.0	3.0
strawberry, mini (*Pepperidge Farm*), 1.4-oz. piece	7.0	1.4

Turtle beans, see "Black beans"

V

	total fat (grams)	saturated fat (grams)
Vanilla extract, 1 tsp.	0	 0
Vanilla flavor drink:		
canned:		
(*Sego* Very Vanilla), 1 can	5.0	.... 1.0
(*Sego* Lite Very Vanilla), 1 can	4.0	.... n.a.
French (*Carnation* Instant Breakfast),		
10 fl. oz.	3.0	5
smooth, creme (*Nestlé Sweet Success*),		
10 fl. oz.	3.0	.... 1.0
refrigerated, French (*Carnation* Instant Breakfast), 8		
fl. oz.	2.5	.... 1.5
Vanilla flavor drink mix, dry, 1 pkt.:		
(*Pillsbury* Instant Breakfast)	0	 0
creamy deluxe (*Nestlé Sweet Success*)	.5	 0
French (*Carnation* Instant Breakfast)	0	 0
Vanilla shake:		
(*Nestlé Killer Shakes*), 1 carton	14.0	.... 8.0
(*Nestlé Quik*), 1 carton	9.0	.... 5.0
Veal, meat only:		
cubed, lean only:		
raw, 1 oz.	.7	2

	total fat (grams)	saturated fat (grams)

Veal, cubed, lean only *(cont.)*

braised or stewed, 9.3 oz. (1 lb. raw)	11.3	3.4
braised or stewed, 4 oz.	4.9	1.5

ground:

raw, 1 oz.	1.9	.8
raw, 1 cup, about 8 oz.	15.3	6.3
broiled, 10.5 oz. (1 lb. raw)	22.6	9.1
broiled, 5.4 oz. (1 cup raw)	11.6	4.7
broiled, 4 oz., about 1 cup diced	8.6	3.4

leg (top round), boneless:

braised, lean and fat, 9.6 oz. (1 lb. raw)	17.2	6.9
braised, lean and fat, 4 oz.	7.2	2.9
braised, lean only, 4 oz.	5.8	2.2
braised, lean and fat, diced, 1 cup	8.9	3.5
braised, lean only, diced, 1 cup	7.1	2.7
roasted, lean and fat, 12.6 oz. (1 lb. raw)	16.7	6.6
roasted, lean and fat, 4 oz.	5.3	2.1
roasted, lean only, 4 oz.	3.8	1.4
roasted, lean and fat, diced, 1 cup	6.5	2.6
roasted, lean only, diced, 1 cup	4.7	1.7

loin:

braised, lean and fat, 1 chop, 2.8 oz. (6.9 oz. raw w/bone)	13.8	5.4
braised, lean only, 1 chop, 2.4 oz. (6.9 oz. raw w/bone and fat)	6.3	1.8
braised, lean and fat, 4 oz.	19.5	7.6
braised, lean only, 4 oz.	10.4	2.9
roasted, lean and fat, 8.1 oz. (1 lb. raw w/bone)	28.3	12.1
roasted, lean only, 8.5 oz. (1 lb. raw w/bone and fat)	14.4	5.4
roasted, lean and fat, 4 oz.	14.0	6.0
roasted, lean only, 4 oz.	7.9	2.9

	total fat (grams)	saturated fat (grams)
rib:		
braised, lean and fat, 6.2 oz. (1 lb. raw w/bone)	22.2	8.9
braised, lean only, 5.75 oz. (1 lb. raw w/bone and fat)	12.7	4.2
braised, lean and fat, 4 oz.	14.2	5.6
braised, lean only, 4 oz.	8.9	2.9
roasted, lean and fat, 8.5 oz. (1 lb. raw w/bone)	33.5	13.0
roasted, lean only, 7.6 oz. (1 lb. raw w/bone and fat)	16.0	4.5
roasted, lean and fat, 4 oz.	15.8	6.1
roasted, lean only, 4 oz.	8.4	2.4
shoulder, whole:		
braised, lean and fat, 6.7 oz. (1 lb. raw w/bone)	19.4	7.2
braised, lean only, 6.4 oz. (1 lb. raw w/bone and fat)	11.1	3.1
braised, lean and fat, 4 oz.	11.5	4.3
braised, lean only, 4 oz.	6.9	1.9
roasted, lean and fat, 9.1 oz. (1 lb. raw w/bone)	21.7	8.8
roasted, lean only, 8.8 oz. (1 lb. raw w/bone and fat)	16.6	6.3
roasted, lean and fat, 4 oz.	9.5	3.9
roasted, lean only, 4 oz.	7.5	2.8
shoulder, arm:		
braised, lean and fat, 1 steak, 6.1 oz. (13.6 oz. raw w/bone)	17.7	6.9
braised, lean only, 1 steak, 5.6 oz. (13.6 oz. raw w/bone and fat)	8.5	2.4
braised, lean and fat, 4 oz.	11.6	4.5
braised, lean only, 4 oz.	6.0	1.7
roasted, lean and fat, 10 oz. (13.6 oz. raw w/bone)	23.3	9.9

	total fat (grams)	saturated fat (grams)
Veal, shoulder, arm *(cont.)*		
roasted, lean only, 9.6 oz. (13.6 oz. raw w/bone and fat)	15.8	6.3
roasted, lean and fat, 4 oz.	9.4	4.0
roasted, lean only, 4 oz.	6.6	2.6
shoulder, blade:		
braised, lean and fat, 5.25 oz. (1 lb. raw w/bone)	18.7	6.8
braised, lean only, 6.1 oz. (1 lb. raw w/bone and fat)	11.3	3.2
braised, lean and fat, 4 oz.	11.4	4.1
braised, lean only, 4 oz.	7.3	2.1
roasted, lean and fat, 8.6 oz. (1 lb. raw w/bone)	21.1	8.4
roasted, lean only, 8.3 oz. (1 lb. raw w/bone and fat)	16.3	6.1
roasted, lean and fat, 4 oz.	9.8	3.9
roasted, lean only, 4 oz.	7.8	2.9
sirloin:		
braised, lean and fat, 7.25 oz. (1 lb. raw w/bone)	26.9	10.6
braised, lean only, 6.5 oz. (1 lb. raw w/bone and fat)	11.9	3.3
braised, lean and fat, 4 oz.	14.9	5.9
braised, lean only, 4 oz.	7.4	2.1
roasted, lean and fat, 9.5 oz. (1 lb. raw w/bone)	28.1	12.1
roasted, lean only, 8.9 oz. (1 lb. raw w/bone and fat)	15.6	6.0
roasted, lean and fat, 4 oz.	11.9	5.1
roasted, lean only, 4 oz.	7.1	2.7
Veal dinner, parmigiana, frozen:		
(*Armour Classics*), 11.25 oz.	22.0	11.0
(*Banquet* Meals), 9 oz.	14.0	5.0
(*Morton*), 8.75 oz.	13.0	4.0

	total fat (grams)	saturated fat (grams)
(*Swanson*), 11.5 oz.	18.0	8.0
Veal entree, parmigiana, frozen:		
(*Banquet* Family), 4.7 oz.	14.0	4.0
w/spaghetti (*Stouffer's* Homestyle), 11⅞ oz.	19.0	4.0
"Veal," vegetarian, frozen		
(*Worthington Veelets*), 2.5-oz. patty	9.0	1.5
Veal variety meats, see specific listings		
Vegetable burger (see also "Burger, vegetarian"), frozen, 1 piece:		
(*Green Giant Harvest Burgers* Original)	6.0	1.5
Italian style (*Green Giant Harvest Burgers*)	7.0	1.5
Southwestern style (*Green Giant Harvest Burgers*)	6.0	1.5
Vegetable chips (*Eden*), 1.1 oz., 50 chips	4.0	1.5
Vegetable dip, 2 tbsp.:		
(*Bernstein's* Savory Ranch)	11.0	1.0
yogurt (*Crowley's*)	2.5	1.5
zesty dill (*Bernstein's*)	12.0	2.5
Vegetable dip mix (*McCormick Collection* Recipe Blend), ⅛ pkg.	0	0
Vegetable entree, canned or packaged:		
stew (*Dinty Moore*), 8 oz.	6.0	2.0
stew (*Knorr*), 1 pkg.	2.0	0
Vegetable entree, frozen:		
w/cheese (*Banquet*), 7 oz.	18.0	8.0
Chinese style, and chicken (*The Budget Gourmet* Light & Healthy), 10 oz.	9.0	1.5
Italian style, and chicken (*The Budget Gourmet* Light & Healthy), 10 oz.	7.0	2.0
lasagna, see "Laságna"		
spicy Szechuan style, and chicken (*The Budget Gourmet*), 10 oz.	9.0	1.5

	total fat (grams)	saturated fat (grams)

Vegetable juice:

all varieties (*R.W. Knudsen Very Veggie*),
8 fl. oz. .... | 1.0 | 0

cocktail:

6 fl. oz. .... | .2 | <.1
(*Mott's*), 10 fl. oz. .... | 0 | 0
all varieties (*"V-8"*), 8 fl. oz. .... | 0 | 0

Vegetable oil, see specific listings

Vegetable pockets, 4.5-oz. piece:

barbecue style (*Ken & Robert's*) .... | 8.0 | .5
broccoli and cheddar (*Ken & Robert's*) .... | 8.0 | 0
Greek style (*Ken & Robert's*) .... | 8.0 | 0
Indian, Oriental, pizza, or Tex-Mex style (*Ken & Robert's*) .... | 8.0 | .5

Vegetable seasoning, (*Perc*), 1 tsp. .... | .1 | 0

Vegetable side dish, frozen (see also "Vegetables, mixed"):

cheddar, English style (*Green Giant* International Mixtures), ½ cup .... | 5.0 | 2.0
Dijon garlic, French style (*Green Giant* International Mixtures), ½ cup .... | 3.0 | 2.0
mandarin (*The Budget Gourmet*), 5.5 oz. .... | 13.0 | 3.0
mushroom, Normandy style (*Green Giant* International Mixtures), ½ cup .... | 3.0 | 2.0
New England recipe (*The Budget Gourmet*), 5.5 oz. .... | 16.0 | 7.0
Parmesan, Italian style (*Green Giant* International Mixtures), ½ cup .... | 2.5 | 1.5
spring, in cheese sauce (*The Budget Gourmet*), 5.5 oz. .... | 10.0 | 5.0
teriyaki, Japanese style (*Green Giant* International Mixtures), ½ cup .... | 0 | 0

Vegetable sticks, breaded, frozen:

(*Schwan's*), 6 pieces, 3.2 oz. .... | 7.0 | 1.0

	total fat (grams)	saturated fat (grams)
(*Stilwell Quik-Krisp*), 5 pieces	9.0	1.5
Vegetables, see specific listings		
Vegetables, mixed, canned or packaged, ½ cup:		
w/liquid	.2	.1
drained	.2	<.1
(*Del Monte*)	0	0
(*Green Giant*)	0	0
(*Green Giant Garden Medley*)	0	0
(*Seneca*)	0	0
(*Stokely*)	0	0
Vegetables, mixed, freeze-dried, ½ cup*:		
(*AlpineAire*)	.4	0
garden (*AlpineAire*)	.5	0
Vegetables, mixed, frozen (see also "Vegetable side dish"):		
10-oz. pkg.	1.5	.3
boiled, drained, ½ cup	.1	<.1
(*Green Giant*), ¾ cup	0	0
(*Green Giant Harvest Fresh*), ⅔ cup	0	0
(*McKenzie's*), ⅔ cup	.5	0
(*Schwan's* Early Garden/Pasta Blend), 1 cup	0	0
(*Schwan's* Summer Garden Pasta Blend), 1 cup	.5	0
all varieties (*Stilwell*), ½ cup	0	0
all varieties, except New England and Western (*Green Giant American Mixtures*)	0	0
in butter sauce (*Green Giant*), ¾ cup	2.0	1.0
California blend (*Schwan's*), 1 cup	0	0
Cantonese (*House of Tsang*), ½ cup	1.0	0
gumbo (*McKenzie's*), ⅔ cup	0	0
Hong Kong (*House of Tsang*), ½ cup	0	0
Italian (*Schwan's* Pasta Blend), 1 cup	.5	0
New England or Western style (*Green Giant American Mixtures*)	1.5	0
soup (*McKenzie's*), ⅔ cup	0	0
stew (*Ore-Ida*), ⅔ cup	0	0

	total fat (grams)	saturated fat (grams)

Vegetables, mixed, frozen *(cont.)*

    stir-fry (*Schwan's*), 1 cup 0 0

    Szechuan (*House of Tsang*), ½ cup 1.0 0

    Tokyo teriyaki (*House of Tsang*), ½ cup 0 0

Vegetables, mixed, pickled:

    (*Krinos* Giardiniera), 3 oz., about ¾ cup 0 0

    (*Zorba* Giardiniera), ½ cup 1.0 0

Vegetarian dishes, canned (see also " 'Beef,'
    vegetarian," "Burger, vegetarian canned"
    and other specific listings):

    (*Loma Linda Nuteena*), 1.9 oz., ⅜" slice .... 13.0 .... 5.0

    (*Loma Linda* Tender Bits), 3 oz., 6 pieces 4.5 5

    (*Loma Linda* Tender Rounds), 2.8 oz. .... 5.0 .... 1.0

    (*Worthington* Savory Slices), 3 oz., 3 slices ...... 9.0 .... 3.5

    (*Worthington Choplets*), 3.2 oz., 2 slices .... 1.5 .... 1.0

    cutlet (*Worthington*), 2.2 oz., 1 slice 1.0 0

    cutlet, multigrain (*Worthington*), 3.2 oz.,
        2 slices 2.0 5

    dinner cuts (*Loma Linda*), 2.4-oz. slice 1.5 5

    stew, country (*Worthington*), 1 cup .... 9.0 .... 1.5

Vegetarian dishes, frozen (see also " 'Beef,' vegetarian,
    frozen" "Burger, vegetarian, frozen," and other
    specific listings):

    (*Natural Touch* Dinner Entree), 3-oz. patty .... 15.0 .... 2.5

    (*Natural Touch* Garden Grain Pattie), 2.3-oz. patty .... 7.0 .... 1.0

    (*Natural Touch* Garden Vege Pattie), 2.4-oz. patty .... 4.0 .... 1.0

    (*Natural Touch* Lentil Rice Loaf), 3.2 oz.,
        1" slice .... 9.0 .... 2.5

    (*Natural Touch* Nine-Bean Loaf), 3-oz. slice ...... 8.0 .... 1.5

    (*Worthington* Dinner Roast), 3 oz., ¾" slice ...... 12.0 .... 2.0

    (*Worthington* FriPats), 2.2-oz. patty .... 6.0 .... 1.0

    (*Worthington Prosage* Roll), 1.9 oz., ⅝" slice .... 10.0 .... 2.0

	total fat (grams)	saturated fat (grams)
croquettes (*Worthington* Golden), 3 oz., 4 pieces	10.0	1.5
Vegetarian dishes, mix (see also specific vegetarian listings):		
dinner loaf (*Loma Linda* Savory), .9 oz., ⅓ cup	1.5	0
dinner loaf (*Natural Touch*), 4 tbsp.	.6	.1
Stroganoff (*Natural Touch*), .8 oz.	3.5	2.0
Venison, meat only, roasted:		
12 oz. (1 lb. raw boneless)	10.8	4.2
4 oz.	3.6	1.4
diced, 1 cup, about 4.9 oz.	4.5	1.8
ground, 1 cup, about 4.1 oz.	3.7	1.5
Vienna sausage, canned:		
(*Libby's*), 3 links	12.0	2.5
(*Hormel*), 2 oz.	13.0	4.0
in barbecue sauce (*Libby's*), 3 links w/sauce	12.0	2.5
beef and pork, 1 oz.	7.1	2.6
beef and pork, 1 link, 2" × ⅞"	4.0	1.5
chicken (*Libby's*), 3 links	8.0	2.5
chicken (*Hormel*), 2 oz.	10.0	3.0
Vine spinach, raw, 1 lb.	1.4	n.a.
Vinegar, all varieties, 2 tbsp.	0	0
Vodka, pure distilled, plain or flavored, 3 fl. oz.	0	0

W

	total fat (grams)	saturated fat (grams)
Waffle, frozen, 2 pieces, except as noted:		
(*Aunt Jemima* Low Fat)	1.5	0
(*Aunt Jemima* Original)	7.0	1.5
(*Downyflake* Crisp & Healthy)	2.0	.5
(*Downyflake* Homestyle), 4 pieces	5.0	1.5
(*Downyflake* Homestyle Jumbo)	4.0	1.0
(*Downyflake* Hot 'n Buttery)	6.0	1.5
(*Eggo* Homestyle)	8.0	1.5
(*Eggo Minis* Homestyle), 3 sets	8.0	1.5
(*Eggo Nutri-Grain*)	6.0	1.0
(*Eggo Special K*)	0	0
(*Schwan's*), 4 pieces	18.0	3.0
apple cinnamon (*Eggo*)	8.0	1.5
apple-cinnamon (*Downyflake* Crisp & Healthy)	2.0	.5
blueberry:		
(*Aunt Jemima*)	7.0	1.5
(*Downyflake*)	4.0	1.0
(*Eggo*)	8.0	1.5
(*Eggo Minis*), 3 sets	8.0	1.5
butter and syrup (*Downyflake*)	4.0	1.0

	total fat (grams)	saturated fat (grams)
buttermilk:		
(*Aunt Jemima*)	6.0	1.5
(*Downyflake*)	4.0	1.0
(*Eggo*)	8.0	1.5
cinnamon (*Aunt Jemima*)	6.0	1.5
cinnamon toast (*Eggo*), 3 sets	9.0	2.0
multibran (*Eggo Nutri-Grain*)	6.0	1.0
nut and honey (*Eggo*)	10.0	2.0
oat bran (*Eggo Common Sense*)	7.0	1.5
oat bran, fruit and nut (*Eggo Common Sense*)	8.0	1.5
oatmeal (*Aunt Jemima*)	7.0	1.0
raisin and bran (*Eggo Nutri-Grain*)	6.0	1.0
strawberry (*Eggo*)	8.0	1.5
whole grain (*Roman Meal*)	14.0	2.0
Waffle breakfast, sticks, w/syrup (*Great Starts Breakfast Blast*), 2.75 oz.	17.0	7.0
Wakame, see "Seaweed"		
Walnut, dried, shelled, except as noted:		
(*Diamond*), 2 oz.	38.5	2.9
black:		
in shell, 4 oz.	15.4	1.0
1 oz.	16.1	1.0
(*Planters*), 2 oz.	31.0	2.0
chopped, 1 cup	70.7	4.5
halves (*Planters*), ⅓ cup	22.0	2.5
ground, fine, 1 cup	43.5	2.9
pieces (*Planters*), 1 oz.	20.0	2.0
English or Persian:		
in shell, 4 oz.	31.6	2.9
1 oz., about 14 halves	17.6	1.6
pieces or chips, 1 cup	74.2	6.7
halves, 1 cup	61.9	5.6
Walnut oil (*Hain*), 1 tbsp.	14.0	1.5
Walnut topping, in syrup (*Smucker's*), 2 tbsp.	10.0	1.0
Wasabi, dry, ¼ oz.	<.1	0

	total fat (grams)	saturated fat (grams)
Water chestnuts, Chinese:		
fresh:		
untrimmed, 1 lb.	.4	n.a.
4 medium, about 1.7 oz.	<.1	0
sliced, ½ cup	.1	0
canned, w/liquid, sliced, ½ cup	<.1	0
Watercress:		
untrimmed, 1 lb.	.4	.1
chopped, ½ cup	<.1	tr.
Watermelon:		
untrimmed, 1 lb.	1.0	n.a.
1" slice, ⅟₁₆ of 10" melon	2.0	tr.
diced, ½ cup	.3	0
Watermelon seeds, dried:		
in hard coat, 4 oz.	19.9	4.1
kernels, 1 oz.	13.5	2.8
kernels, 1 cup	51.2	10.6
Wax bean:		
fresh, see "Green beans"		
canned (*Seneca*), ½ cup	0	0
Wax gourd:		
raw, untrimmed, 1 lb.	.6	.1
raw, cubed, ½ cup	.1	<.1
boiled, drained, ½ cup	.2	<.1
Welsh onion, see "Onion, Welsh"		
Welsh rarebit, frozen (*Stouffer's* Side Dish), ¼ cup	9.0	4.0
Wendy's, 1 serving:		
burgers and sandwiches:		
bacon cheeseburger, Jr.	25.0	8.0
Big Bacon Classic	36.0	13.0
cheeseburger, Jr. or Kid's Meal	13.0	5.0
cheeseburger deluxe, Jr.	20.0	7.0
chicken, grilled	7.0	1.5
chicken, breaded	20.0	4.0
chicken club	25.0	6.0

	total fat (grams)	saturated fat (grams)
hamburger, single, plain	15.0	6.0
hamburger, single, w/everything	23.0	7.0
hamburger, Jr. or Kid's Meal	9.0	3.0
chicken nuggets, 6 pieces	20.0	5.0
chicken nuggets sauce, 1 pkt.:		
barbecue, honey, or sweet-sour	0	0
sweet mustard	1.0	0
chili and chili sides:		
chili, small, 8 oz.	6.0	2.5
chili, large, 12 oz.	9.0	4.0
cheddar, shredded, 2 tbsp.	6.0	3.0
saltine crackers, 2 pieces	.5	0
baked potato, 1 piece:		
plain	0	0
plain, w/1 pkt. sour cream	6.0	4.0
plain, w/1 pkt. whipped margarine	5.0	1.0
bacon and cheese	18.0	4.0
broccoli and cheese	14.0	2.5
cheese	23.0	8.0
chili and cheese	24.0	9.0
sour cream, w/chives	6.0	4.0
salads to go, w/out dressing:		
Caesar salad, side	5.0	2.0
chicken salad, grilled	8.0	1.5
garden salad, deluxe	6.0	1.0
side salad	3.0	.5
taco salad	30.0	11.0
salad dressing, 2 tbsp.:		
blue cheese	19.0	3.0
celery seed	7.0	1.0
French	11.0	1.5
French, fat free	0	0
French, sweet red	10.0	1.5
Hidden Valley Ranch	10.0	1.5
Hidden Valley Ranch, reduced fat /calorie	5.0	1.0

	total fat (grams)	saturated fat (grams)

Wendy's, salad dressing *(cont.)*

Italian, golden	7.0	1.0
Italian, reduced fat/calorie	3.0	.5
Italian Caesar	16.0	2.5
Thousand Island	13.0	2.0

side dishes:

fries, small	12.0	2.5
fries, medium	17.0	4.0
fries, Biggie	20.0	4.0
soft breadstick, 1 piece	3.0	.5

superbar:

Alfredo sauce, ¼ cup	1.5	0
cheese sauce, ¼ cup	1.0	0
macaroni and cheese, ½ cup	6.0	2.5
Parmesan cheese, grated, 2 tbsp.	5.0	3.0
picante sauce, 2 tbsp.	0	0
refried beans, ¼ cup	3.0	1.0
rice, Spanish, ¼ cup	1.0	0
rotini, ½ cup	2.0	0
sour topping, 2 tbsp.	5.0	5.0
spaghetti sauce, ¼ cup	0	0
spaghetti meat sauce, ¼ cup	1.5	.5
taco chips, 8 pieces	7.0	1.0
taco meat, 2 tbsp.	4.0	1.0
taco sauce, 2 tbsp.	0	0
taco shell, 1 piece	4.0	.5
tortilla, flour, 1 piece	2.5	.5

desserts:

chocolate chip cookie	13.0	4.0
frosty, small	10.0	5.0
frosty, medium	13.0	7.0
frosty, large	17.0	9.0

West Indian cherry, see "Acerola"

Western dinner, frozen:

(*Banquet* Meals), 9.5 oz.	20.0	9.0

	total fat (grams)	saturated fat (grams)
(*Morton*), 9 oz.	16.0	7.0
Wheat, whole grain:		
(*Arrowhead Mills*), ¼ cup	1.0	0
durum, 1 cup	4.7	.9
hard red spring, 1 cup	3.7	.6
hard red winter, 1 cup	3.0	.5
hard white, 1 cup	3.3	.5
soft red winter, 1 cup	2.6	.5
soft white, 1 cup	3.3	.6
Wheat, parboiled, see "Bulgur"		
Wheat, sprouted, 1 cup	1.4	.2
Wheat bran:		
(*Arrowhead Mills*), ¼ cup	.5	0
crude:		
1 oz.	1.2	.2
1 cup	2.6	.4
2 tbsp.	.3	<.1
Wheat flour:		
white:		
all purpose, 1 cup	1.2	.2
all varieties, except whole wheat (*Pillsbury*), ¼ cup	0	0
bread, 1 cup	2.3	.3
cake, 1 cup	.9	.1
pastry (*Arrowhead Mills*), ¼ cup	.5	0
self-rising, 1 cup	1.2	.2
self-rising, enriched (*Aunt Jemima*), 3 tbsp.	0	0
tortilla mix, 1 cup	11.8	4.6
unbleached or whole grain (*Arrowhead Mills*), ¼ cup	.5	0
whole grain, 1 cup	2.2	.4
whole wheat (*Pillsbury's Best*), ¼ cup	2.0	0
whole wheat (*Arrowhead Mills*), ¼ cup	.5	0
Wheat germ:		
(*Arrowhead Mills*), 3 tbsp.	.5	0

	total fat (grams)	saturated fat (grams)

Wheat germ *(cont.)*

crude, 1 oz. 2.8 5

crude, 1 cup .... 11.2 .... 1.9

crude, 1 oz., about ¼ cup 3.0 5

toasted, 1 cup .... 12.1 .... 2.1

Wheat pilaf mix (*Near East*), 1 cup* .... 4.5 .... 1.0

Wheat "nuts," see "Wheat snack"

Wheat salad, see "Tabbouleh"

Wheat snack (see also "Snack mix"):

(*Sonoma* Wheat Nuts), .5 oz., 2 tbsp. 3.0 0

chips (*Zings*), 1.8-oz. bag .... 11.0 .... 2.0

tortillas, see "Corn chips and similar snacks"

wheat "nuts":

unflavored, 1 oz. .... 16.4 .... 2.5

macadamia flavored, 1 oz. .... 16.1 .... 2.4

all other flavors, 1 oz. .... 17.7 .... 2.7

Whelk, meat only, raw, 4 oz. .... .5 .... <.1

Whey:

acid:

fluid, 1 cup, about 8.7 oz. 2 1

dry, 1 oz. 2 1

dry, 1 cup, about 2 oz. 3 2

sweet:

fluid, 1 cup, about 8.7 oz. 9 6

dry, 1 oz. 3 2

dry, 1 cup, about 5.1 oz. .... 1.6 .... 1.0

Whipped topping, see "Cream topping"

Whiskey, pure distilled, 3 fl. oz. 0 0

Whiskey sour mixer:

(*Holland House*), 4 fl. oz. 0 0

(*Mr. & Mrs. "T"*), 4 fl. oz. 0 0

White beans, ½ cup:

dried:

raw 9 2

boiled 3 1

	total fat (grams)	saturated fat (grams)
small, raw	1.3	.3
small, boiled	.6	.1
canned (*Stokely*)	.5	0
canned, w/liquid	.4	.1
White Castle, 1 serving:		
cheeseburger	11.2	n.a.
chicken sandwich	7.5	n.a.
fish sandwich, w/out tartar sauce	5.0	n.a.
hamburger	7.9	n.a.
sausage sandwich	12.3	n.a.
sausage w/egg sandwich	22.0	n.a.
side dishes:		
french fries	14.7	n.a.
onion chips	16.6	n.a.
onion rings	13.4	n.a.
White flowered gourd, see "Gourd"		
White sauce mix:		
(*Durkee*), ¼ pkg.	.5	0
(*Knorr* Classic Sauces), ⅛ pkg.	1.0	.5
Whitefish, mixed species, meat only:		
raw, 4 oz.	6.7	1.0
smoked, 4 oz.	1.1	.3
Whiting, mixed species, meat only:		
raw, 4 oz.	1.5	.3
baked, broiled, or microwaved, 4 oz.	1.9	.4
Wiener, see "Frankfurter"		
Wild rice:		
raw, 1 cup	1.7	.2
cooked, 1 cup	.6	.1
freeze-dried (*AlpineAire*), ½ cup*	.3	0
Wild rice entree, freeze-dried, pilaf, w/almonds		
(*AlpineAire*), 1⅓ cups*	6.0	n.a.
Wild rice mix (see also "Rice dishes, mix"), and		
country vegetables (*Spice Islands*), 1 pkg.	0	0
Wine, all varieties, 4 fl. oz.	0	0

	total fat (grams)	saturated fat (grams)
Wine, cooking, all varieties (*Holland House*), 2 tbsp.	0	0
Winged bean:		
raw, untrimmed, 1 lb.	3.9	1.1
raw, 1 pod, .6 oz.	.1	<.1
boiled, drained, ½ cup	.2	.1
Winged bean, dried:		
raw, ½ cup	14.9	2.1
boiled, ½ cup	5.0	.7
Winged bean leaves, trimmed, 1 oz.	.3	.1
Winged bean tuber, trimmed, 1 oz.	.3	<.1
Winter squash (see also specific squash listings):		
all varieties:		
raw, untrimmed, 1 lb.	.7	1
raw, cubed, ½ cup	.1	<.1
baked, cubed, ½ cup	.6	.1
Wolf fish, Atlantic, meat only, raw, 4 oz.	2.7	.4
Wonton rolls, frozen, pizza flavor (*Schwan's*), 5 pieces	16.0	6.0
Wonton wrapper (*Nasoya*), 1.2 oz., 5 pieces	0	0
Worcestershire sauce:		
(*Lea & Perrins*), 1 tsp.	0	0
(*Trappey's* Chef Magic), 1 tsp.	0	0

Y

	total fat (grams)	saturated fat (grams)
Yam:		
fresh:		
raw, untrimmed, 1 lb.	.7	.1
raw, cubed, ½ cup	.1	<.1
baked or boiled, ½ cup	.1	<.1
canned or frozen, see "Sweet potato"		
Yam, mountain, Hawaiian:		
raw, untrimmed, 1 lb. or 1 medium	.4	.1
raw, cubed, ½ cup	.1	<.1
steamed, cubed, ½ cup	.1	<.1
Yam bean tuber:		
raw, untrimmed, 1 lb.	.1	0
boiled, drained, 4 oz.	.1	0
Yam patties, frozen:		
(*McKenzie's*), 2 oz. piece	0	0
(*Stilwell*), 2 pieces	1.0	0
Yardlong bean:		
fresh:		
raw, untrimmed, 1 lb.	1.7	.5
raw, sliced, ½ cup	.2	<.1
boiled, drained, sliced, ½ cup	.1	<.1

	total fat (grams)	saturated fat (grams)

Yardlong bean, fresh *(cont.)*
| dried, raw, ½ cup | 1.1 | .3 |
| dried, boiled, ½ cup | .4 | .1 |

Yeast, baker's, ¼ oz. or ¼ tsp. — 0 0

Yellow bean, dried:
| raw, ½ cup | 2.6 | .7 |
| boiled, ½ cup | 1.0 | .2 |

Yellow squash:
fresh, see "Crookneck squash"
| frozen, breaded (*Stilwell*), 6 pieces | 0 | 0 |
| frozen, sliced (*McKenzie's*), ⅔ cup | 0 | 0 |

Yellow bean, see "Wax bean" and "Green bean"

Yogurt:
plain, 1 cup, except as noted:
whole milk	7.4	4.8
whole milk (*Axelrod/Crowley*)	9.0	5.0
whole milk (*Stonyfield Farm*), 8 oz.	9.0	6.0
low fat	3.5	2.3
low fat (*Axelrod/Crowley*)	2.5	1.5
low fat (*Colombo*)	4.5	2.5
low fat (*Dannon*)	4.0	2.5
low fat (*Dannon*), 8-oz. container	4.0	2.0
low fat (*Friendship*)	3.0	1.5
nonfat, all brands	0	0
skim milk	.4	.3

all flavors, 8 oz., except as noted:
(*Axelrod/Crowley* Nonfat)	0	0
(*Axelrod/Crowley* Swiss Lowfat)	2.5	1.5
(*Axelrod/Crowley* Swiss Nonfat)	0	0
(*Breyer's* Lowfat 1%)	2.5	1.5
(*Breyer's* Lowfat 1.5%)	3.0	2.0
(*Colombo* Fat Free/*Light 100*)	0	0
(*Dannon* Light /Light 'N Crunchy Nonfat)	0	0
(*Dannon* Fruit on the Bottom Lowfat)	3.0	1.5
(*Dannon* Danimals Lowfat), 4.4 oz.	2.0	1.0

	total fat (grams)	saturated fat (grams)
(*Dannon Sprinkl'ins* Lowfat), 4.1 oz.	2.5	.... 1.5
(*Light n' Lively*), 6 oz. or 4.4 oz.	0	 0
(*Knudsen*)	0	 0
(*Weight Watchers Ultima 90*)	0	 0
except banana berry and grape (*Light n' Lively* Kidpack Lowfat 1%), 4.4 oz.	1.0	5
except raspberry and strawberry (*Light n' Lively* Multipack Lowfat 1%), 4.4 oz.	1.0	5
banana berry and grape (*Light n' Lively* Kidpack Lowfat 1%), 4.4 oz.	1.0	.... 1.0
blueberry or strawberry banana (*Friendship* Fruit Crunch), 5.5 oz.	3.5	.... 1.5
cherry, w/honey grahams (*Dannon Sprinkl'ins Crazy Crunch* Lowfat), 4.4 oz.	3.0	.... 1.5
coffee:		
(*Dannon* Lowfat), 1 cup	3.5	.... 2.0
(*Dannon* Lowfat), 8-oz. container	3.0	.... 2.0
(*Friendship*), 1 cup	3.0	.... 1.5
cranberry-raspberry (*Dannon* Lowfat), 8-oz. container	3.0	.... 2.0
w/fruit topping, all flavors (*Dannon Double Delights* Lowfat), 6 oz.	2.5	.... 1.5
grape, w/chocolate grahams (*Dannon Sprinkl'ins Crazy Crunch* Lowfat), 4.4 oz.	2.5	.... 1.5
lemon (*Dannon* Lowfat), 1 cup	3.5	.... 2.0
lemon (*Dannon* Lowfat), 8-oz. container	3.0	.... 2.0
peach (*Friendship* Fruit Crunch), 5.5 oz.	4.5	.... 1.5
raspberry, red (*Light n' Lively* Multipack Lowfat 1%), 4.4 oz.	1.0	.... 1.0
strawberry (*Friendship* Fruit Crunch), 5.5 oz.	4.5	.... 1.5
strawberry (*Light n' Lively* Multipack Lowfat 1%), 4.4 oz.	1.0	.... 1.0
vanilla:		
(*Breyer's* Lowfat), 1 cup	3.0	.... 2.0
(*Dannon* Lowfat), 1 cup	3.5	.... 2.0

	total fat (grams)	saturated fat (grams)

Yogurt, vanilla *(cont.)*

(*Dannon* Lowfat), 8-oz. container	3.0	2.0
French (*Colombo* Low Fat)	4.0	2.5
w/chocolate grahams (*Dannon Sprinkl'ins Crazy Crunch* Lowfat), 4.4 oz.	2.5	1.5
w/honey grahams (*Dannon Sprinkl'ins Crazy Crunch* Lowfat), 4.4 oz.	3.0	1.5

Yogurt, frozen, ½ cup:

all flavors:

(*Ben & Jerry's* Nonfat)	0	0
(*Blue Bell* Nonfat)	0	0
(*Crowley* Silver Premium Nonfat)	0	0
(*Dannon Light*)	0	0
(*Edy's* Fat Free)	0	0
all fruit flavors (*Crowley* Silver Premium)	2.0	1.5
"banana cream pie" (*Dannon Light 'n Crunchy*)	1.0	0
banana strawberry (*Häagen-Dazs*)	4.0	2.0
Brownie Nut Blast (*Häagen-Dazs Exträas*)	9.0	4.0
candy bar swirl (*Crowley* Silver Premium)	4.0	2.0
cherry, black (*Schwan's* Lowfat)	2.5	2.0
cherry chocolate cherry (*Dannon Pure Indulgence*)	3.0	1.0
Cherry Garcia (*Ben & Jerry's*)	3.0	2.0

chocolate:

(*Crowley* Silver Premium)	2.5	1.5
(*Edy's*)	3.0	1.5
(*Häagen-Dazs*)	4.0	2.0
(*Schwan's* Lowfat)	3.0	2.0
triple (*Dannon Light 'n Crunchy*)	0	0
chocolate brownie chunk (*Edy's*)	4.0	1.5
chocolate chip (*Crowley* Silver Premium)	4.0	2.5
chocolate chip cookie dough (*Crowley* Silver Premium)	3.5	2.0
chocolate chunk, double (*Blue Bell* Lowfat)	3.0	2.0
chocolate fudge brownie (*Ben & Jerry's*)	4.0	2.0
chocolate nut, crunchy (*Dannon Pure Indulgence*)	3.0	0

	total fat (grams)	saturated fat (grams)
citrus heights (*Edy's*)	2.5	1.5
coco-nut fudge (*Dannon Pure Indulgence*)	3.0	1.5
coffee (*Crowley* Silver Premium)	2.5	1.5
coffee (*Häagen-Dazs*)	4.0	2.0
coffee almond fudge (*Ben & Jerry's*)	7.0	2.0
cookies and cream:		
(*Blue Bell* Lowfat)	3.0	2.0
(*Dannon Pure Indulgence*)	3.0	2.0
(*Edy's*)	4.0	1.5
English toffee crunch (*Ben & Jerry's*)	6.0	2.5
espresso, crunchy (*Dannon Pure Indulgence*)	3.0	2.0
fudge swirl (*Crowley* Silver Premium)	2.0	1.5
Heath toffee crunch:		
(*Crowley* Silver Premium)	3.5	2.0
(*Dannon Pure Indulgence*)	3.0	1.5
(*Edy's*)	4.0	2.0
marble fudge (*Edy's*)	3.0	1.5
mocha chocolate chunk (*Dannon Light 'n Crunchy*)	1.0	0
Neapolitan (*Crowley* Silver Premium)	2.5	1.5
Orange Tango (*Häagen-Dazs Exträas*)	2.0	1.0
orange vanilla swirl (*Edy's*)	2.5	1.5
peach:		
(*Häagen-Dazs*)	4.0	2.0
(*Schwan's* Lowfat)	2.5	1.5
perfectly (*Edy's*)	2.5	1.5
peanut chocolate crunch (*Dannon Light 'n Crunchy*)	0	0
pecan praline and cream (*Blue Bell* Lowfat)	2.0	1.0
Praline Pandemonium (*Häagen-Dazs Exträas*)	9.0	4.0
praline and cream (*Crowley* Silver Premium)	4.0	1.5
raspberry (*Edy's*)	2.5	1.5
Raspberry Rendezvous (*Häagen-Dazs Exträas*)	2.0	1.0
raspberry vanilla swirl (*Edy's*)	2.5	1.5
rocky road (*Edy's* Lactose Reduced)	10.0	5.0

	total fat (grams)	saturated fat (grams)

Yogurt, frozen *(cont.)*

(*Starburst* Lowfat)	2.0	1.0
strawberries and cream (*Edy's* Lactose Reduced)	8.0	5.0
strawberry:		
(*Edy's*)	2.5	1.5
(*Häagen-Dazs*)	4.0	2.0
(*Schwan's* Lowfat)	2.5	2.0
strawberry cheesecake (*Blue Bell* Lowfat)	2.0	1.0
Strawberry Cheesecake Craze (*Häagen-Dazs Exträas*)	7.0	3.0
strawberry chocolate chip (*Edy's*)	4.0	2.0
vanilla:		
(*Blue Bell* Lowfat)	2.0	1.0
(*Crowley* Silver Premium)	2.5	1.5
(*Edy's*)	2.5	1.5
(*Häagen-Dazs*)	4.0	2.0
(*Schwan's* Lowfat)	3.0	2.0
vanilla almond crunch (*Häagen-Dazs*)	6.0	2.0
vanilla blueberry swirl (*Dannon Light 'n Crunchy*)	1.0	0
vanilla chocolate twist (*Blue Bell* Lowfat)	2.0	1.0
vanilla raspberry truffle (*Dannon Pure Indulgence*)	3.0	2.0
"Yogurt," tofu, ½ cup:		
all flavors, except chocolate and vanilla fudge (*Tofutti*)	1.0	0
chocolate fudge (*Tofutti*)	2.0	1.0
vanilla fudge (*Tofutti*)	2.0	0
Yogurt bar, frozen, 1 piece:		
cherry chocolate fudge (*Häagen-Dazs*)	12.0	7.0
Cherry Garcia (*Ben & Jerry's*)	16.0	10.0
chocolate almond (*Frozfruit*)	4.0	1.0
chocolate fudge (*Edy's*)	15.0	n.a.
coffee or vanilla chocolate crunch (*Häagen-Dazs*)	11.0	2.0

	total fat (grams)	saturated fat (grams)
orange, piña colada, or strawberry daiquiri (*Häagen-Dazs*)	1.0	<1.0
peach or raspberry (*Häagen-Dazs*)	1.0	0
peach, strawberry, or strawberry-banana (*Frozfruit*)	0	0
strawberry or raspberry (*Schwan's Push 'Ems*)	2.5	1.5
strawberry or raspberry (*Starburst*)	1.0	.5
toffee crunch (*Edy's*)	14.0	n.a.
vanilla and almonds (*Edy's*)	15.0	n.a.
Yogurt cup, 1 cup:		
(*Blue Bell* Lowfat Snack Cups)	1.0	1.0
(*Starburst* Lowfat Cups)	1.5	1.0
Yogurt dip, see specific listings		
Yokan, 1 oz.	<.1	0

Z

	total fat (grams)	saturated fat (grams)
Ziti, see "Pasta"		
Ziti dishes, frozen, in marinara sauce (*The Budget Gourmet* Side Dish), 6.25 oz.	10.0	4.0
Zucchini:		
fresh:		
raw, untrimmed, 1 lb.	.6	.1
raw, sliced, ½ cup	.1	<.1
boiled, drained, sliced, ½ cup	.1	tr.
canned, ½ cup:		
(*Progresso* Italian Style)	2.0	0
in tomato juice	.1	<.1
in tomato sauce (*Del Monte* Italian Style)	0	0
frozen:		
10-oz. pkg.	.4	.1
boiled, drained, 4 oz. or ½ cup	.1	<.1
sliced (*Stilwell*), ⅔ cup	0	0
breaded (*Empire* Kosher), 2.9-oz. piece	0	0

Corinne T. **Netzer**

SHE KNOWS WHAT'S GOOD FOR YOU!

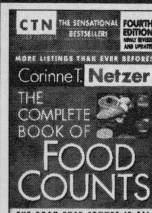